COSMETIC SCIENCE
Volume 1

COSMETIC SCIENCE

Volume 1

*On behalf of the Society
of Cosmetic Chemists of
Great Britain*

Edited by

M. M. BREUER

Biomedical Department, Gillette Research Institute,
Rockville, Maryland, USA

1978

ACADEMIC PRESS

London   New York   San Francisco

A Subsidiary of Harcourt Brace Jovanovich, Publishers

ACADEMIC PRESS INC. (LONDON) LTD.
24/28 Oval Road, London NW1 7DX

United States Edition published by
ACADEMIC PRESS INC.
111 Fifth Avenue, New York, New York 1003

Library of Congress Catalog Card Number: 77–74374
ISBN: 0–12–133001–X

Printed in Great Britain by
William Clowes & Sons Limited
London, Beccles and Colchester

12/17/84

CONTRIBUTORS

P. BILEK   *Forschungsabteilung (Research Department) Greiter AG, A-3400 Klosterneuburg-Weidling, Elisabethstrasse 51–53, Austria*

E. L. CUSSLER   *Department of Chemical Engineering, Carnegie-Mellon University, Pittsburgh, Pennsylvania 15213, USA*

W. B. DAVIS   *Beecham Products Research Department, Leatherhead, Surrey, England*

S. DOSKOCZIL   *Forschungsabteilung (Research Department) Greiter AG, A-3400 Klosterneuburg-Weidling, Elisabethstrasse 51–53, Austria*

N. FUKUHARA   *Shiseido Co. Ltd, 5–5 Ginza 7 Chome, Chuo-Ku, Tokyo, Japan*

MAX GLOOR   *Department of Dermatology, Universitats-Hautklinik, Heidelberg, West Germany*

F. GREITER   *Forschungsabteilung (Research Department) Greiter AG, A-3400 Klosterneuburg-Weidling, Elisabethstrasse 51–53, Austria*

J. J. MURRAY   *Department of Children's Dentistry, Institute of Dental Surgery, Eastman Dental Hospital, 256 Gray's Inn Road, London WC1X 8LD*

COLIN PROTTEY   *Unilever Research Laboratory, Port Sunlight, Wirral, Merseyside L62 4XN, England*

I. D. RATTEE   *Department of Colour Chemistry, University of Leeds, Leeds LS2 9JT, England*

LINDA SHAW   *Department of Children's Dentistry, Institute of Dental Surgery, Eastman Dental Hospital, 256 Gray's Inn Road, London WC1X 8LD, England*

G. B. WINTER   *Department of Children's Dentistry, Institute of Dental Surgery, Eastman Dental Hospital, 256 Gray's Inn Road, London WC1X 8LD, England*

PREFACE

The preparation of cosmetics, although one of the most ancient of human activities, remained an empirical pursuit until the end of the Second World War. During the last decades, however, the manufacture of cosmetic and toiletry products has developed into a major industry supplying millions of consumers all over the world with standardized, high quality products. The change from a craft practised by individual artisans into a manufacturing industry dominated by large international concerns with facilities for mass production and mass marketing, necessitated the establishment of systematic research and development programs, new manufacturing technologies and highly reliable quality assurance procedures.

In the early stages of its evolution, the cosmetic industry relied mainly on the knowledge and technology which it borrowed from mature, established scientific disciplines and industries (e.g. dermatology, biochemistry, textile and leather industries). The situation has now changed; the scientific methods and industrial processes used today are becoming more and more specific to the area of cosmetics and toiletries. We are witnessing the emergence of a new branch of the applied sciences: Cosmetic Science.

The appearance of "Cosmetic Science" is a manifestation of the emergence of this new scientific and technological discipline. In publishing this series, our aim was to provide a vehicle for authoritative articles reviewing the current state of knowledge in scientific and technological areas that are of particular interest to the Scientists, Managers, Medical Practitioners, Cosmetologists and Technologists who are active in the development of more effective products and processes with the aim to provide better personal care.

Cosmetic Science is an applied discipline which utilizes the results of fundamental physical, biological and social sciences, it is practiced on all continents and has many diverse problems. Therefore, it is appropriate that the contributors to the first and subsequent volumes of this series should represent many different backgrounds and nationalities.

I firmly believe that the future of the cosmetic and toiletries industry depends on its ability to provide new products with substantially improved consumer benefits. The industry will only be able to meet the challenge which this task represents if it will utilize all the available knowledge that science and technology can offer. The principal task of "Cosmetic Science" is to facilitate this process.

I should like to take this opportunity and express my appreciation to the authors of the various chapters for their excellent contributions. Also, I should like to thank the council and the officers of the Society of Cosmetic Chemists of Great Britain, who have helped and encouraged the creation of this Series. My particular thanks go to Mr G. A. C. Pitt, and Ms A. E. Young, past presidents of the Society who have played an active role in nurturing this venture along its early path, and to Mrs Pat Salzedo, the General Secretary of the Society, without whose help and suggestions "Cosmetic Science" would never have left the ground.

Rockville, Maryland   M. M. BREUER
USA
January 1978

CONTENTS

COSMETICS AND DENTAL HEALTH
G. B. Winter, J. J. Murray and Linda Shaw

THE CLEANING, POLISHING AND ABRASION
OF TEETH BY DENTAL PRODUCTS
W. B. Davis

COSMETIC MARKET AND TECHNOLOGY IN JAPAN
Nobukazu Fukuhara

PREDICTING SKIN FEEL
E. L. Cussler

CURRENTLY USED SUNSCREEN MATERIALS— FORMULATION AND TESTING

F. Greiter, S. Doskoczil and P. Bilek

COLOUR IN COSMETICS

I. D. Rattee

DETERMINATION AND ANALYSIS OF SEBUM ON SKIN AND HAIRS
Max Gloor

THE MOLECULAR BASIS OF SKIN IRRITATION
Colin Prottey

COSMETICS AND DENTAL HEALTH

G. B. Winter, J. J. Murray and Linda Shaw
Institute of Dental Surgery,
Eastman Dental Hospital,
London, England

I. INTRODUCTION

From a cosmetic point of view, probably the most important aspect of dental health is the colour and integrity of a persons teeth. Sparkling white teeth are generally considered aesthetically pleasing, whereas discoloured, decayed and broken down teeth are socially disadvantageous. Although the general public tend to focus mainly on the hard tissues of the teeth, the dental profession has always been aware of the effect of gum health on an individual's appearance, and in recent years a greater emphasis has been placed in commercial advertising on the cosmetic importance of reducing gingivitis (inflammation of the gums) and destructive periodontal disease (destruction of the supporting structures of the teeth).

Teeth can be discoloured because of intrinsic or extrinsic stains. Intrinsic stains are built into the tooth and can only be treated by bleaching or masking the discolouration with a restoration. Extrinsic stains can be removed by a dentist or dental hygienist carrying out a professional prophylaxis, and by the individual adopting good oral hygiene habits, involving the correct application of a toothbrush in conjunction with a dentifrice, and where appropriate the use of dental floss and wood sticks. Good oral hygiene has a marked effect on reducing gingivitis: gums which are red, swollen and bleed easily can be improved over a period of 2–4 weeks if all debris and plaque is removed, until the gingivae become firm and pink and are closely adapted to the necks of the standing teeth. When the deeper periodontal structures are inflamed periodontal therapy is required to remove plaque which has become embedded between the teeth and gums. In many cases the plaque has calcified to form calculus and this can only be removed by a thorough scaling and polishing by a dentist or a hygienist. In some cases the gums have to be re-contoured to eliminate pocketing so as to give the patient the opportunity of maintaining the periodontal tissues in good health. Many therapeutic agents have been added to dentifrices in an effort to improve their cleaning power and to help to reduce inflammation.

In this chapter the main causes of intrinsic discolouration and extrinsic tooth stain will be considered, and the mechanical and chemical methods of controlling dental plaque will be reviewed.

II. INTRINSIC DISCOLOURATION

Once a tooth has erupted normally into the mouth, its colour will remain essentially unchanged, unless the tooth is attacked by caries or traumatized, and providing the vitality of the pulp is maintained (Fig. 1).

A. Dental Caries

Dental caries is one of the commonest chronic diseases of civilized man. Often the first clinical sign is a change in the colour of the tooth; the enamel appears white and chalky due to demineralization of tooth structure. As the lesion progresses the tooth appears dark and discoloured, a sign that tooth tissue has been irreversibly destroyed (Plate 1). The enamel which covers teeth has no powers of regeneration. The only course of action is for the caries to be removed and a restoration inserted. As far as anterior teeth are concerned, the aesthetic appearance of the finished restoration is extremely

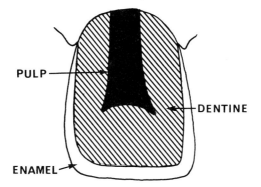

Fig. 1.   Anatomy of the dental tissues. Diagram of the crown of an upper central incisor showing enamel, dentine and pulp.

COLOUR PLATES

Plate 1. Gross caries with discolouration in upper and lower incisor teeth.

Plate 2. Patient, aged 14 years, with non-vital upper right central and lateral incisor teeth—darkening of these teeth is apparent.

Plate 3. The same patient as in Plate 2 following the placement of crowns on the non-vital teeth, and on the upper left lateral incisor to improve the aesthetic appearance.

Plate 4. Intrinsic staining of the teeth as a result of a prolonged course of tetracycline therapy during their formation.

Plate 5. Chalky pitted appearance of upper central incisor teeth attributed to an excess of fluoride in the drinking water.

Plate 6. Hereditary enamel defect known as amelogenesis imperfecta. Inadequate acrylic crowns have been placed on the upper central incisors and lower left incisors.

Plate 7. The same patient as in Plate 6, with porcelain crowns on anterior teeth, and gold crowns on posterior teeth.

Plate 8. Hereditary opalescent dentine (dentinogenesis imperfecta), showing disobvious gingivitis.

Plate 9. Extrinsic staining of incisor, canine and premolar teeth following one months' use of a dental gel containing chlorhexidine.

Plate 10. Gross plaque and calculus formation on the lower incisor teeth with obvious gingivitis.

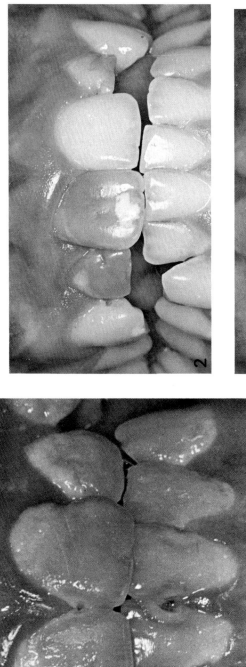

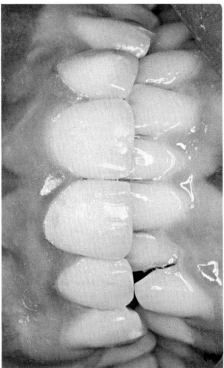

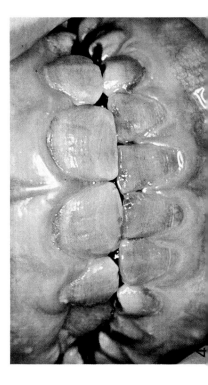

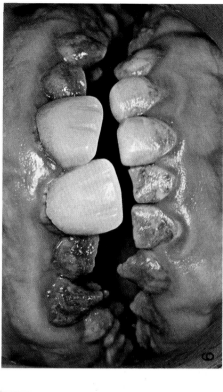

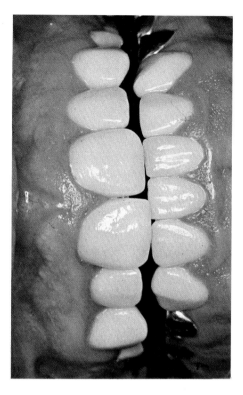

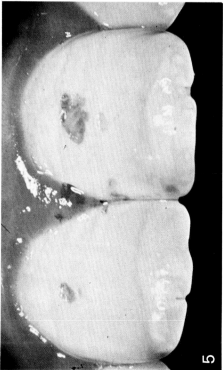

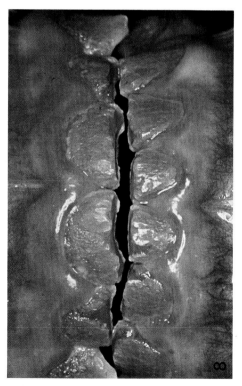

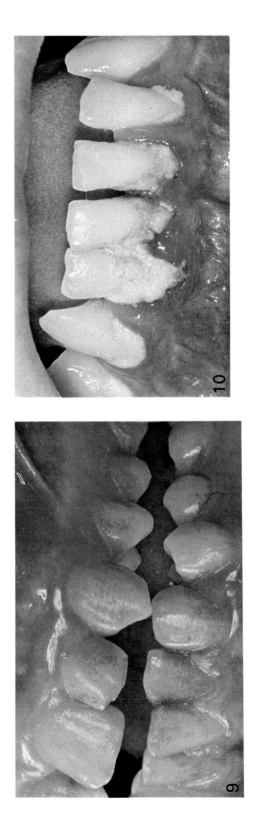

important. For many years silicate cement has been used to restore anterior teeth. This material is marketed in a range of shades so that the colour of the tooth can be matched very closely and the aesthetic results are very pleasing initially. However, silicates have a much higher coefficient of expansion than tooth enamel, and are very much softer, so that over a period of time silicate restorations, in some patients' mouths particularly, deteriorate and have to be replaced. More recently a tremendous interest has been shown in developing new anterior composite restorations, based on the substance bis-phenol glycidyl methacrylate. These new materials are much harder than silicate cements, and in consequence are more difficult to polish and adapt to the margins of the tooth cavity. Over a period of time they tend to lose their surface sheen, although they do not wear away as quickly as silicate restorations. These new materials, particularly when they are bonded onto the enamel using an acid-etch technique, have opened up new horizons for the dental surgeon, in particular with respect to the aesthetic appearance of restorations in anterior teeth, but more research is needed to improve the long term cosmetic properties of these materials.

The prevalence of dental caries is high in advanced industrialized societies where sucrose is an important ingredient in the diet. In developing countries which originally had a very low prevalence of caries, the intro-duction of foods containing sucrose and fermentable carbohydrates has been associated with an increase in the amount of tooth decay. Dental plaque, which mainly consists of aggregations of bacteria and their products on the tooth surface, produces acid in the presence of sucrose, and if the tooth surface is susceptible, dental caries results. If the teeth can be kept scrupulously clean and free from plaque, very few lesions occur, although it is doubtful whether the average person can achieve a situation where plaque is completely absent from their mouth and for this reason a regular thorough professional prophylaxis is usually necessary in addition to an individual's own oral hygiene regime.

In areas with approximately 1 mg fluoride ions per litre naturally present in the drinking water, the prevalence of dental caries has been found to be markedly reduced (Fig. 2). Although fluoride is naturally present in all water supplies, sometimes in concentrations well above 1 mg/l or 1 ppm, in the majority of cases the fluoride concentration is lower than this figure, and many communities have adjusted the fluoride content of their drinking water to 1 mg/l by adding sodium fluoride or hydrofluosilicic acid at the pumping stations. Studies have shown that these communities benefited from this measure (Fig. 3) and as a result the World Health Organization has recommended all member states to implement water fluoridation wherever possible and that it should be regarded as the cornerstone of any national programme for dental caries prevention.

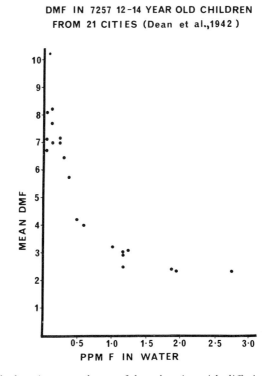

DMF IN 7257 12-14 YEAR OLD CHILDREN
FROM 21 CITIES (Dean et al.,1942)

Fig. 2.   Graph showing prevalence of dental caries with differing water fluoride levels. Caries expressed as mean number of decayed, missing and filled teeth (DMF) per child.

Fluoride has also been added to dentifrices, usually in the form of sodium monofluorophosphate or stannous fluoride, to yield 1000 ppmF. Regular use of a fluoride dentifrice has been shown to have a beneficial effect in reducing the number of new cavities occurring and this benefit has been observed in areas with low and optimum concentrations of fluoride in the public water supplies.

B. Pulp Changes

The pulp is the vital part of the tooth and contains cells, blood vessels, nerves and connective tissue. One of the major causes of pulp death is untreated dental caries, whereby the enamel and dentine are destroyed thus allowing bacteria from the mouth easy access to the pulp, causing infection

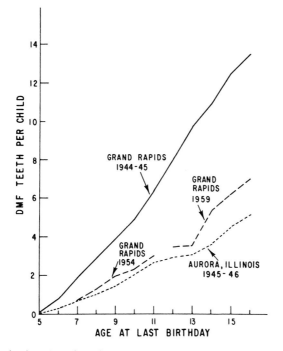

Fig. 3. Graph showing dental caries in Grand Rapids children after 10 and after 15 years of artificial fluoridation, compared with the natural fluoride area of Aurora, Illinois.

and destroying vital pulp tissue. Trauma to teeth, particularly anterior teeth, is another important cause of pulp death, either by rupturing the blood vessels at the apical foramen or by fracturing the crown of the tooth and so exposing the pulp to bacteria. A tooth with a non-vital pulp slowly darkens and the enamel and dentine become more brittle. In these cases endodontic treatment is necessary to remove the non-vital pulp tissue, a root filling is inserted and the colour of the tooth improved by placing a crown, usually made of porcelain, onto the tooth (Plates 2 and 3).

C. Disorders During Tooth Development

Dental caries and trauma may affect a tooth once it has erupted into the mouth, but a tooth is very susceptible to injury during the whole period of its development. The first permanent molar tooth and the incisor teeth begin to mineralize around the time of birth and the crowns of these teeth are completed by the fourth year of life. These teeth erupt into the mouth usually from the age of five or six onwards and therefore disturbances to their development during these early years can result in discoloured or badly formed teeth. Some people suffer from rare genetic conditions in which the enamel or dentine is incorrectly formed. Teeth affected in this way may have a very poor appearance, and are usually treated by restoration with crowns to improve aesthetics.

Altogether nearly 100 different factors may be associated with defects of enamel; these are listed in Table I, and can be divided into two main groups: those which cause localized defects limited to one or a few teeth and those which cause generalized defects, affecting most or all teeth. Localized defects may be caused by trauma, infection or irradiation. Generalized defects may be due to environmental or inherited conditions. Generalized defects caused by environmental factors may occur in the prenatal, neo-natal or post-natal periods and may be due to infection, endocrine and nutritional disturbances, haemolytic disorders, exogenous intoxications and cardiac, renal and gastrointestinal disturbances. Inherited disorders may affect the teeth alone or may be one manifestation of a more generalized condition. The following examples show how the appearance of a tooth can be affected by disorders during development.

1. *Infection*

If a carious primary tooth is left untreated, the pulp is inevitably involved and an abscess frequently forms. In some instances, particularly in premolar teeth which develop in close proximity to the roots of the primary molar teeth, the abscess connected with the primary tooth affects the development of the succeeding permanent tooth. A serious systemic infection in young children, for example broncho-pneumonia or gastroenteritis, can affect developing ameloblasts which lay down the enamel matrix, causing a disturbance of enamel formation or mineralization during the period of the illness and may be seen as a line or groove on a number of teeth.

2. *Drugs and Diet*

Many serious infections require antibiotic therapy, but one of the side effects of the tetracycline group of drugs is that they bind to the calcifying portions of the teeth and prolonged therapy can produce disfiguring yellow, yellow-brown or grey teeth (Plate 4). This condition is irreversible and although it may be possible to improve the appearance by bleaching or coating the surfaces with composite resins the final treatment is usually to crown the anterior teeth with porcelain jacket crowns. Doctors have therefore been advised that tetracycline therapy should be avoided if

Table I
Causes of enamel hypoplasia and intrinsic discolourations of teeth

Localized	Generalized				
	Environmental			Hereditary	
	Prenatal	Neonatal	Post-natal	Tooth only	Accompanied by general disease
Acute trauma to primary teeth	Rubella	Haemolytic disease	Otitis media	Autosomal dominant thin and smooth hypoplasia	Kinky hair syndrome
Extraction of primary teeth	Congenital syphilis	Prematurity	Measles		Ectodermal dysplasia
			Scarlet fever	Autosomal dominant thin and rough hypoplasia	Oculoectodermal dysplasia
Cleft palate repair	Alloxan diabetes	Neonatal asphyxia	Chickenpox		Epidermolysis bullosa dystrophica
Gunshot jaw wounds	Thalidomide	Breech presentation	Bulbar polio	Autosomal dominant randomly pitted hypoplasia	Focal dermal hypoplasia
	Fluoride	Twinning	Whooping cough		
Electric burn to mouth	Maternal Vit. A deficiency	Caesarian section	Smallpox	Autosomal dominant localized hypoplasia	Hurler's syndrome
			Pneumonia		

Table I—*continued*
Causes of enamel hypoplasia and intrinsic discolourations of teeth

Localized	Generalized				
	Environmental			Hereditary	
	Prenatal	Neonatal	Post-natal	Tooth only	Accompanied by general disease
Irradiation	Maternal Vit. D deficiency	Prolonged labour	Tuberculosis	X-linked dominant rough hypoplasia	Hunter's syndrome
Ankylosis	Congenital allergies	Intrapartum haemorrhage	Diphtheria		San Filippo's syndrome
Jaw fracture	Maternal hypoxia	Bronchopulmonary infection	Vit. A deficiency	Autosomal dominant hypocalcification	Morqui–Ullrich syndrome
Periapical infection of primary teeth		Neonatal hypocalcaemia	Vit. C deficiency		Ehlers-Danlos syndrome
Acute osteomyelitis		Meningitis	Vit. D deficiency	X-linked recessive hypomaturation	Lipoid Proteinasis syndrome
	Pregnancy toxaemia		Vit. D intoxication		Juvenile hyperuricaemi syndrome
	Cardiac disease		Fluoride	Autosomal recessive pigmented hypomaturation	Marshall syndrome
	Kidney disease		Lead intoxication	Snow capped teeth	Oculomandibulocephaly
	Anaemia		Tetracyclines	Autosomal dominant hypomaturation with occasional	Down's syndrome

Popliteal Pterygium syndrome

Rieger's syndrome

Mandibulofacial dysostosis syndrome

Congenital facial diplegia syndrome

Orodigitofacial dysostosis syndrome

Cleidocranial dysostosis

Ichthyosis Vulgaris

Phenylketonuria

Infantile allergy syndrome

Prader-Willi syndrome

Porphyria

Pseudo-hypoparathyroidism

Congenital haemolytic anaemia

Nephrotic syndrome

Hypothyroidism

Hypoparathyroidism

Hypogonadism

possible, unless there is an overriding medical reason, below the age of eight years.

Some babies who are bottle fed may be at risk from hypocalcaemia during the first few weeks of life possibly due to the relatively high phosphate content of cow's milk. If hypocalcaemia occurs it is possible for the development of primary teeth to be affected, but permanent teeth are rarely involved in these cases.

Although an optimum level of fluoride in drinking water is beneficial in reducing dental caries, an excess of fluoride can cause staining and/or pitting of teeth. In fact it was the presence of this stain on the teeth of inhabitants of Colorado Springs which stimulated a dentist, Frederick McKay, in 1902, to study this problem. It was not until 1931 that fluoride was isolated from the public water supplies. In conjunction with Trendley Dean he showed that at 1 ppmF mottling was of no public health significance, but as the fluoride concentration increased beyond this an increasing proportion of the population had noticeable stains on their teeth which was intrinsic and could not be removed (Plate 5).

3. *Genetic Conditions*

Hereditary enamel defects unassociated with evidence of systemic disease are collectively known under the title of amelogenesis imperfecta. At least ten types of amelogenesis imperfecta have been described (Winter and Brook 1975). All these conditions are rare in the community and amelogenesis imperfecta of all types has been estimated to occur about 1:14 000 in the general population. Most common is the autosomal dominant hypocalcification type which occurs about 1:20 000. This anomaly affects both dentitions. The teeth erupt with a dull, lustreless, opaque white, honey coloured or light brown surface. In the more severely affected teeth the soft enamel rapidly wears away leaving a rough, discoloured and highly sensitive dentine exposed within a few months of eruption (Plate 6). The posterior teeth must be protected with full veneer gold crowns: anterior teeth are treated initially with "basket crowns" – gold crowns with a tooth coloured acrylic facing – which can be replaced by porcelain crowns when the child reaches the age of 16 years approximately (Plate 7).

There are a number of hereditary defects of dentine in some of which the enamel may be affected to a variable degree, but in which the underlying dentine is always incorrectly formed and the teeth may be discoloured as a result (Plate 8). Furthermore in some of these cases restorative treatment may be complicated because of poor root formation.

III. EXTRINSIC STAINS

Extrinsic stains are produced by deposition on the surface of the teeth. Some individuals accumulate both stains and calculus much more rapidly than others. Certain factors predispose to this accumulation, including roughness of the enamel, irregularity of the teeth, poor oral hygiene and a high mucin content of saliva. Following prophylaxis of the teeth with an abrasive paste, a complete film of salivary glycoproteins is redeposited on the surface enamel within hours. This pellicle is macroscopically invisible but may readily pick up stain if a toothpaste without an abrasive is used. Bacteria, fungi, desquamated epithelial cells and food debris accumulate on the tooth surface and, in the absence of mechanical tooth cleaning procedures, a bacterial plaque is formed. If the surface enamel is intact it is the superficial pellicle, plaque and calculus which become stained, but if there is any hypoplastic or hypomineralized enamel or exposed dentine then stain may penetrate these areas.

A. "Chromogenic Bacteria"

Many of the stains seen on children's teeth have been classically described as being due to the presence of certain bacteria in plaque.

1. *Green Stain*
Green stain is common in children of all ages and particularly affects a crescent close to the gingivae in upper anterior teeth. The surface enamel is often irregular in this region, but it has been suggested that the membrane remnants that covered the tooth before eruption also act as a nidus for the multiplication of bacteria. Bacillus pyocyaneus, Penicillium glaucum and Aspergillus have all been suggested as causative organisms. This stain tends to recur after removal.

2. *Black Stain*
Occasionally, in both children and adults, a fine black line running about 1 mm from the gingivae on both lingual and buccal surfaces of the teeth is seen. This is known as the mesenteric line and is said to be associated with a low caries incidence (Shourie, 1947). Its aetiology is obscure but it is often particularly pronounced near the excretory ducts of salivary glands, and it has been suggested that chromogenic bacteria deposit pigment in areas of increased mucin production.

3. *Brown Stain*

Brown stains are found at any age, but particularly in children. The lingual surfaces of the maxillary posterior teeth, close to the gingivae, are often involved. Stones (1962) stated that its presence usually indicated a susceptibility to caries, but the evidence for this is somewhat scant.

4. *Orange Stain*

Orange stain occurs in approximately 3% of children and although many bacteria, including Bacillus roseus, Sarcina rosea and Micrococcus roseus, have been isolated from it, there is no doubt that it is associated with poor oral hygiene. It is rapidly removed by dental prophylaxis and will not recur if good oral hygiene is maintained.

B. Nicotine

By far the most common stain in adults is produced by nicotine deposition. The colour, intensity, amount and distribution of tobacco stains varies with the type and quantity of tobacco used and the degree and length of exposure, but is also related to oral hygiene and individual susceptibility. More extensive staining is often found on the lingual aspects of the teeth indicating the importance of oral hygiene in its prevention. On undamaged enamel surfaces the tobacco staining is only superficial, but if there is any exposed dentine, it penetrates the tubules. Many investigators have found that the formation of calculus is significantly increased in tobacco smoking (Pindborg, 1949).

C. Dentifrices and Drugs

Stain deposits caused by dentifrices are not a problem for most patients, but a relationship has been demonstrated between the presence of stannous fluoride in a dentifrice and the production of yellow-brown staining. Naylor and Emslie (1967), James and Anderson (1967) and Fanning *et al.* (1968) all showed increased staining with the use of a stannous fluoride paste.

Chlorhexidine, both when incorporated into a dentifrice and when used as a mouthwash, has also been shown to produce discolourations. The stain is deposited on the surface of natural teeth, silicate fillings, and artificial teeth and is said not to penetrate the surface. It is not, however, easy to remove and often requires polishing with a prophylactic paste by a dentist or hygienist for complete elimination (Plate 9). The origin, nature and mechanism of formation are essentially unknown and no definite relationship has been found with smoking or the intake of certain food-stuffs. Although the anti-plaque effectiveness of chlorhexidine has been demonstrated in many clinical trials (Löe, 1973) the main problem associated with its use remains its propensity to form stain.

Other substances used for treating various conditions within the mouth may also discolour the teeth. Iodine, silver nitrate and essential oils such as Eugenol will stain exposed dentine. Potassium permanganate has been incorporated into mouthwashes and black deposits of hydrated manganese dioxide may occur. Mouthwashes formulated with inorganic and organic mercury compounds, and mercurial salts used as antiseptics such as mercurochrome and metaphen, yield black, green and orange discolourations.

Certain drugs administered for systemic medical conditions cause staining. Iron is occasionally given in liquid form for the treatment of anaemia. This results in a black iron sulphide deposit. Para-amino salicylic acid was extensively used in the treatment of pulmonary tuberculosis and yellow-brown tooth discolourations were observed.

D. Food Substances

Some food substances, such as certain red wines, black cherries, raspberries and other fruits, produce transitory staining of the surface pellicle. However, there are many other foodstuffs with the ability to produce more persistent staining. Coffee, tea and cola drinks give brownish discolourations, and highly spiced foods containing saffron, red pepper, turmeric etc. leave red and yellow stains. The habit of chewing betel nut, areca and liquorice results in an intense brown stain which is extremely difficult to remove.

E. Metallic Deposits

Various metals and metallic preparations can stain the teeth. This is a superficial deposit unless the enamel is hypoplastic or exposed dentine is present. Apart from those compounds used for medicinal purposes, metallic stains result from inhalation of dust or fumes by workers in the manufacturing industries. Amongst metals capable of producing tooth discolourations are copper, nickel, iron, silver, manganese, antimony, tin, chromium and cadmium.

IV. MECHANICAL CONTROL OF PLAQUE

If the enamel surface is intact then pellicle, plaque or calculus formation must be present for the build up of extrinsic stain. With established severe staining it is usually necessary for a professional prophylaxis with an abrasive paste and a rotary brush to be carried out to remove all the deposit. However, it is then up to the individual to practise oral hygiene methods aimed at preventing plaque formation.

Epidemiological investigations have shown a strong correlation between the amount of plaque and the severity of periodontal disease (Greene, 1966). In a series of classical studies Löe and his co-workers (Löe et al., 1965; Theilade et al., 1966) showed that when all oral hygiene procedures were discontinued plaque accumulated and gingivitis developed. These clinical investigations confirmed the intimate association between the state of oral hygiene and the health of the periodontium. Since dental plaque is the ultimately important factor causing periodontal disease, preventive methods should aim at its removal and reduction in formation.

At one time it was commonly believed that eating coarse fibrous foods had a natural cleansing effect. Many workers have now shown that eating considerable quantities of foods such as carrots has no effect on plaque accumulation in gingival areas. Plaque develops even in the absence of food in the mouth; the consistency and type of diet affects only the quantity and biochemistry of the developing plaque.

A. Toothbrushing—Types of Toothbrush

Many studies have attempted to determine the relative effectiveness of different types of toothbrush. Short term trials have indicated the superiority of powered brushes over manually operated brushes, but once the novelty effect of electric toothbrushing has worn off, in the long term tests have shown that they are both equally effective (Greene, 1966; Crawford et al., 1975; McAllan et al., 1976). Powered brushes may well be of value for the physically or mentally handicapped.

Toothbrushes vary widely in size and shape, and in the type and configuration of bristles. There is much conflicting evidence as to their influence on cleaning effect. Kardel et al. (1971) claimed that the size and shape of the brush head had no significant effect on cleansing ability whereas Scully and Wade (1970) showed that short headed brushes were more efficient. Recently published work (Scopp et al., 1976) indicated that a new contoured toothbrush was significantly better at plaque removal than conventional commercially available toothbrushes. However, although statistically significant differences have been demonstrated between shapes of brushes the clinical significance is probably limited.

Misconceptions have developed about the bristle material itself but there is now almost universal agreement that nylon bristles are preferable. Natural bristles deteriorate much more rapidly than their nylon counterparts due to water absorption and there is no conclusive evidence that differences exist between them as far as plaque removal and abrasivity are concerned (Wade, 1953; Mooser, 1959).

There is also disagreement on the relative merits of soft, medium and hard textured brushes. Bergenholtz *et al.* (1967) claimed that there was no difference in cleansing efficiency between hard and soft bristles whilst Scully and Wade (1970) found that hard textured bristles were superior. Hine (1950) showed that hard bristles of one brand could correspond to medium or soft of another.

No difference in efficacy of plaque removal was observed between the space-tufted and multitufted toothbrushes in studies by Bergenholtz *et al.* (1969) and Kardel *et al.* (1971). A trial carried out by Bay *et al.* (1967), however, reported a better cleaning effect with multi-tufted toothbrushes.

At present it must be inferred that there is no clear indication of the superiority of any particular toothbrush design, shape or texture.

B. Methods of Toothbrushing

Greene (1966) listed seven methods of toothbrushing:

1. Vertical
2. Horizontal
3. Roll technique
4. Vibratory techniques (Charters, Stillman and Bass)
5. Circular technique
6. Physiological technique
7. Scrub-brush method

Many workers have shown no statistical differences between the different techniques according to plaque removal effectiveness (Frandsen *et al.*, 1970; Hansen and Gjermo, 1971). Later work by Frandsen *et al.* (1972) indicated that the Charter's and Scrub-brush methods were more effective than the roll technique in removing plaque, but they also stated that the effectiveness of a particular technique depended partly on the instructor. The relative effectiveness of the different methods is difficult to determine because of the many variables involving the patient and the dentition. In some adults with gingival recession, the horizontal method of brushing may increase the degree of root dentine abrasion and lead to V-shaped notches in the teeth. However, it is probable that no one technique is suitable for everyone and the choice should be individually determined.

C. Frequency of Toothbrushing

More frequent toothbrushing has been shown to lead to better plaque control and less gingivitis (McKendrick *et al.*, 1970). Stanmeyer (1957) found that brushing twice a day was sufficient to maintain oral health, but brushing a third time produced no additional benefit. Most unsupervised and uninstructed individuals do not achieve complete plaque removal with a toothbrush (Lindhe and Koch, 1966). Löe (1969) demonstrated that gingivae can remain clinically healthy with complete removal of plaque once every second day. It must therefore be concluded that efficiency of toothbrushing is more important than frequency of toothbrushing.

D. Toothbrushing Without Toothpaste

Several investigators have found that adequate cleansing could be achieved by the use of toothbrush alone and that removal of plaque and debris depends more on brushing technique and time than on the dentifrice (Mooser, 1959; Moss, 1971). An evaluation of most clinical trials led the American Dental Association Council on Dental Therapeutics (1970) to conclude that although some individuals could clean their teeth with brush and water alone, most individuals required some abrasive to assist in removing materials that tended to accumulate on teeth. Since this report Badersten and Egelberg (1972) and Wong Lee (1974) have also confirmed this by showing that brushing with paste is more effective in removing or reducing plaque than brushing with water. There is considerable evidence to suggest that if a dentifrice is not used an aesthetically objectionable brown stained pellicle develops on the teeth of 90% of the population within a four week period (Manly, 1943; Robinson, 1969; Hefferen, 1974; Davis and Rees, 1975).

Perhaps the most important property of a toothpaste can be assessed by preventing its use. In many clinical trials where toothbrushing has been carried out without a toothpaste many of the participants withdrew or expressed dissatisfaction at being prevented from using a dentifrice. The use of toothpaste is an important motivating aspect of toothbrushing and most people would either not brush their teeth at all, or not brush them as effectively if a dentifrice was not employed (Dudding *et al.*, 1960; Wong Lee, 1974).

E. Toothbrushing with Toothpaste

The primary objective in using a dentifrice is to aid the cleansing of accessible tooth surfaces and make toothbrushing more pleasant. The most important constituents of a dentifrice in relation to its mechanical cleansing properties are the abrasives and surface active agents.

1. *Abrasives*

In 1974 the British Standards Institute published a specification for toothpastes (BS 5136:1974) in which particular attention was focused on the subject of excessive abrasion of the dental tissues. It was stated in this report that abrasion could conceivably represent a harmful property of toothpaste which cannot easily be recognized by the user. Wear of the tooth substance may well be as much due to faulty brushing technique as to the abrasivity of the dentifrice, but nevertheless the B.S.I. stressed that reasonable control should be exercised over the abrasive properties. A radio-isotope tracer technique, originally used by Grabenstetter *et al.* (1958), was described as the recommended method of determining abrasion. This system of measurement gives an ordinal value for a given test product in relation to a specified standard reference paste rather than assigning an absolute numerical value. A mass of information detailing *in vitro* abrasion tests on enamel and dentine by various abrasive components of dentifrices is now available. However, the question posed by Kitchin and Robinson in 1948 "How abrasive need a dentifrice be?" remains largely unanswered.

The American Dental Association's report on the abrasivity of current dentifrices (1970) stated that a dentifrice should be no more abrasive than is necessary to keep the teeth clean, that is free of accessible plaque, debris and superficial stain. Considering the removal of plaque and debris, the evidence for the effectiveness of abrasives is equivocal. Several studies have been carried out comparing the plaque removing abilities of high, moderate, low and non-abrasive dentifrices and no statistical or clinical differences have been shown between pastes (Bergenholtz, 1971; Toto and Rapp, 1972). Reference has already been made to the fact that when toothbrushing is carried out without toothpaste extrinsic staining of the teeth develops. The level of toothpaste abrasivity required to prevent and remove stain has been difficult to evaluate. McCauley *et al.* (1946) and Bergenholtz (1971) reported that insufficiently abrasive dentifrices favoured the production of pigmented pellicle but did not suggest any threshold levels. Gerdin (1970), however, disputes whether any abrasive is necessary at all. His studies of the effect of a non-abrasive dentifrice containing polymethyl methacrylate spherical granules compared with a conventional abrasive dentifrice in children showed that the total frequency of discoloured stains was somewhat lower in the non-abrasive group. It should be noted that there were a considerable number of complaints from adults using the non-abrasive paste on the unacceptable levels of staining. Moreover, even in children, there have been reports of excessive staining with the use of low abrasive dentifrices (Forsman 1974).

There will obviously be considerable individual variation in the need for an abrasive related to the different propensities for the development of extrinsic stain, but as yet there is no accurate indication as to just how abrasive a toothpaste should be.

2. *Surface Active Agents*

Essentially all dentifrices now marketed contain surface active agents. These are usually synthetic detergents such as sodium lauryl sulphate and sodium N-lauroyl sarcosinate which produce the foaming property of the toothpaste. Surface active detergents can lower the surface tension, penetrate and loosen surface deposits, and emulsify or suspend the debris which the toothbrush removes from the tooth surface. Their principal contribution may be the effect on consistency, foaming properties, or other physical characteristics of the mixture. The surface active agent concentration in a dentifrice is also important in that it can modify the characteristics of the abrasive. For example, the abrasiveness of a slurry of calcium carbonate is diminished by approximately half when a substantial quantity of

Table II
Clinical fluoride dentifrice trials

Agent	Number of studies	Number showing statistically significant reductions in caries increment
Sodium fluoride	10	6
Acidulated phosphate fluoride	4	2
Potassium fluoride	1	1
Stannous fluoride	33	28
Sodium monofluorophosphate fluoride	19	19
Amine fluoride	2	2

sodium alkyl sulphate is present (Gershon and Pader, 1972). Thus abrasiveness must be determined not only of that material added for its specific abrasive character but of the total dentifrice formulation.

F. Other Mechanical Aids to Plaque Control

Hansen and Gjermo (1971) found that toothbrushing did not significantly remove interdental plaque even in patients with wide open interdental spaces. Such adjuncts to plaque removal as woodpoints and dental floss have been shown to be effective in removing plaque in these areas, but the main problem in their use is adequate motivation of the patient.

V. CHEMICAL CONTROL OF PLAQUE

Nearly forty substances with potential therapeutic activity have been incorporated in dentifrice formulations. These agents are summarized in Tables II and III. The majority of them are specifically anti-plaque agents but the mode of action of some substances is still unknown. A similar number of potential "active agents" have been incorporated into mouthrinses etc., but have not yet been incorporated into a dentifrice (Table IV).

A. Fluorides (Table II)

The caries reducing effect of fluoride compounds in dentifrices is extremely well documented and requires no further enlargement. It has also been reported by Lobene and Soparkar (1974) that brushing with a 1·66% amine fluoride toothpaste for seven days showed a 20% reduction in plaque and a 37% reduction in gingivitis in the test group over the control.

B. Antibiotics

Eight antibiotics have been used in clinical toothpaste trials. These are penicillin, vancomycin, streptomycin, kanamycin, bacitracin, tyrothricin, macrolide CC 10232 and gramicidin. Any medically useful wide-spectrum antibiotic should not be used for dental application. Repeated topical applications may give rise to the development of resistant strains of bacteria,

Table III
Clinical dentifrice trials of potential therapeutic agent formulations

Group	Name of active agent	Number of studies using toothpaste	Number of studies showing reductions in:		
			(a) Plaque	(b) Gingivitis	(c) Caries
1. ANTIBIOTICS	Penicillin	7			1
	Vancomycin	9	7	4	
	Streptomycin	1			
	Kanamycin	3	3	2	
	Bacitracin	2			
	Tyrothricin	4			2
	Macrolide CC 10232	3	3	1	
	Gramicidin	1			
2. SURFACTANTS					
(a) Cationic amines	Urea (i) Low content	3			1
	(ii) High content	8			6
	Urea peroxide	6	1	1	
	Quaternary ammonium compounds	1	4		
	Long chain primary amines: tetradecylamine	4	1		4
	Bisguanides: chlorhexidine	11	9	5	1
(b) Anionic	Sodium oxalate and sodium dehydroacetate	2			2

		10	9	2
	cellulase etc.			2
	Acids	2		
	Chelating Agents:			
	Sodium hexametaphosphate	1	1	
	Ex 347 (Extar)	3	3	
	Disodium etidronate (polyphosphonate)	4	4	
	Cariostatic phosphates:			
	inorganic phosphate	1		
	Calcium saccharose phosphate	1		1
	Zinc salts	1	1	1
	Hexachlorophene	1		
	Organic ammonium iodide (Stark Jod Kaliklora)	1		1
	Vitamin toothpastes	1		
	Chloroform	2		
	Hypertonic sea-salt	1		1
	Anti-hypersensitivity Agents:			
	Formalin	7		
	Strontium chloride	8		
	Potassium nitrate	1		
	Chlorophyll	6		2

4. CRYSTAL GROWTH INHIBITORS

5. MISCELLANEOUS

Table IV
Studies of potential therapeutic agents not yet tested in dentifrice formulations

Group	Name of active agent	Number of studies	In vitro	In vivo Animal	In vivo Man	Total micro-organisms	Plaque	Gingivitis	Caries
1. ANTIBIOTICS	Chloramphenicol	1			1				1
	Aureomycin	3	2		1			1	2
	Tetracycline	1			1		1		
	Spiramycin	2			2			2	
	Erythromycin	1			1		1		
	Neomycin	2			2				
	Polymixin B	2			2		2		
	Actinobolin	2	2		2	2			
2. SURFACTANTS									
(a) Cationic amines	Quaternary ammonium compounds:								
	Cetylpyridinium chloride	4			4		3		
	"with Domiphen bromide"	3			3		2	2	
	"with Dequalinium acetate"	1			1				
	Benzalkonium chloride	5	2		3	2	1		
	Benzethonium chloride	3			3		2		
	Dequalinium chloride	1			1				
	Domiphen bromide	2			2		1		
	Phemerol	1							
	Damol	1							
	D301	1			1		1		
	Long chain primary								

Phosphoramidates:

Victamine C and chlormethyl analogues	5	2				3
3. ENZYMES						
Dextranase	10		4	6		3 (animal)
Mutanase	3		2	1		2
4. CRYSTAL GROWTH INHIBITORS Cariostatic phosphates:						
Dibasic Calcium phosphate	5		3			4
Tricalcium phosphate	2		2	2		2
Sodium metaphosphate	1		1			1
Calcium glycerophosphate	3		1	2	2	1
Ion exchange resins	6	4		2	4 (in vitro)	
Ascoxal (ascorbic acid+H_2O_2)	7		7		3	
Zinc salts	8		8		7	
Fluoro-salicylanilides	2	2	2			2
Anti-ureas	1	1	1		1	
5. MISCELLANEOUS						
Quinine	2		2	1		
Erythrocin	2	2		2		
Iodine	6		6	2	2	
Dodecyldiamoethyl-glycine	1	1		1		
Essential oils, e.g. thymol	1		1			

hypersensitivity reactions and alteration of the oral flora with fungal over-growth. Many antibiotics also have toxic side-effects, for example tyro-thricin, gramicidin and streptomycin have been associated with haemolytic damage. The only antibiotics which have shown effectiveness against plaque and gingivitis and are relatively safe are vancomycin and macrolide CC 10232. These both require further extensive long term clinical studies before their use can be recommended.

C. Surface Active Agents (Surfactants)

The contribution of the synthetic detergent surfactants to physical cleansing has already been referred to. Surfactant molecules contain a hydrophobic water repellent non-polar grouping and a hydrophilic water attracting grouping. They arrange themselves at liquid interfaces so as to reduce surface tension. Their affinity for cell surfaces makes them toxic to bacteria.

1. *Cationic Amines*

Urea and urea peroxide have been incorporated in toothpastes since 1935. Low content urea pastes have proved ineffective as therapeutic agents and higher amounts are extremely unpalatable. However, the use of urea peroxide in gel form has shown promising results in the control of plaque and gingivitis and justifies further trials (Kaslick *et al.*, 1975).

Many quaternary ammonium compounds such as cetylpyridinium chloride and benzalkonium chloride have been used extensively and effectively in mouthwashes, but there is only one report of one of these compounds being tested in a dentifrice (Harrap, 1974). Plaque was shown to be inhibited over a 16-hour period.

Long straight chain primary amines have been investigated as potential cariostatic and anti-plaque compounds in clinical trials in New Zealand. Despite early beneficial results, a later study with more rigorous control and better statistical assessment by Ludwig (1963) showed no effects. *In vitro* work by Turesky (1972) demonstrated anti-plaque effectivity.

The most promising group of therapeutic agents to be investigated recently is the bisguanides, and in particular chlorhexidine. Schroeder (1969) first studied their plaque inhibitory potential. Chlorhexidine was found to be the most effective *in vivo* and the least toxic of the compounds tested. Eleven clinical trials have been reported of its formulation as a toothpaste, and all demonstrated some reduction in plaque, gingivitis or caries.

2. *Anionic Surfactants*

Soap and synthetic detergents not only have surface active properties but also inhibit glycolytic enzymes essential in the Embden–Meyerhof cycle for the glycolysis of sucrose in plaque. Soaps have largely been replaced in toothpaste by synthetic detergents because of their precipitation with calcium salts, high alkalinity and unpleasant taste.

The anti-plaque effectiveness of synthetic detergents has not been accurately measured as clinical trials testing such substances as sodium-N-lauroyl sarcosinate and sodium lauryl sulphate have not used a true placebo. There have been 13 clinical studies of sarcosinate containing dentifrices, of which four showed no reductions in plaque, caries or the maintenance of pH when compared with other pastes. Sodium ricinoleate and its sulphonate have undergone ten clinical trials; all except one demonstrated plaque and calculus reduction. However, the Council on Dental Therapeutics of the American Dental Association regarded the evidence in support of antibacterial activity of surfactants as controversial and stated that their usefulness in caries control had not been adequately established. They are important in the formulation of the correct physical properties of a toothpaste.

D. Enzymes

Proteolytic enzymes incorporated into dentifrices have been assessed in ten clinical trials. Theoretically their action is to reduce mucin deposition and to inhibit or soften calculus deposits. In nine studies significant differences in plaque and calculus levels were found in the test group when compared with the control group. No reductions in caries incidence have ever been reported. There are problems in the formulation of any enzyme compound due to their instability.

Later research in this field concentrated on the dextran and laevan groups of the complex muco-polysaccharides synthesized by the oral bacteria which constitute an important part of dental plaque. Fitzgerald *et al.* (1968) reported the results of *in vitro* and animal studies with the enzyme dextranase which stimulated six clinical trials of a dextranase mouthwash and proposed studies with dentifrices. However, the results in man were extremely disappointing as all six clinical trials demonstrated no benefits with the use of the mouthwash. Further work is being carried out on another enzyme, mutanase, which has shown good potential in animal experiments (Guggenheim *et al.*, 1972) but there is no published work on its use in man.

E. Crystal Growth Inhibitors

Many substances have been incorporated into dentifrices with the potential ability to remove calculus and prevent its formation.

If plaque is allowed to remain in the mouth for long periods it may gradually calcify and be converted into calculus. Plaque from different individuals varies greatly in its tendency to calcify. It has been reported that the saliva of rapid calculus producers has a high concentration of protein and ammonia, but the wide variations in calculus formation from one person to another are not clearly understood. Chronic inflammation of the gums induced by plaque eventually results in the formation of periodontal pockets. Calculus may then be deposited in these pockets and is known as sub-gingival calculus. This is a secondary phenomenon as the plaque is considered to be the primary agent in the aetiology of periodontal disease. Both sub- and supra-gingival calculus provide irregular surfaces for the retention of dental plaque and contribute to the displacement of attached epithelium and the progression of periodontal disease.

When chronic gingivitis progresses to chronic periodontitis, and other tissues supporting the teeth are inflamed, then the condition is no longer completely reversible and requires the intervention of a dentist or dental hygienist. Treatment may simply involve scaling and polishing the teeth, but a considerable variety of surgical and conservative procedures may be necessary to prevent further progression of the disease. However, although the task of physically removing old sub- and supra-gingival calculus remains in the hands of the dentist or hygienist, much work has been directed towards chemical control of calculus formation (Plate 10).

Any substance used in the chemical control of dental plaque and all mechanical oral hygiene procedures will have some effect on calculus deposition. Crystal growth inhibitors interfere with the calcification of established plaque and thus inhibit calculus formation.

Prior to the 1930s acids such as hydrochloric and sulphuric were employed in an effort to dissolve calculus with attendant disastrous results. Chelating agents were then investigated; these can dissolve crystalized calcium salts to form stable soluble compounds. Sodium hexametaphosphate, Ex 347, and mono- and tri-ethanolamine diglycolate are all chelating agents that have been used in man and have been shown to dissolve calculus. Their use has been discontinued, as it would appear that selective dissolution of calculus is not a safe approach. It is so similar in mineral content to cementum and dentine that it seems virtually impossible to appreciably dissolve its mineral content without also affecting the dental hard tissues themselves.

Disodium etidronate has been shown to inhibit crystal growth of hydroxyapatite but has a relatively low chelating ability at a physiological pH. Sturzenberger *et al.* (1971) incorporated a 3% concentration of this substance into a suitable dentifrice and showed its effectiveness in reducing calculus formation in a six month clinical study. Another crystal inhibitor, Victamine C, and its chlormethyl analogue has also shown *in vivo* anti-calculus activity. The clinical trials so far concluded have involved limited numbers of participants and further study is necessary (Fischmann *et al.*, 1973).

Anti-calculus and anti-plaque activity has also been claimed for a variety of zinc salts. Of the eight clinical trials so far reported only one has used zinc acetate in a dentifrice, the remaining seven employed zinc salts in the form of mouthwashes. The study by Compton and Beagrie (1973) showed no significant calculus reduction in the group using the zinc mouthwash when compared with the group on the control mouthwash, but all the other studies demonstrated some plaque and/or calculus reduction.

F. Miscellaneous

Chlorophyll was first used in a dentifrice in 1949 following claims for caries preventive, gingivitis reducing and deodorizing properties. Five clinical trials have been reported, three gave negative findings and the results of the other two studies must be regarded as inconclusive. Its use in toothpaste has been discontinued.

Hexachlorophene has been used for many years as a toothpaste additive. A clinical trial reported by Anerud (1970) demonstrated no significant differences between groups using test or control pastes. A Scandinavian toothpaste is commercially available which contains 0·75% of an organic iodide with which Fiedler (1934) showed clinical benefits in patients with gingivitis. Systemic absorption and hypersensitivity reactions have been described.

Quinine derivatives have also been incorporated into toothpastes; *in vitro* anti-plaque activity has been demonstrated but the hypersensitivity reactions associated with the use of quinine render it an undesirable dentifrice additive. Vitamin toothpastes appear to be ineffective *in vivo* as chemotherapeutic agents against oral flora.

Recently chloroform has been incorporated into many brands of toothpaste as an organic solvent and to enhance the flavour. However, Allen *et al.* (1975) investigated its action on the oral mucosa and found inflammation, ulceration, necrosis and intra-epithelial abscesses.

The benefits of a natural saline paste in periodontal therapy were reported by Morgues *et al.* (1965). The results with this sea-salt dentifrice are difficult to interpret due to subjective assessments and inadequate control groups.

Essential oils have been incorporated into toothpastes primarily as flavouring agents, but Gomer *et al.* (1972) observed considerable plaque reduction with thymol and eucalyptol mouthrinses. These oils are found in one commercially available dentifrice.

Other therapeutic agents formulated in toothpastes are those specifically effective against increased sensitivity from exposed root dentine and include formalin, strontium chloride and potassium nitrate. Many clinical trials have been carried out but more objective methods of testing are required before an accurate evaluation of their effects can be made.

VI. CLINICAL METHODS USED IN EVALUATING DENTAL PRODUCTS

Any potential therapeutic agent is tested initially *in vitro* and then followed by extensive animal studies. However, the final evidence as to effectiveness can only be obtained from a controlled clinical trial on human volunteers. The protocol for carrying out controlled clinical trials has been established and is now closely followed in most studies (W.H.O. Oral Health Surveys, Basic Methods 1971; F.D.I. Technical Report No. 1, 1974). The evaluation of agents or procedures which are potentially useful in the control and prevention of caries, plaque, gingivitis and extrinsic staining requires that each of these parameters should be accurately measured.

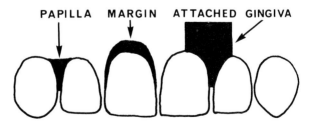

Fig. 4.   Diagram showing the different parts of the gum margin defined by Massler *et al.* (1950), namely, Papilla, Margin and Attached gingiva (PMA index). Note that these units are not distinct from one another: the margin encroaches into two papillae and the attached gingiva involves one papilla, part of the two adjacent margins and extends apically.

Epidemiological surveys and clinical trials have been restricted in the past due to the lack of objective evaluation techniques. A specific index has been developed for use in caries diagnosis which is now almost universally accepted, but there is no comparable definitive index for plaque, gingivitis and staining measurement. Any system of measurement should be simple to use and permit the study of a large number of people in a minimum amount of time. It must be highly reproducible both within and between examiners and yet be sufficiently sensitive and accurate to detect small changes in the condition. Early attempts at formulating indices tended to be either very subjective and thus open to wide variations in examiner interpretation, or else too insensitive for use in clinical trials.

A. Evaluation of Oral Hygiene

Arbitrary descriptions such as good, fair and poor were initially used to describe oral hygiene. Ramfjord (1959) later developed an index to measure plaque and calculus which was further modified by Greene and Vermillion (1964), to become the Oral Hygiene Index. This can be used in both epidemiological surveys and clinical trials, but assesses plaque and calculus according to the area of tooth surface covered rather than in relation to the gingival crevice area which would be more relevant to the aetiology of periodontal disease.

Silness and Löe (1964) described a plaque scoring system in which measurements were restricted to the gingival region. Deposits on individual tooth surfaces are recorded. This has proved to be a very useful index when combined with the gingival index and is now used in many clinical trials.

B. Measurement of Gingivitis

The multiplicity of indices used for diagnosing gingivitis and periodontal disease indicates that none of them are entirely satisfactory. The early signs of gingivitis depend particularly on a subjective colour differentiation on which many examiners find it impossible to agree. The first recording systems were very subjective and lacked precise definition but a more exact scoring was devised by Massler et al. (1950) and considered the degree of gingivitis in three areas. These were the papillae (P), the margin (M) and the attached gingivae (A), and it thus became known as the PMA index (Fig. 4).

Russell (1956) developed an index which has been used in epidemiological surveys but was too insensitive for clinical trials. It measured not only gingivitis but also the irreversible destruction of the periodontal tissues. Criteria were accepted only on positive indications of disease and consequently scores were an underestimation.

The Gingival Index of Löe and Silness (1963) expressed inflammation and location separately. Their scoring criteria were clearly defined and based on the ease with which bleeding was elicited from the gingivae around each of four surfaces of the tooth. This system was related directly to their system for measuring plaque and thus enabled the location of aetiological agents to be correlated with inflammation. It has been found to be very useful in clinical trials, and consistency both between and within examiners is high.

C. Assessment of Staining

One of the most difficult aspects of assessing the abilities of different tooth-pastes to remove and prevent stain is that there is no satisfactory objective way to measure stain *in vivo*. The first attempt at an accurate and detailed evaluation of stain diagnosed clinically was made by Lobene (1968). This index, with minor modifications, was also used by Van Abbe *et al.* (1971). However, a major disadvantage of the method is that Lobene stated that moderately to highly stained teeth were necessary to permit statistical verification of results. Davis and Rees (1975) developed a technique assessing the percentage area of each tooth that was stained. Shaw and Murray (1977) utilized a standardized grid system to record and measure the percentage of stained areas (Fig. 5). This system was found to be extremely sensitive in measuring low levels of stain and detecting small changes in area. After an initial training period the examiners involved were able to consistently reproduce their diagnoses and there was a high level of agreement between examiners as to the presence of stain and the area involved when assessing the same patients.

Lobene (1968) and Davis and Rees (1975) showed that the stain removal powers of commercially available dentifrices differed significantly from one another. Shaw and Murray (1977) carried out a study involving the use of a low and moderate abrasive dentifrice and found that the low abrasive paste resulted in the accumulation of increased extrinsic stain. The distribution of stain was also different when compared with the moderate abrasive paste as significantly more staining was found on the labial surfaces of the teeth in the group of people using the low abrasive paste. There was, however, only one serious complaint about the aesthetic-ally unacceptable stain and it may be that the general adult population accept some staining of the teeth as inevitable or are not even aware of its

LABIAL

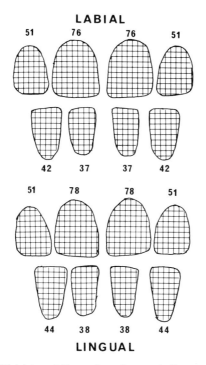

LINGUAL

Fig. 5.   Outlines of labial and lingual surfaces of all incisor teeth with super-imposed standardized grid-system. This chart is used to record and measure the extent of extrinsic tooth stains. (Shaw and Murray, 1977.)

presence. It is probably necessary, therefore, to determine not only the level of abrasivity in a paste which will keep the teeth free from stained pellicle, but also the level of staining which is acceptable to the general public, and this requires an accurate and reproducible method of measuring stain.

VII. IMPROVING ATTITUDES TO DENTAL HEALTH

Although there seems to be an increasing awareness on the part of the general public concerning the importance of dental health, nevertheless staining, plaque and mild gingivitis are often unrecognized and largely ignored. Despite the massive advertising campaigns of dentifrice manu-facturers, it is apparent that not all people brush their teeth regularly. In Great Britain it has been estimated that 70% of toothpastes are used in 30%

of homes, but it is also estimated that toothpaste sales have increased 25% over the last five years. Motivation is necessary to stimulate the practice of good oral hygiene habits which must be instituted early in life. Many dental health education studies have shown that considerable improvements in oral hygiene can be obtained following instruction. The greatest reduction in gingivitis and plaque indices in children is observed when toothbrushing is supervised daily, but effective home care is not carried on when the supervision is stopped. It is therefore essential that more efficient and effective means of communication and motivation are developed.

The aim of dental health education is not only to increase knowledge but to change a person's behavioural pattern so that a permanent improvement in oral hygiene habits is achieved. A recent National Dental Health Action Campaign attempted to show people that with a little effort, care and attention they can keep their teeth for life. The Campaign encouraged thorough and effective cleaning of teeth and gums and emphasized the fact that preventive dentistry plays an important role in the home as well as the dentist's surgery.

SUMMARY

In general over the past decade there has been an increasing awareness concerning the important contribution that good dental health makes to a person's general appearance. Dental treatment to restore carious or unsightly teeth, to remove extrinsic stain and calculus by careful scaling and prophylaxis, and to re-contour gums and eliminate pockets by periodontal surgery, can play an important part in achieving a good cosmetic effect.

It is apparent that mechanical cleaning of teeth and gums by brushing is the most important factor in removing plaque and maintaining good oral health. A pleasant tasting, well formulated dentifrice certainly makes toothbrushing more pleasant for the vast majority of people who are prepared to carry out daily oral hygiene measures. Attempts have been made to control plaque chemically, but the multiplicity of so-called "active agents" incorporated into dentifrices in an attempt to inhibit plaque growth and reduce or eliminate gingivitis suggests strongly that no ideal agent has yet been discovered. A 1972 Workshop on Antimicrobial Agents and Caries, held by National Institute of Dental Research, recommended as possible candidates for extended clinical trials the antibiotics vancomycin (a glycopeptide), kanamycin (an aminoglycoside of the streptomycin group), CC 10232 (a macrolide without generic name), spiramycin (a macrolide), and actinobolin; and the synthetic antibacterial chemicals chlorhexidine and Alexidine[R] (bisbiguanides), Victamines[R] (cationic surface active organic phosphoamidates), and several organic amine fluorides (Carlos 1974).

However, there is no doubt that a positive attitude on the part of the patient and a willingness to carry out simple oral hygiene measures regularly is absolutely essential to the maintenance of good oral health.

REFERENCES

Allen, A. L., Hawley, C. E., Cutright, D. E. and Seibert, J. S. (1975). An investigation of the clinical and histologic effects of selected dentifrices on human palatal mucosa. *J. Periodont.*, **46**, 102–112.

American Dental Association (1970). Abrasivity. *J. Am. dent. Ass.*, **81**, 1177.

Anerud, A. (1970). The effect of preventive measures upon oral hygiene and periodontal health. Thesis, Univ. Oslo.

Badersten, A. and Egelberg, J. (1972). Plaque removing effects of brushing with a dentifrice. *Tandlak.*, **64** (**23**), 770; *Oral Res. Abst.*, 1974, **9**, 1531.

Bay, I., Kardel, K. M. and Skougaard, M. R. (1967). Quantitative evaluation of the plaque-removing ability of different types of toothbrushes. *J. Periodont.*, **38**, 526–533.

Bergenholtz, A., Hugoson, A. and Sohlberg, F. (1967). Den plaqueavlagsnande formagan hos nagra munhygieniska hjalpmedel. *Svensk Tandläk. Tidskr.*, **60**, 447.

Bergenholtz, A., Hugoson, A. and Lundgren, D. (1969). The plaque removing ability of various toothbrushes used with the roll technique. *Svensk Tandläk. Tidskr.*, **62**, 15–25.

Bergenholtz, A. (1971). Mechanical cleaning in oral hygiene. *In* "Oral Hygiene" (Ed. A. Frandsen) 27–60 Munksgaard

British Standards Institute (1974). Specifications for toothpastes. BS 5136

Carlos, J. P. (1974). Quoting: 1972 workshop on antimicrobial agents and caried held by National Institute of Dental Research. Prevention and Oral Health, Bethesda, N.I. of Dent. Res., DHFW publication No. N1H 74–707.

Compton, F. H. and Beagrie, G. S. (1975). Inhibitory effect of benzethonium and zinc chloride mouthrinses on human dental plaque and gingivitis. *J. Clin. Periodont.*, **2**, 33–43.

Crawford, A. N., McAllan, L. H., Murray, J. J. and Brook, A. H. (1975). Oral hygiene instruction and motivation in children using manual and electric toothbrushes. *Community dent. oral Epidemiol.*, **3**, 257–261.

Davis, W. B. and Rees, D. A. (1975). A parametric test to measure the cleaning power of toothpaste. *J. Soc. Cosmetic Chemists*, **26**, 217–225.

Dudding, N. J., Dahl, L. O., Muhler, J. C. (1960). Patient reaction to brushing teeth with water, dentifrice or salt and soda. *J. Periodont.*, **31**, 386–392.

Fanning, E. A., Gotjamanos, T., Vowles, N. J. and van der Wielen, I. (1968). The effects of fluoride dentifrices on the incidence and distribution of stained tooth surfaces in children. *Archs oral Biol.*, **13**, 467–469.

Federation Dentaire Internationale (1974). "Principal requirements for controlled clinical trials of caries preventive agents and procedures", (Eds. H. S. Horowitz, L. J. Baume, O. Backer-Dirks, G. N. Davies, G. L. Slack), Techn. Rep. No. 1.

Fiedler, H. (1934). Klinische Beitrage zur Jodtherapie in der operation zahnheilkindhe. Inaugural Discussion, Liepzig.

Fischman, S. L., Picozzi, A., Cancro, L. P. and Pader, M. (1973). The inhibition of plaque in humans by two experimental oral rinses. *J. Periodont.*, **44**, 100–103.

Fitzgerald, R. J., Spinell, D. M. and Stoudt, T. H. (1968). Enzymatic removal of artificial plaques. *Arch. oral Biol.*, **13**, 125–128.

Forsman, B. (1974). Studies on the effect of dentifrices with low fluoride content. *Community dent. Oral Epidemiol.*, **2**, 1–10.

Frandsen, A. M., Barbano, J. P., Suomi, J. D., Chang, J. J. and Burke, A. D. (1970). The effectiveness of the Charters', scrub and roll methods of toothbrushing by professionals in removing plaque. *Scand. J. dent. Res.*, **78**, 459–463.

Frandsen, A. M., Barbano, J. P., Suomi, J. D., Chang, J. J. and Houston, R. (1972). A comparison of the effectiveness of the Charters, scrub and roll methods of toothbrushing in removing plaque. *Scand. J. dent. Res.*, **80**, 267–271.

Gerdin, P. O. (1970). Studies in dentifrices. I. Abrasiveness of dentifrices and removal of discoloured stains. *S.T.T.*, **63**, 275.

Gershon, S. D. and Pader, M. (1972). *In* "Cosmetics, Science and Technology" (Eds. M. S. Balsam and E. Sagarin), Chapter 14. Wiley Interscience.

Gomer, R. M., Holroyd, S. V. and Feidi, P. F. (1972). The effect of oral rinses. *J. Am. Soc. Prev. Dent.*, **2**, 6–7.

Grabenstetter, R. J., Broge, R. W., Jackon, F. L. and Radike, A. W. (1958). Measurement of abrasion of human teeth by dentifrice abrasion: a test utilizing radio-active teeth. *J. dent. Res.*, **30**, 1060.

Greene, J. C. (1966). Oral health care for the prevention and control of periodontal disease. *In* "World Workshop in Periodontics" (Eds S. P. Ramfjord, D. A. Derr, M. Ash), 399. University of Michigan, Michigan.

Greene, J. C. and Vermillion, J. R. (1964). The simplified oral hygiene index. *J. Am. dent. Ass.*, **68**, 7–13.

Guggenheim, B., Muhlemann, H. R. and Regolati, B. (1972). Caries and plaque inhibition in rats by mutanase. *Caries Res.*, **6**, 253 (pre-printed abstract).

Hansen, F. and Gjermo, P. (1971). The plaque-removing effect of four toothbrushing methods. *Scand. J. Dent. Res.*, **79**, 502–506.

Harrap, G. J. (1974). Assessment of the effect of dentifrices on the growth of dental plaque. *J. Clin. Periodont.*, **1**, 166–174.

Hefferen, J. J. (1974). How abrasive should a toothpaste be? *Pharmacy Times*, 50–52.

Hine, M. K. (1950). Use of the toothbrush in the treatment of periodontitis. *J. Am. dent. Ass.*, **41**, 158–168.

James, P. M. C. and Anderson, R. J. (1967). Clinical testing of a stannous fluoride-calcium pyrophosphate dentifrice in Buckinghamshire schoolchildren. *Brit. dent. J.*, **123**, 33–39.

Kardel, K. M., Olesen, K. P. and Bay, I. (1971). Mechanical cleaning in oral hygiene. *In* "Oral Hygiene" (Ed. A. Frandsen), 34. Quoted by Bergenholtz, A. Munksgaard.

Kaslick, R. S., Shapiro, W. B. and Chasens, A. I. (1975). Studies on the effect of a urea peroxide gel on plaque formation and gingivitis. *J. Periodont.*, **46**, 230–232.

Kitchin, P. C. and Robinson, H. B. G. (1948). How abrasive need a toothpaste be? *J. dent. Res.*, **27**, 501–506.

Lindhe, J. and Koch, G. (1966). The effect of supervised oral hygiene on the gingiva of children – progression and regression of gingivitis. *J. Period. Res.*, **1**, 260.

Lobene, R. R. (1968). Effect of dentifrices on tooth stains with controlled brushing. *J. Am. dent. Ass.*, **77**, 849–855.

Lobene, R. R. and Soparkar, R. M. (1974). Effect of amine fluorides on human plaque and gingivitis. I.A.D.R. Abstract No. 369.

Löe, H. (1969). A review of the prevention and control of plaque. *In* "Dental Plaque: a symposium held in the University of Dundee" (Ed. W. D. McHugh), 259. Livingstone, Edinburgh.

Löe, H. (1973). Does chlorhexidine have a place in the prophylaxis of dental diseases? *J. Periodont. Res.*, **8**, Suppl. 12, 93–99.

Löe, H. and Silness, J. (1963). Periodontal disease in pregnancy. I. Prevalence and severity. *Acta. odont. Scand.*, **21**, 533–551.

Löe, H., Theilade, E. and Jensen, S. (1965). Experimental gingivitis in man. *J. Period.*, **36**, 177.

Ludwig, T. G. (1963). Clinical trial of a dentifrice containing tetradecylamine. *N.Z. dent. J.*, **59**, 220–223.

Manly, R. S. (1943). A structureless recurrent deposit on teeth. *J. dent. Res.*, **22**, 479–486.

Massler, M., Schour, I. and Chopra, B. (1950). Occurrence of gingivitis in suburban Chicago schoolchildren. *J. Periodont.*, **21**, 146–164.

McAllan, L. H., Murray, J. J., Brook, A. H. and Crawford, A. N. (1976). Oral hygiene instruction in children using manual and electric toothbrushes: benefits after six months. *Brit. dent. J.*, **140**, 51–56.

McCauley, H. B., Sheehy, M. J., Scott, D. B., Keyes, P. H. Fanale, S. J. and Dale, P. P. (1946). Clinical efficacy of powder and paste dentifrices. *J. Am. dent. Ass.*, **33**, 993–997.

McKendrick, A. J. W., Barbenel, L. M. H. and McHugh, W. D. (1970). The influence of time of examination, eating, smoking and frequency of brushing on the oral debris index. *J. Periodont. Res.*, **5**, 205–207.

Mooser, M. (1959). Abrasive action of toothbrushes with natural and synthetic bristles and of toothpastes. *Paradontologie*, **13**, 131–133.

Morgues, F. (1965). Hypertonic salt paste as a habitual dentifrice and as a therapeutic agent of gingivitis. *Chir. dent. France*, **25**, 39–45.

Moss, A. (1971). Abrasive effect of selected dentifrices and toothbrushes. Quoted by Wictorin, L. *Acta. odont. Scand.*, **30**, 383–395.

Naylor, M. N. and Emslie, R. D. (1967). Clinical testing of stannous fluoride and sodium monofluorophosphate dentifrices in London schoolchildren. *Brit. dent. J.*, **123**, 17–23.

Pindborg, J. J. (1949). Tobacco and gingivitis. II. Correlation between consumption of tobacco, ulceromembranous gingivitis and calculus. *J. dent. Res.*, **28**, 460–463.

Ramfjord, S. P. (1959). Indices for prevalence and incidence of periodontal disease. *J. Periodont.*, **30**, 51–59.

Robinson, H. B. G. (1969). Individualizing dentifrices: the dentists responsibility. *J. Am. dent. Ass.*, **79**, 633.

Russell, A. L. A. (1956). A system of classification and scoring for prevalence surveys of periodontal disease. *J. dent. Res.*, **35**, 350–359.

Schroeder, H. E. (1969). "Formation and Inhibition of Dental Calculus". 129–162. Huber, Stuttgart.

Scopp, J. W., Cohen, G., Cancro, L. P. and Bolton, S. (1976). Clinical evaluation of a newly designed contoured toothbrush. *J. Periodont.*, **47**, 87–90.

Scully, C. M. and Wade, A. B. (1970). The relative plaque removing effect of brushes of different length and texture. *Dent. Pract.*, **20**, 244–248.

Shaw, L. and Murray, J. J. (1977). A new index for measuring extrinsic stain in clinical trials. *Community Dent. Oral Epidemiol.*, **5**, 116–120.

Shourie, K. L. (1947). Mesenteric line or pigmented plaque: a sign of comparative freedom from caries. *J. Am. dent. Ass.*, **35**, 805–807.

Silness, J. and Löe, H. (1964). Periodontal disease in pregnancy. II. Correlation between oral hygiene and periodontal condition. *Acta. odont. Scand.*, **22**, 121–135.

Stanmeyer, W. R. (1957). Measure of tissue response to frequency of toothbrushing. *J. Periodont.*, **28**, 17–22.

Stones, H. H. (1962). "Oral and Dental Diseases", 4th ed., 489–493. Livingstone, Edinburgh and London.

Sturzenberger, O. P., Swancar, J. R. and Reiser, G. (1971). Reduction of dental calculus in humans through the use of a dentifrice containing a crystal growth inhibitor. *J. Periodont.*, **42**, 416–419.

Theilade, E., Wright, W. H., Jensen, S. B. and Löe, H. (1966). Experimental gingivitis in man. II. A longitudinal clinical and bacteriologic investigation. *J. Periodont. Res.*, **1**, 1–13.

Toto, P. D. and Rapp, G. W. (1972). A clinical comparison of a new low abrasive dentifrice with intermediate and high abrasive dentifrices. *J. Periodont.*, **43**, 492–494.

Turesky, S., Glickman, I. and Sandberg, R. (1972). *In vitro* chemical inhibition of plaque formation. *J. Periodont.*, **43**, 263–269.

van Abbé, N. J., Bridge, A. J., Ribbons, J. W., Dean, P. M. and Lazarou, J. A. (1971). The effect of dentifrices on extrinsic tooth stains. *J. Soc. Cosmet. Chem.*, **22**, 457.

Wade, A. B. (1953). Clinical assessment of the relative physical properties of nylon and bristle brushes. *Brit. dent. J.*, **94**, 260–264.

Winter, G. B. and Brook, A. H. (1975). Enamel hypoplasia and anomalies of the enamel. *Dent. Clin. North America*, **19**, 3–24.

Wong-Lee, T. K. (1974). The role of a dentifrice in toothbrushing. Thesis submitted in partial fulfilment for the degree of Master of Science in periodontology.

World Health Organisation (1971). Oral Health Surveys, Basic Methods.

THE CLEANING, POLISHING
AND ABRASION OF TEETH
BY DENTAL PRODUCTS

W. B. Davis
Beecham Products Research Department,
Leatherhead, Surrey, England

I. INTRODUCTION

A dentifrice is a preparation (paste, powder cake or liquid) which aids in the removal of debris from tooth surfaces. Such a definition is a little too narrow because the cleaning, abrasion and polishing of teeth are three inter-related functions of the particulate components of dentifrices which may remove material that is more strongly adhering than the word "debris" implies.

The cleaning of teeth has two facets: clinically it is beneficial to remove all the plaque, materia alba and sugary food remains from the teeth and gums at least once a day; and from the cosmetic viewpoint it is required that the teeth be kept free of stain and other visible deposits. Apart from fulfilling these cleansing requirements, dentifrices may also be used as carriers of therapeutic ingredients such as fluoride and of flavouring agents which act as breath fresheners which may, in some cases, slow down plaque growth. In the oral cavity we have in essence two basic types of tissue in an aggressive environment: enamel and the gingivae. A particularly vulnerable area is the gingival margin where hard, mainly inorganic tissues meld with the vital soft tissues of the gums. Between the teeth and the gums and between each tooth and its neighbour lie small zones of saliva and tissue with very little physical disturbance. Add to this situation a multitude of microorganisms and a regularly replenished supply of protein and carbohydrates: We have the potential hazards of caries and gingivitis.

The present treatment of cleaning, polishing and abrasion is from a physical/mechanical viewpoint but the clinical and chemical interaction of the oral hygiene regimen, the oral environment and the diet must be borne in mind in order to keep the mechanical parameters in their true perspective.

The most obvious, short-term benefits of using a dentifrice during toothbrushing are cosmetic and psychological whereas the clinical benefits are of a long-term nature and not so obvious to the user. There are a few benefits associated with the use of dentifrices which are often ignored: For instance

(a) The pleasing mouth-freshening sensation encourages people to brush their teeth more often than they would with a brush only.

(b) Dentifrices reduce the build up of microorganisms in the toothbrush bristles.

(c) Dentifrices are ideal carriers of topical therapeutic treatments in the mouth.

(d) There is evidence accumulating which suggests that some of the ingredients of dentifrices inhibit the reformation and growth of plaque colonies.

(e) The credit for the increased public awareness of the benefits of good oral hygiene and fluoride is mainly due to the advertising efforts of the large competitive dentifrice manufacturers; who are also carrying out or helping to finance valuable research activities.

The magnitude of the research effort with respect to the abrasion of teeth can be appreciated from Fig. 1.

The cleaning, polishing and abrading operations are basically abrasion processes involving the distortion, movement, or complete removal of material constituting, or deposited on the exposed part of the teeth. Both

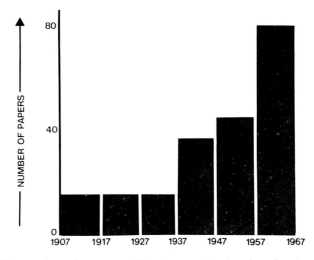

Fig. 1.   The number of papers published on work related to abrasive particles in dentifrices.

dentine and (to a lesser extent) enamel can be made to flow slightly under compressive loads but their ductility is many times less than that of metals. Furthermore, heating caused by friction cannot melt or improve the flow characteristics of dentine or enamel as can happen with metals. Therefore the normal wear and polishing factors associated with flow, melting and the formation of a Beilby layer, well documented with respect to metals, (Barrett, 1952) cannot be applied to the behaviour of the hard dental tissues.

II. HISTORY

The history of dentistry is a vast subject mainly outside the terms of reference of the present treatment. But certain items of historical nature are necessary to set the scene for today's intensive research activities in dentifrices.

The history of dentifrices is conveniently considered in three sections extending 2500 and 2000 years back. Foulk and Pickering (1935) noted that various forms of calcium carbonate had been used since very early times [over 2000 years ago according to Hippocrates (400 B.C.)] on account of its mild abrasive action. Today despite many alternatives to calcium carbonate it is still a major constituent of many successful dentifrices, but we assume that the perfect particulate ingredient has yet to be discovered. Aids to tooth cleaning such as the fibrous sticks mentioned by Manley et al. (1975) are being used today by many "primitive" people quite effectively; while in the Western hemisphere one still hears of people using salt, bicarbonate of soda and soot as aids to toothbrushing.

The dentifrices used 2000 years ago were usually whitish powders, of crushed coral, marble, or the ashes of burnt animal and vegetable material. They were used very infrequently, for cosmetic purposes, by very few people. Some 500 years ago dentifrices were still basically the same sort of powders but were used more frequently, often with claims for therapeutic benefits although their efficacy left much to be desired.

Around 20 years ago therapeutic efficacy for dentifrices became more possible and toothpastes came into general everyday use by a larger fraction of the Western world.

During the 2000 years or so of its development the main physically active ingredient of a dentifrice has been the solid particulate ingredient referred to in modern formulations as "The Abrasive". Tables I and II list typical ancient and modern abrasives and flavouring agents. The main differences between the two columns are purity and abrasivity level. Because modern dentifrices are intended for twice daily usage for brushing

W. B. DAVIS

Table I
Ancient and modern dentifrice abrasives

Year	Abrasive
400 B.C.	Powdered marble or whitestone Ash of head of hare
A.D. 130	Vegetable ashes Powdered sea shells Powdered cuttlefish bones Pumice Powdered coral
14th century	Burnt eggshells Charcoal Soot Salt Bicarbonate of soda Magnesia

20th century	Dicalcium phosphate
	    (dihydrate)
	Dicalcium phosphate
	    (anhydrous)
	Insoluble sodium metaphosphate
	Calcium pyrophosphate
	Calcium carbonate
	Precipitated silica
	Zirconium silicate
	Calcium silicate
	Alpha alumina trihydrate
	Calcined alumina
	Titanium dixoide
	Polymers such as polyethylene
	Sodium bicarbonate
	Dehydrated silica gel
	Sodium alumino silicate
	Magnesium aluminium silicate

periods of up to two minutes the abrasivity, with respect to both dentine and enamel must be carefully selected. Earlier dentifrices were used infrequently, probably to remove substantial accumulations of plaque, stained pellicle and calculus.

Table II
Flavouring agents

Year	Flavouring
14th and 15th century	Cane sugar
	Rose water
	Honey
	Cinnamon
20th century	Anise oil
	Cinnamaldehyde
	Cinnamon oil
	Clove oil
	Peppermint oil
	Eucalyptol
	Spearmint oil
	Menthol
	Saccharin
	Methyl salicylate
	Vanilla

In the fourteenth century many enthusiastic claims were made for dentifrices and mouthwashes but little evidence was available to substantiate any of the claims. Indeed; with our present knowledge on the subject it is obvious that many treatments were not only unpleasant to use, but also positively harmful to the teeth and oral mucosa. (Vinegar, acetic acid and even sulphuric acid were used as teeth whiteners.)

It has been suggested, that in our modern society where teeth "suffer" from affluence, most of the things that we enjoy are immoral, illegal, or cariogenic: Using a properly formulated fluoride toothpaste is none of these ills and is a very enjoyable pastime, particularly before breakfast. Toothbrushing with a dentifrice will leave the mouth free of odour and acid-forming microorganisms, will impart a fresher feeling to the user and help protect the teeth against attack during and after subsequent meals.

Today one is constantly reminded of the need for an "aid" to toothbrushing; the intention of which is to reduce the time required to maintain an adequate level of oral hygiene bearing in mind the modern, processed diet. Time is the overriding factor in many peoples treatment of their oral hygiene requirements. While dentists recommend several brushings per day, each lasting around 2 mins; many of those who own a toothbrush use it less than once a day and would be surprised how long 2 mins brushing

would seem. According to Heath and Wilson (1974) a force of approximately 5N is applied during this short treatment period when toothbrushes and dentifrices are required to function as well as an extended
brushing period with a toothbrush and water alone. Thus the speed of
action of therapeutic ingredients and the cleansing aids formulated into
modern dentifrices are of paramount importance. This is particularly true
in cases where cumulative damage or unsightly stains will build up if
incomplete cleansing is an individual's normal habit.

The flavour, colour and therapeutic activities of the present generation
of dentifrices are being intensively investigated by academic, professional
and industrial organizations. Recent research activities on the bio-avail-
ability and effectiveness of fluoride have been very successful. Improved
dentifrice formulations can now reduce the incidence of caries in children
by up to 40% in a period when they are very susceptible to caries and are
likely to develop a fear of regular visits to the dentist, if on each occasion
restorative treatment is required.

According to manufacturers claims and authorities such as the ADA
and the BDA; such resistance to dental caries can be achieved by the use of
correctly formulated fluoride-containing toothpastes even when used in the
home under non-supervized conditions. Indeed Peterson et al. (1975) have
shown that significant improvements in caries resistance can be achieved
even when children are living in an area where the drinking water contains a
near-optimum level of fluoride. As Forward (1973) has shown that the
fluoridation of surface layers of enamel from a dentifrice is almost instan-
taneous, it is not surprising that a typical, short-duration brushing period is
sufficient to significantly improve the caries resistance of exposed enamel.
(The duration of exposure to the fluoride treatment from dentifrices is
longer in interstitial areas than on more exposed aspects of the dentition
because of incomplete clearing of the dentifrice from such sites. These
interstitial sites are, of course, also more vulnerable to caries because of the
poor clearance of plaque and food debris.)

Historically dentifrices have been mildly abrasive formulations, more
recently with detergent power, and more recently still with flavouring
additives and therapeutically active ingredients.

III. THE TISSUES AND MATERIALS ENCOUNTERED IN THE ORAL CAVITY

Having briefly mentioned the relation of teeth to their unusually hostile
environment the first thoughts on their structural and mechanical status

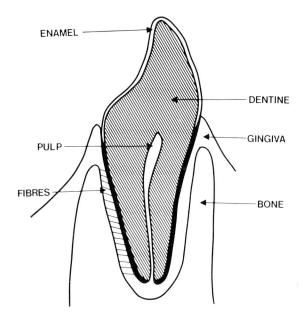

ENAMEL

DENTINE

GINGIVA

PULP

FIBRES

BONE

Fig. 2.   The essential mechanical constituents of the teeth and supporting tissues.

must surely be of sheer admiration. The teeth are chemically, physically and mechanically ideal for the functions they carry out (Fig. 2).

Each tooth is shaped and located within the dentition to cut and or chew with maximum efficiency. Each tooth is firmly anchored to its base via a rigid, but nevertheless shock-absorbent system of fibres. Each tooth is crowned with a hard, protective, wear resistant, layer of enamel. (Which is the hardest tissue in the body.) The tooth is normally bathed in a fluid super-saturated with respect to calcium and phosphate ions; thus the occasional chemical attack encountered when eating low pH foodstuffs is probably corrected without interference.

A. Enamel

Enamel is basically a continuous inorganic matrix which can most simply be described as mainly micro-crystalline hydroxyapatite (Fig. 3) the remainder being amorphous hydroxyapatite, a little water and very little organic material. The matrix consists of interlocking keyhole-like section prisms of regular crystalline orientation (Fig. 4).

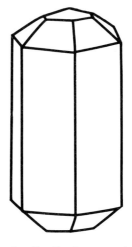

Fig. 3.   The fundamental unit cell of hydroxyapatite crystals within dentine and enamel.

The microstructure of enamel and other hard tissues has been well illustrated by Mjor and Pindborg (1973) and Scott and Symons (1971) and been shown to consist of horseshoe or fish-like section prisms 4–6 μm diameter comprised of uniform arrays of crystallites. The crystallites tend to adopt the hexagonal section of the unit cell of hydroxyapatite. They are approximately 1/6 μm long and 1/40 μm diameter and tend to lie along the axis of the prism in the "head" and normal to the axis in the "tail" region. Johnson (1971) showed that the dissolution rates for the centres of prisms differs considerably from the peripheral areas but the overall resistance to acid dissolution of enamel from the diet is less than that for dentine. When enamel is etched in dilute hydrochloric acid the prism perimeters are most resistant to attack. When etched with neutral ethylene diamine tetraacetic acid the prism perimeters are least resistant to attack. This work suggests greater permeability at prism perimeters and brings attention to complexing as a second mechanism for the loss of enamel. When enamel is immersed in fresh orange juice the prism perimeters are preferentially etched (Fig. 4). Approximately 95% by weight of enamel is of inorganic nature, 1% is organic proteinaceous material and 4% is water (Fig. 5).

Treating the exposed enamel surface as pure hydroxyapatite is an oversimplification in chemical terms particularly as there is likely to be a high frequency of hydroxyl ion replacement by fluoride ions in surface layers. This replacement is a result of the high affinity that fluoride ions, (available in the diet or from oral care products), have for hydroxyapatite.

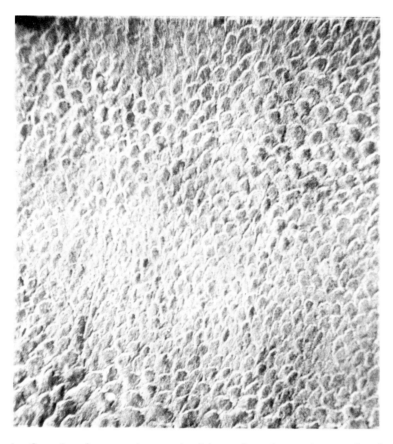

Fig. 4.   Scanning electron micrograph of the surface of enamel exposed to fresh orange juice for ten minutes. The horseshoe-like sections of enamel prisms are clearly visible. (× 800.)

In practice, as will be later expanded, freshly-exposed enamel becomes coated with a tenacious, amorphous film of salivary muco-protein free of microorganisms within hours of exposure (pellicle). This thin film, initially in the order of 1 μm thick, is invisible and resistant to toothbrushing and the abrasive action of the diet. Pellicle forms a membrane over the enamel crown and will continuously thicken and become discoloured unless controlled with the aid of an effective dentifrice.

The hardness of well mineralized enamel is near that of natural apatite. (That is 5 on the Moh's scale.) The hardness of a material is its resistance to scratching or indentation by a harder material. The original Moh's hardness scale (later modified to include certain very hard minerals) is based on the

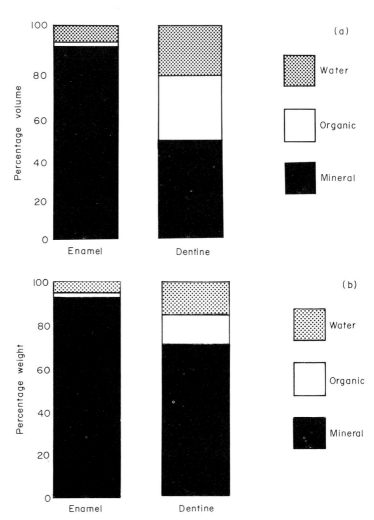

Fig. 5(a).   The composition of dentine and enamel by volume.
(b).   The composition of dentine and enamel by weight.

mineralogist's method of identifying minerals by scratching them, or attempting to scratch them with known minerals. The hardness of enamel, dentine and several important minerals are listed in Table III on the Moh's hardness scale and with their Knoop Hardness Numbers (KHN). The Moh's hardness numbers are dimensionless whereas the Knoop hardness number is effectively the pressure sustained by the flat polished surface of substrate when it is supporting a diamond pyramid indentor.

Table III
The hardness of minerals and tissues

Material	Moh's hardness	Knoop hardness number $Kg\ mm^{-2}$
Wax	0·2	32
Talc	1	—
Ice	1.5	—
Gypsum	2	—
Sodium chloride	2	32
Dentine	2–2.5	50–60
Brushite	2·5	—
Calcite	3	135
Morelite	3.5	—
Fluorite	4	163
Enamel	4–5	300
Magnesia	4–5	370
Apatite	5	430
Calcium pyrophosphate	5	—
Amorphous silca	5	—
Pumice	6	—
Feldspar	6	560
Crystalline silica	7	820
Topaz	8	1340
Tungsten carbide	9	1800
Alumina	9–10	2100
Diamond	10	7000

Enamel is hard and wear resistant with regard to foodstuffs and is indeed harder than most mineral powders used in dentifrices. Thus its wear resistance will cope with the physical attacks normally encountered except for large thermal and mechanically induced loads.

If tensile stresses are built up within the bulk of the enamel, any defect such as a microcrack near the surface will easily propagate through the enamel because it is a brittle material. Fortunately the enamel only acts as a protective crown to the bulk of the tooth. Any crack propagating through enamel towards the central portion of the tooth is very likely to be arrested at the interface between the dentine and enamel. At the junction the stresses are dispersed within the plane of the junction and in cases where this dispersal is insufficient to stop the crack propagating into the dentine it is likely to become arrested because plastic deformation of the dentine absorbs the energy driving the crack forward through the tooth.

B. Dentine

The bulk of the root and body of the tooth is composed mainly of dentine with a central pulpal chamber. Dentine has a lower inorganic mineral content than enamel but the mineral portion once again approximates to hydroxyapatite, present as plate-like crystallites up to $1/10$ μm diameter $1/300$ μm thick.

Dentine, unlike enamel, is initially a vital tissue which can be repaired and reinforced by tissue replacement and calcification from sources within the overall regenerative system of the body. The hydroxyapatite crystallites form a matrix of highly mineralized tubules (Fig. 6) approximately 5 μm in diameter.

The organic content of dentine (15–20%) [see Fig. 5], is distributed within the central column of the tubules and to a lesser extent within the highly mineralized tubule walls. According to Eastoe (1967) the organic portion is largely tough collagen fibrils of diameter 0.1–0.2 μm of indefinite length which are very similar to the matrix within which the inorganic crystallites were laid down. The collagen contributes to the toughness and mechanical strength of the dentine. As the dentine matures in adults there is a tendency for further mineralization to occur, particularly if the outer regions become exposed to the oral environment or damaged (for example by caries attack or during restorative treatment).

The dentine gradually increases in mineral content with age as a result mainly of deposition of apatite on the tubule walls which ultimately leads to the complete closure of the tubules. This is observed as a progressive change from opaque to more translucent dentine. The degree of translucency can be used to estimate the age of a tooth and is generally thought to be accompanied by a decrease in the plasticity of dentine i.e. it becomes more brittle with age.

The hardness of dentine is much more variable than the hardness of enamel but tooth to tooth variations in hardness do not appreciably affect wear resistance (Fig. 7). It varies with position within a single tooth and with the age of a tooth because of changing degrees of mineralization.

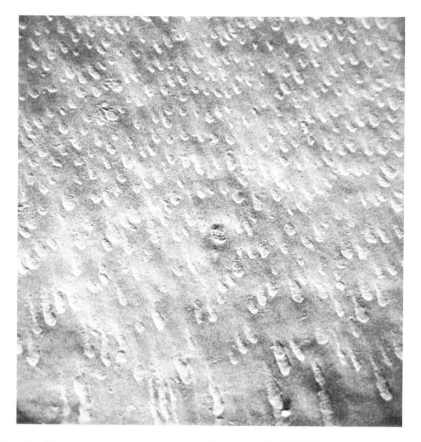

Fig. 6.   Dentine exposed to the oral environment. ($\times$ 500.) When gum recession exposes root dentine to the oral environment acid attack by dietary insult (despite the remineralization of surface layers from salivary calcium and phosphate ions), a progressive loss of dentine and the surface architecture reflects the underlying tissue microstructure. The cores of dentine tubules are preferentially eroded by dietary insult.

C. Cementum

Cementum is a relatively soft calcified tissue thinly covering the hard tooth tissue below the initial gum margin. The wear resistance of the thin layer of cementum is low, therefore the survival of any cementum that becomes exposed to the oral environment as a result of gum recession is so short that it is considered of no significance in protecting the underlying dentine.

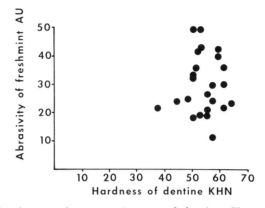

Fig. 7. The hardness and wear resistance of dentine. Twenty-four dentine specimens were found to vary little in hardness but were very variable with respect to their wear resistance when brushed with a toothpaste/water slurry.

D. Gingiva

The soft tissues of the gums, the gingivae, are not often mentioned with respect to abrasion and wear processes. Gum recession is generally attributed to the soft tissues response to toxins produced by the plaque and other inflammatory influences. However, rapid gum recession can be caused by misuse of toothbrushes, toothpicks and dental floss. Recession can lead to the exposure of dentine. Subsequent damage or loss of dentine may then be wrongly attributed to the choice of dentifrice.

E. Salivary deposits (cuticle)

1. *Acquired Pellicle*
When an enamel crown first enters the oral cavity it is covered with a primary cuticle. The primary cuticle is the last product of the ameloblasts. The primary cuticle is 1–10 μm thick and is rapidly worn off; to be replaced by the acquired pellicle formed by the precipitation of glycoproteins from the saliva. The formation of pellicle on enamel and dentine, re-exposed to the saliva by wearing off the existing pellicle, is a rapid process. A complete film is formed within hours.

Unless a sufficiently abrasive dentifrice is used in an effective brushing routine; Saxton (1973) showed that the pellicle increases in thickness at a rate near 1 μm per week. Davis and Rees (1975) (Fig. 8) showed that in a period of 4 weeks the colour of the stained pellicle (usually brown) becomes obvious unless the toothpaste has adequate abrasivity. The pellicle film is structureless, continuous with the subsurface cuticle and free of micro-organisms.

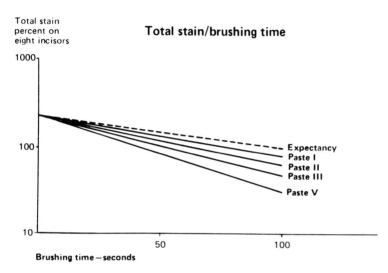

Fig. 8.   The cleaning powers of toothpastes. The cleaning powers of tooth-pastes can be varied with careful control of the ingredients, and exceed the cleaning powers of a toothbrush and water even when the observers expectancy is taken into account in clinical trials.

It was established by Manly (1943), Robinson (1969), and Hefferen (1974) that a toothbrush and water alone cannot remove pellicle. A simple experiment to determine the mechanical resistance of pellicle can be carried out at home in front of a mirror:

After brushing thoroughly with a toothbrush and water, an easily accessible, stained pellicle area is selected; a soft plastic or wooden cocktail stick is used to try and remove the stain. However, if a steel instrument or a particularly hard plastic is used the stain can be scratched, exposing white underlying enamel. Removal of a thin area of pellicle by scratching in this way is a suggested method of estimating the thickness of the pellicle film.

2. Plaque

Several hours after a thorough cleansing of the teeth and gums, colonies of bacteria in the order of 1 mm across will be accumulating. Such colonies comprise the major part of the soft loosely adhering film known as plaque.

Plaque is made readily visible to the naked eye by painting the teeth and gums, or rinsing the mouth, with a staining solution such as erythrocin. Plaque disclosing tablets are also available which when chewed and rinsed around the mouth disclose the location and extent of plaque. (Such tablets can be used as an aid to train patients in correct oral hygiene practice. They are instructed to use a suitable brushing technique, in combination with a disclosing agent, until all plaque is removed.)

McHugh (1970) showed that plaque is a sticky tenacious mass of extra-cellular polysaccharides and micro-organisms such as cocci and rods which can synthesize carbohydrates to form acids. Such microorganisms multiply to form colonies on the teeth and gums which can be removed using a toothbrush and water alone. Plaque removal is not thought to be aided by the use of a dentifrice but it is likely that the more inaccessible areas have an increased probability of being cleared when the detergent action of a toothpaste is invoked. Furthermore, minute remnants of a plaque colony that may not be readily visible could act as immediately active nuclei for the reformation of plaque colonies. The more thorough cleansing action imparted by the detergent and abrasive constituents of dentifrices may inhibit the reformation of plaque because of the cleansing efficacy.

It is uncertain at the present time which ingredient or function of denti-frices is responsible for inhibiting the re-formation of plaque colonies, but plaque inhibition is a real benefit indicated by clinical observers. In the early stages of the development of a colony of plaque, rods and cocci are predominant but in more mature plaque (3–4 days old) the balance changes somewhat and the sticky mass contains an increased amount of cellular debris and filamentous organisms. Mature plaque is thought to be more pathogenic to the gingivae than fresh plaque because of this change in microflora. Complete cleansing of the teeth at least every 2–3 days is thus necessary to limit gingivitis.

3. Calculus

As the plaque becomes even more mature there is a tendency for calcifica-tion to be nucleated within the mass of the plaque. The source of minerals for such calcification being the calcium and phosphate ions within the saliva. The net result of continuous calcification of the plaque being calculus which can physically irritate the soft tissues at the gingival margin; leading eventually to gingivitis if left unattended. On occasional visits to the dentist patients prone to calculus are given a prophylaxis treatment to eliminate the calculus. However, prevention is better than cure. Prevention of calculus build-up can best be achieved by regular, effective tooth brushing.

IV. TOOTHBRUSH DESIGN

Today's toothbrush designs are making relatively small steps forward in efficiency. Toothbrushes, as such, are relatively modern; apparently appearing in Europe in forms resembling modern articles about 200 years ago. In 1780 William Addis produced a bristle toothbrush with a bone handle. There was little change in design until the beginning of the twentieth century when synthetic handles, and eventually plastic bristles replaced the previously used natural materials. The advantages of modern materials were entirely from the manufacturing viewpoint and until recently, natural bristle brushes were widely thought to be most satisfactory. Today it is difficult to obtain a bristle brush and there is no reason to treat one as superior. The function of the toothbrush is to clean teeth, but the essential gingival cleaning and massage should be inseperably identified with an effective toothbrush design. The intention of the toothbrush is to cause a shearing action across the hard and soft tissue surfaces, with a dentifrice increasing the friction and helping to float away debris dislodged by the bristles. Natural bristles obtained from the backs of swine have rather variable physical properties depending on factors such as geographical location and the season during which they are collected. Natural bristle diameters 0·007–0·010 in. are ideal but the range within a brush usually extends well beyond this range.

Modern toothbrushes have toothbrush handles made of polymers such as polystyrene, polymethyl methacrylate and bristles made of nylon, usually 0·008–0·015 in. diameter. The length and number of bristles to each tuft and the numbers of tufts to each brush vary considerably with shape and description such as "oval", "tufted end" and "straight trim" being used. Two or more parallel rows of tufts normally employed with the bristles all lying normal to the brushing plane. There are many patents registered for serrated, converging and diverging bristles. Even though the toothbrush design has held a mysterious fascination for inventors it is probably fair to say that there is no major advantage in using a brush other than a medium grade, flat-trim type.

Toothbrush stiffness has been the subject of much dispute amongst the manufacturers: "Soft" graded brushes of one manufacturer have been found to be measurably stiffer than the "stiff" graded brushes of another, even if softening by water uptake is accounted for. It is likely that an international standard of grading stiffness will be issued within the next decade, as recommended by Heath and Wilson (1971), McFarlane (1971) and Hillier (1972), but even then it will be possible to vary the stiffness by changing the diameter, length, modulus of elasticity or packing density of the individual filaments.

V. THE REMOVAL OF ORAL DEBRIS

The parameters controlling toothpaste abrasion of hard tooth tissues also control the removal of softer accumulations from the tooth surfaces. The factors governing removal are somewhat tempered by the low resistance of accumulations. (Except in the case of calculus which is probably similar in behaviour to dentine.)

Wilkinson and Pugh (1970) suggested a direct relationship between enamel abrasivity and the cleaning performance of toothpastes, Robinson (1969) Pfrengle (1964) and Davis and Rees (1975) consider that dentine abrasivity values rank closer to stain removal power than enamel abrasivity. Stained pellicle and dentine can both be removed from the tooth by scratching with a hard plastic instrument whereas plastic will make no mark whatsoever on the enamel surface. As previously mentioned, the abrasive power of mineral particles is critically controlled by the relative hardnesses of the powder mineral and the substrate. After allowing for the difference in hardness between dentine and stained pellicle, the other parameters such as size and concentration affect the cleaning power performance in the same sense as dentine abrasivity.

Having briefly mentioned the deposits that accumulate on the teeth and gums and indicated the consequences thereof; the reasons for regularly cleaning the teeth and gums become self evident. It is essential for clinical reasons to control plaque growth and regeneration particularly in the more inaccessible areas. To do this takes approximately 2 min. brushing, followed by cleaning of the spaces between the teeth (inaccessible to the toothbrush) using dental floss or an interdental wood stick. (Misuse of a wood stick can lead to damage of the soft tissues.)

In practice stiff toothbrushes are popular, presumably because the user feels that increasing the brush stiffness beyond a grade that is comfortable to use will compensate, in part, for missed brushing sessions.

The brushing methods known as the roll, the vibratory, the physiological downstrokes and the Bass technique are frequently recommended, all of which when applied properly give adequate cleansing of the teeth in clinical terms according to Macphee and Cowley (1969) and Suomi (1971). If, however, an adequate brushing method such as one of the above listed methods is applied using a toothbrush and water without an effective toothpaste (or if the toothpaste used is not sufficiently abrasive with regards to pellicle); the pellicle layer covering the crowns will thicken and become more easily visible. After 3 or 4 weeks of effective toothbrushing with a non-abrasive dentifrice 90% of the population will have accumulated a pellicle layer sufficiently thick and pigmented to be visible as a dark brownish stain covering at least a small portion of their teeth. Obviously such stained areas are cosmetically undesirable. To remove and prevent the reformation of stained pellicle it is necessary to carry out adequate tooth-brushing with an effective dentifrice.

VI. THE MEASUREMENT OF DENTIFRICE PERFORMANCE PARAMETERS

A discussion of dentifrice efficacy must be based on reproducible perform-ance data, (preferably objective) related to *in vivo* events. The design of reproducible laboratory experiments of more or less linear sensitivity to changes of varying magnitude such as abrasion is relatively simple. However, there are two major problems associated with attempts to relate *in vitro* experimental data to every day performance in the oral cavity.

(i) Reproducing, in a shortened period of time, the mechanical, chemical and biological changes occurring over a long period of time.
(ii) Proving the relation between low variance laboratory results and performance in the very variable population whose eating and oral hygiene habits vary considerably.

The parameters to be considered are (1) abrasion, (2) polish and (3) stain-removal power. The above sequence is the same as the order of ease of measurement, which has unfortunately resulted in an abundance of abrasivity data (in particular dentine abrasivity) and the almost complete absence of stain-removal power data for commercial dentifrices.

A. Abrasion

As will be discussed in more detail later the mechanisms of wear such as scratching or fatigue apply to metals, ceramics or biological tissues to differing degrees of importance, depending on the relative mechanical properties (e.g. hardness and plasticity) of the abrasive and substrate materials as shown by Wright (1969). Therefore dentine, enamel and synthetic substitutes will be considered separately as the substrate to allow a closer consideration of the test parameters.

Gravimetric methods such as those of Smith (1935) and Wright and Finske (1937) involve measuring weight changes of substrate blocks before and after abrasion has taken place. Two basic methods simulating, in the laboratory, the sequence of *in vivo* brushing with a toothpaste have evolved: (a) Whole brush and (b) Single tuft. Basically the substrate is immersed in a slurry containing 25–75% by weight of toothpaste, the remainder being water or a thicker, inert diluent such as a solution of carboxymethyl cellulose, or glycerol. The abrasion is then carried out by pressing (at a fixed load) a whole brush or single tuft onto the substrate surface and causing shear movements of circular or oscillatory nature for 1000–10 000 strokes. Such a treatment lasts for up to 1 hr and causes as much abrasive wear as 6–12 months' routine toothbrushing.

In gravimetric test methods the abrasivity of dentifrices are ranked according to the weight losses effected by accelerated brushing.

Radiotracer methods such as those of Bull *et al.* (1968), Grabenstetter *et al.* (1958) and Wright and Stephenson (1967) are basically the same as gravimetric methods except in that the loss of substrate caused by abrasion is quantified by initially making the tooth tissues radioactive and then using the activity of the abrasive slurry (induced by the transfer of abraded, radioactive tissue from the substrate to the abrasive slurry) as a measure of the relative abrasivities of the dentifrices tested.

The radiotracer techniques are more sensitive than gravimetric methods and are not subject to variations caused by the gain and loss of water; however the irradiation of dentine and enamel (and the consequential damage to the tissues) is at present an inadequately defined area of experimental procedure.

Surface profile methods such as those of Ashmore *et al.* (1972), Davis and Winter (1976), Padbury and Ash (1974) and Cordon (1971) measure the volume of material removed by a standard brushing sequence rather than the mass; thus avoiding errors caused by variation in density within the bulk of the substrate. High sensitivity surface profilometers enable the simultaneous measurement of the volume of material abraded from the substrate and the quality of the surface finish effected by the abrasion process (i.e. the absence of deep scratches which is the clinically significant parameter loosely related to "polish") to be carried out.

VII. POLISH

Synthetic substitutes for dentine and enamel such as antimony, silicon and copper are unsuitable as substitutes for abrasion tests; but are particularly unsuitable for tests designed to quantify the polishing power of dentifrices because of the great differences in flow and melting properties between dental tissues and substitutes.

In surface profilometer tests the degree of polish can be measured from the magnified traces of the abraded area and quoted either as average

Table IV
Classification of polishing power

Maximum scratch depth	Polishing power
$< 1/4\ \mu m$	Very good
$1/4–1\ \mu m$	Good
$1–2\ \mu m$	Fair
$2–5\ \mu m$	Poor
$> 5\ \mu m$	Bad

scratch depth, maximum scratch depth (see Table IV) or in a more general engineering term such as the Centre Line Average (CLA) which is a commonly used roughness parameter in engineering.

At the present time the reflectivity of dry tooth surfaces is a more popular parameter used to measure the polishing powers of dentifrices. Tainter *et al.* (1947) adapted a paint gloss measuring method for *in vitro* tests. Schiff and Shaver (1971) developed a similar method that could be used *in vivo* for polish determination which had also been used in quantifying the removal of stained pellicle by the abrasive action of dentifrices. (An area of research of more realistic use of reflection parameters.) The reasons for scepticism about the significance of polish data are that (a) teeth are normally viewed wet and shiny, and (b) optical reflectivity is associated with surface asperities of an order of magnitude smaller than the microorganisms thought to be responsible for caries and gingivitis.

Manly *et al.* (1975) developed an interesting abrasion/smoothness measurement apparatus which measures surface smoothness (in units of length similar to the CLA readings of profilometer) by quantifying the scatter of a laser beam as it is transmitted through a replica of the abraded enamel surface.

VIII. CLEANING POWER

The cleaning power of dentifrices with respect to plaque removal have not been shown to differ significantly, but Lobene (1968) showed that the stain-removal powers of commercially available dentifrices differed significantly from one another. In this test naturally stained, lay volunteers were brushed under laboratory controlled conditions and after each brushing period the remaining stain was classified according to the colour intensity and coverage of the gingival arc. Davis and Rees (1975) confirmed the presence of differences in the stain-removal powers of dentifrices (Fig. 8) by a technique similar to that of Lobene (1968) except that the stain present during the test sequence of brushings was quoted as the percentage area of each tooth that was stained, regardless of the colour or intensity of the stained area.

Wilkinson and Pugh (1970) similarly disregarded the colour and intensity of stain in their stain-removal test: After a prophylaxis treatment volunteers use a test paste for two weeks and present themselves for examination and a photographic record to be made. The photographic records are then ranked by a panel of judges in order to rank the cleaning powers of test dentifrices.

In vitro stain-removal tests have been developed, in order to make data easier to obtain in a reproducible form, which involve coating a substrate with materials such as waxes or lacquers which are brushed off under test slurries.

IX. *In vivo* ABRASION TEST METHODS

In vitro tests have always suffered from the fact that the data cannot be used with any degree of confidence until they are checked against the findings of *in vivo*, or at least *in situ* tests. The intention of such a comparison is to show, if possible, that *in vitro* data give a true indication of the practical changes that occur under real-life conditions. Davis (1975) and Wright (1975) showed that radio-tracer dentine abrasion tests, if used to estimate real-life abrasion, could suggest that abrasion would occur at up to twice the rate found in practice (Fig. 9).

Rees and Davis (1975) showed, from an *in situ* test, that dentine and enamel abrasion caused by the toothbrush and toothpaste are not the major causes of tissue loss: A flattened dentine/enamel insert, set in the labial surface of an upper incisor, porcelain crown was examined periodically by taking replicas of the test area. Whilst the volunteer was on a low acid diet; the dentine of the insert, and the soft part of the composite restorative (used to fix the insert in place) were observed to be preferentially lost, but no abrasion scratches were observed (Fig. 10). When the food and drink intake was changed to a high acid diet the composite restorative and porcelain crown were unaffected but the microstructures of both the dentine and enamel became pronounced and there was an increased rate of loss of tissue. (The junction area shown in Fig. 11 suggests that this was particularly true at the dentine/enamel junction.) *In vitro* data to support this *in vivo* test (Tables V and VI) show that acids typical of those consumed in normal Western diet dissolve dentine and enamel as fast or even faster than

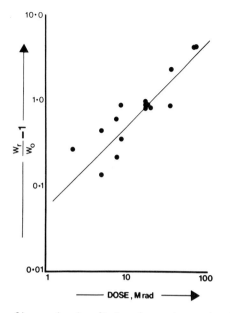

Fig. 9.   The effects of increasing irradiation dose prior to the abrasion testing of hard dental tissues. (W_0 is the wear rate of samples prior to irradiation, W_r is the wear rate of samples after receiving up to 100 Mrads of irradiation.)

these tissues can be abraded with a toothbrush and paste. (Exposure of the teeth to dietary acids is much longer than the exposure time to tooth brushing.)

Cowell (1974) used gold, circumferential clasps cemented to lower premolars for *in vivo* studies; 2 mm square sections cut from the cemento–enamel junction of extracted teeth were examined after exposure to the oral environment.

Brasch *et al.* (1969) recorded changes in the surface topography of enamel caused by prophylaxis, toothbrushing and dietary factors, by taking cellulose acetate replicas from the labial aspects of the incisors. They showed that the damage, in the form of scratches caused by pumice or zirconium silicate, was not obliterated even after six months' toothbrushing with calcium carbonate or dicalcium phosphate dihydrate toothpaste.

In vivo methods involving uncontrolled exposure to toothbrushing and acidic foodstuffs are very difficult to operate and can lead to more un-certainties than facts. Thus, in the past the notching of teeth such as that indicated in Plate 1 has been credited to gum recession, erosion, tooth-paste abrasion of dentine and bad brushing techniques. Without examining each case individually it is likely that two or more factors are involved. For

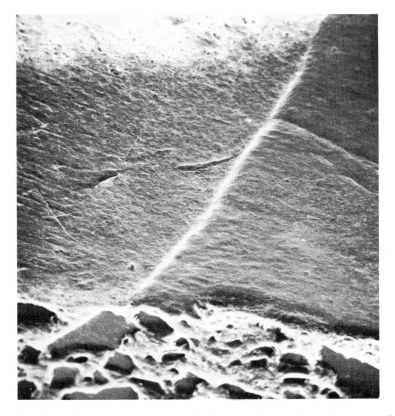

Fig. 10.   Scanning electron micrograph of dentine/enamel junction exposed to dietary insult and repair mechanisms in the mouth whilst a low-acid diet is consumed. (× 200.) The dentine (left) and the polymer matrix of a composite restorative material (bottom) have been lost at a greater rate than enamel (right) and the composite restorative filler particles.

instance it is highly likely that tooth notching near the cemento–enamel junction will be accelerated if:

(i)   The tooth tissues are low in fluoride ions.

(ii)   Low pH foods are regularly eaten.

(iii)   Toothbrushing with a highly abrasive dentifrice is carried out after a low pH meal.

(iv)   Over-zealous toothbrushing is practised, particularly if the back and forth "scrubbing" action is used.

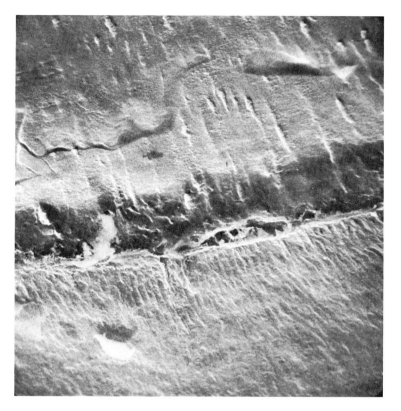

Fig. 11. The dentine (top)/enamel (bottom) junction when a high fruit diet is being consumed. (Scanning electron micrograph × 500.)

Table V
Erosion data generated by surface profilometer technique after 10-min immersion in agitated test solution

Erosive liquid	Rate of enamel loss (μm/min)	Rate of dentine loss (μm/min)	Enamel:dentine ratio
Fresh orange juice	0·6	0·6	1:1
Fresh apple juice	0·3	0·3	1:1
Citric acid buffered to pH 4·6	2·0	0·9	2:1
Cola type beverage	0·3	0·4	3:4
Neutral EDTA	0·5	1·0	1:2

Table VI
Abrasivity data generated by surface profilometer techniques (1 E.A.U.= 1/50 nm of tissue removed per brushing stroke)

Base	Enamel abrasivity	Dentine abrasivity	Dentine/enamel ratio
Zirconium silicate	500–750	11 600	15–23
Pumice	561–700	8000–10 000	11–16
Silica	58–61	1000–2000	200
Calcium pyrophosphate	35–70	2000–3000	30–90
Calcium carbonate	10–40	2000–4000	100–200
Dicalcium phosphate	3–5	1300–1900	250–650
Acrylic	<0·2	100	500+

X. MODERN DENTIFRICE FORMULATIONS

Historically dentifrices have improved the efficacy of toothbrushing in one way or another (at least claims were made about efficacy in certain areas) but it is the intention of modern dentifrices to aid toothbrushing in all ways possible without involving any risks of irritancy, damage or undesirable flavours.

There are other formulation factors related to manufacture, such as colour, syneresis, stability, corrosion and viscosity, which must be controlled to create a saleable product. However, the detergent and solid particulate matter which control the cleaning, polishing and abrasion characteristics of a formula are of paramount importance as shown by differences in cleaning power that are available.

The functional ingredients of toothpastes are essentially

(1) Abrasives (or fricative agent)   (6) Active ingredient
(2) Liquid carrier   (7) Anti corrosive
(3) Detergent   (8) Binder
(4) Humectant   (9) Colouring
(5) Flavouring

Typical recently introduced formulations containing such ingredients are:

    1. *Clear gel toothpaste*
(UK Patent 1972, 1264292)

	Weight (%)
Dehydrated silica gel	20·0
Sodium lauryl sulphate + glycerine	7·0

Sorbitol	70·0
Chloroform	0·75
Flavour	1·15
Colourant	0·5
Sodium carboxymethyl cellulose	0·25
Saccharin	0·2
Sodium benzoate	0·08

2. *Plaque and calculus inhibiting toothpaste*
(UK Patent, 1974, 1373001)

	Weight (%)
Water	36·9
Glycerol	30·0
Silica	19·0
Zinc citrate	10·0
Sodium lauryl sulphate	1·5
Flavour	1·0
Thickener	0·9
Titanium dioxide	0·5
Saccharin	0·2

3. *Low abrasive stain-removing toothpaste*
(US Patent 1972, 3,703,578)

	Weight (%)
Dicalcium phosphate dihydrate	40·0
Polyoxyethyleneglycol 400	23·275
Glycerin	23·275
Polyoxyethyleneglycol 4000	5·0
Aluminium octoate	5·0
Sodium lauryl sulphate	1·5
Flavouring	1·0
Sodium saccharin	0·75
Esters of parahydroxy benzoic acid	0·2

4. *Improved anti-caries fluoride toothpaste*
(UK Patent, 1975, 1384375)

	Weight (%)
Calcium carbonate	48·0
Glycerol	26·0
Sodium lauryl sulphate	2·0
Sodium carboxymethylcellulose	0·9
Magnesium aluminium silicate	0·75
Sodium monofluorophosphate	0·8
Calcium glycerophosphate	0·2
Calcium silicate	0·2
Flavouring and saccharin	0·1

XI. ABRASIVE PARTICLES AND WEAR PROCESSES

Some of the types of particles used in such modern dentifrices are seen in Figs 12–15. Much research energy has been expended seeking the mineral particles which will cause the removal of plaque and stained pellicle without contributing significantly to the loss of hard dental tissues. Spherical polymer particles (Fig. 12) display virtually no abrasive action above that of the toothbrush and water only. A commercial everyday-use dentifrice based on this type of solid particulate matter was thought by Larson (1969) to have been unable to prevent the accumulation of stained pellicle.

In Fig. 13 the low density of an expanded silica particle is clearly apparent. Silica particles, as such, are very hard, sharp and abrasive towards dentine and enamel; however, a synthetic, amorphous, porous silica particle with a very fine elementary particle size (50 nm) very loosely linked into agglomerates in the order of 10 μm diameter is claimed to be a safe, effective

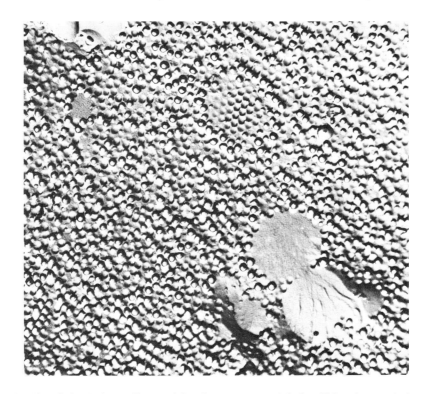

Fig. 12. Spherical acrylic particles in a commercial dentifrice (transmission electron micrograph of a freeze-fracture replica × 7000).

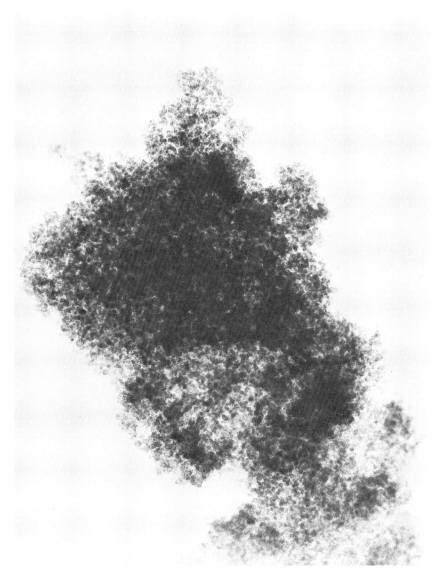

Fig. 13.   The ultra-fine structure of an expanded silica particle (transmission electron micrograph × 120 000).

abrasive. Such loose agglomerates of silica do not have an excessively abrasive action to dentine or enamel when correctly formulated into dentifrices. Figs 14 and 15 show chalk particles of very different abrasivities

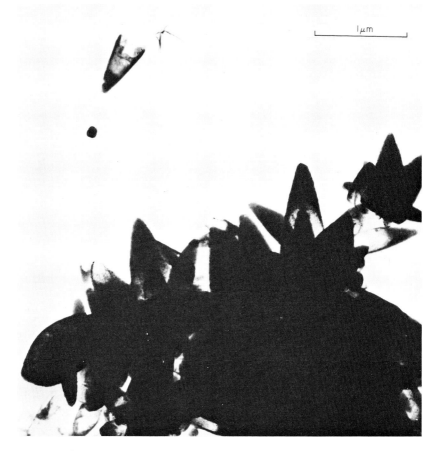

Fig. 14. The type of precipitated chalk particles used as the base of the British Standards Reference paste (transmission electron micrograph ×25 440).

(2:1) that could be used in dentifrices. When particles such as those mentioned above are incorporated into toothpastes their abrasive, polishing and cleaning actions depend on many interrelated factors.

A. Particle Hardness

The hardness of a particle (Table III) relative to a test substrate is the decisive factor controlling the abrasion process ("Abrasion", by definition, is the removal of material from the bulk of the substrate, during relative

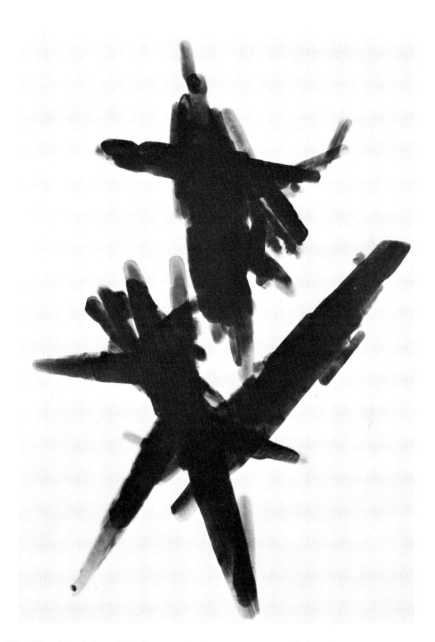

Fig. 15. Precipitated chalk particles from a commercial dentifrice (transmission electron micrograph × 36 920).

movement of the abrasive and substrate, thus the term can be extended to include the removal of surface films coherent with the substrate, such as pellicle). If a potentially abrasive particle is significantly softer than the substrate to be abraded the particle will deform when pressed against the substrate. To cause penetration and damage to the substrate; stress sufficient to cause permanent damage must be applied via the abrasive particles. (This may not be strictly true for fatigue-type wear processes which are one or two orders of magnitude slower than scratching or plastic shearing wear processes.) Deformation of soft (low elastic modulus) particles will spread the applied load over bigger substrate areas thus decreasing the load per unit area (stress) consequently decreasing the possibility of causing damage to the substrate.

Wright (1969) showed that abrasive particles of materials with hardnesses approaching 0·8 of the substrate hardness can cause appreciable wear by a scratching process. The reason for this is that as the abrasive particles

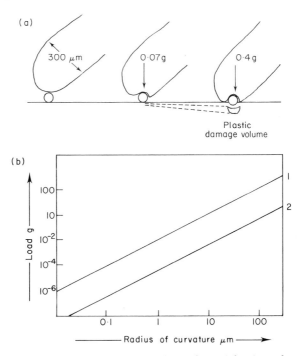

Fig. 16(a). The elastic penetration of spherical particles into dentine and the onset of permanent, plastic deformation at increasing applied loads.
(b). A computation of the loads at which plastic deformation is initiated in dentine (1) and enamel (2) when hard spherical particles, of various radii of curvature, are pressed into flat surfaces.

COLOUR PLATES

Plate 1. Clinically observed notching of exposed dentine near the gum margin.

Plate 2. Scratches formed when enamel is brushed under a water-base slurry containing pumice particles such as those used in prophylaxis pastes. (Optical micrograph under interference conditions × 200.)

Plate 3. Scratches formed by hard particles are removed when enamel is brushed under a water-base slurry containing precipitated chalk particles. The surface texture reflects details of the underlying enamel tissue. (Optical micrograph under interference conditions.)

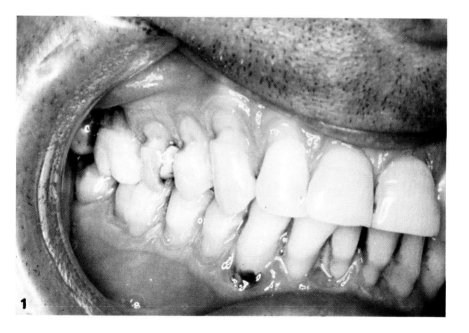

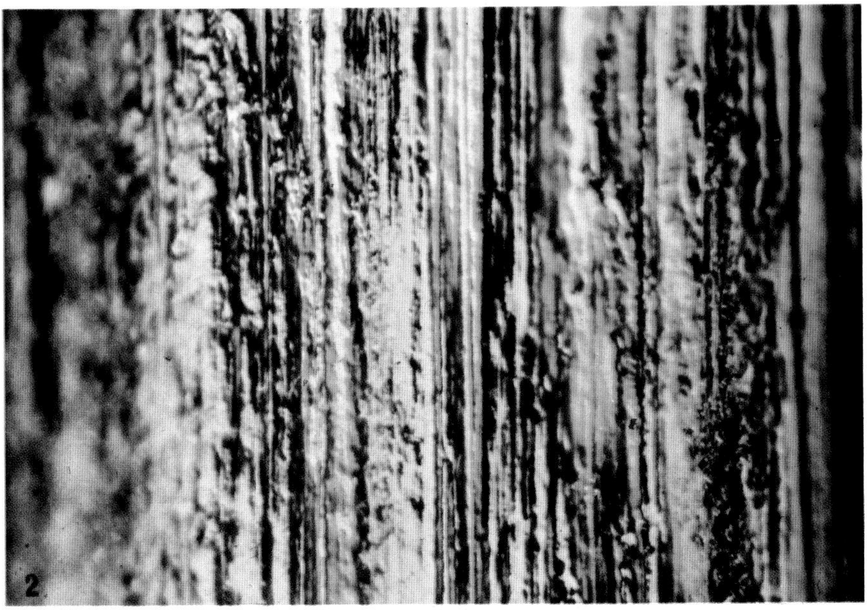
2

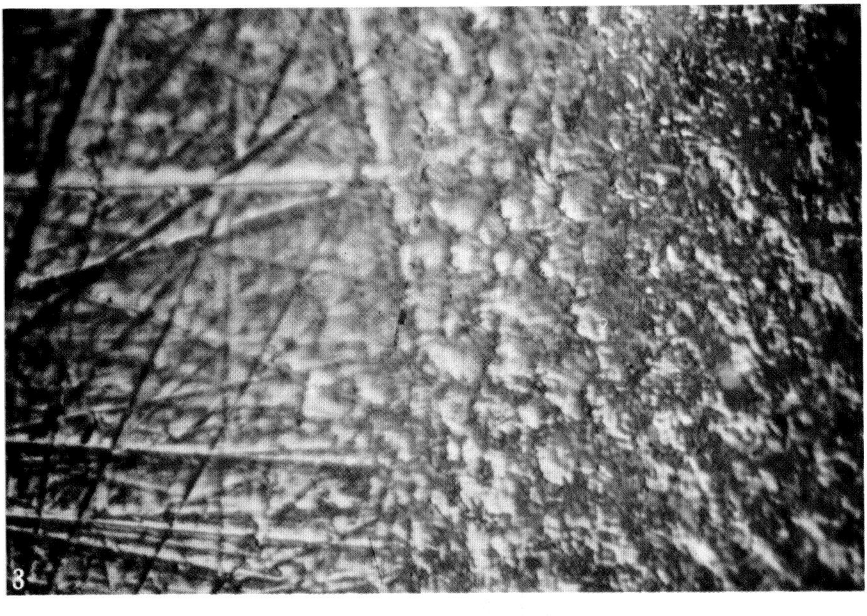
8

deform they can work-harden to a hardness greater than that of the substrate. Thus after a certain degree of spreading they resist further distortion and if the applied loads are sufficient they can penetrate the substrate and behave as harder particles.

The scratching abrasive wear of hard tooth tissues is the result of particles penetrating the surface layers to such an extent that plastic damage occurs. When a particle is partly embedded in the substrate by a normal load and then drawn across the surface by applying a shear load, subsurface damage occurs (Figs 16a and b), or in more extreme cases; scratches can be produced extending along the path of particle movement. (Figs 17a and b.) Plate 2 shows scratches caused when pumice particles typical of those used in prophylaxis pastes are brushed across enamel. Pumice particles are harder than dentine or enamel and therefore maintain their shape when loaded. Softer particles, such as those of hydrated dicalcium phosphate, chalk and polymers, deform when pressed against enamel so that scratches are rarely produced in enamel when such materials are used in dentifrices.

Softer particles, or lightly loaded hard particles, cause plastic deformation a little below the surface with the surface layer only elasticly distorted (i.e. fully recoverable). Repeated exposure to stresses which cause such subsurface damage results in cumulative damage and the ultimate, local failure of the subsurface region. Loss of material will eventually occur when a flake of material is lost from the substrate. Wear caused by this process is termed "fatigue wear" and the flake-loss is termed "spalling". Fatigue wear differs from scratching wear in that the dimensions of the flakes are affected by the microstructure of the substrate. Plate 3 illustrates how the prism structure of enamel is reflected in the surface architecture of an area abraded with a single nylon tuft and soft mineral slurry.

The abrasive processes, scratching and fatigue, outlined above are applicable to various substrates, plaque, pellicle, dentine and enamel although scratching may form tears in more fibrous tissues. For a given combination of abrasive and substrate; removal will occur by fatigue and scratching depending on the relative hardnesses. The efficacy of removal by the scratching process depends on the size, shape, relative hardness, strength and concentration of the abrasive particles. If any of these factors is lacking the process will be slow.

B. Particle Shape

The shape parameter is rather difficult to define but the degree of roundness is important because spherical particles will tend to roll and even if dragged

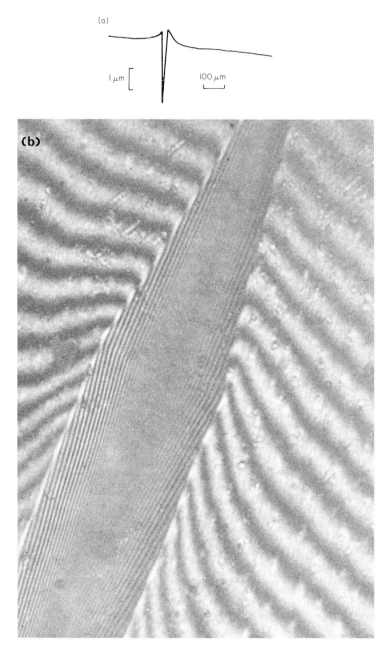

(a)

1 μm   100 μm

Fig. 17(a).   A surface profilometer trace of the surface topography of scratched enamel. The vertical magnification being 100 times the horizontal magnification distorts the true profile of scratches which generally have shallow inclined sides. (b).   An optical interference micrograph of a similar scratch in dentine. Once again the profile is distorted to carry out detailed studies of deformation and material loss.

across a surface the angle of contact with the surface is not amenable to scratching as shown by Dean and Doyle (1975), Powers and Craig (1972) and Lindhe (1964).

The sharpest edges or points of dentifrice particles can be given a radius of curvature defining them. Finer radii of the corners of particles or surface protuberances mean sharper cutting actions and easier penetration of the substrate provided that the particle does not deform or break. Sharp asperities on the surface of large particles increase the abrasive potential and make relations very difficult to define.

C. Elasticity and Strength of Particles

In practice the strength and elasticity of a particle is deduced from its hardness. This is an acceptable practice with regard to stiffness because the elastic modulus of a material is a major contributory factor to its hardness. Particle strength is however not necessarily related to hardness and is critical with respect to abrasion because a particle must be able to withstand the applied stresses without fracturing, during the abrasive process if it is to be effective. Weak particles such as expanded silica particles break down when stressed.

D. Mode of Fracture of Particles

If abrasive particles tend to be blunted by deformation, or by many minute chips falling away from the cutting edges; the abrasivity decreases considerably with usage. If particles fail by brittle fracture, leaving (or even producing) sharp edges; the abrasivity will decrease only slowly with usage as the overall particle size becomes reduced.

E. Particle Size

The particle size and the size distribution of particles in toothpastes are two important factors in the control of abrasion, polishing and stain-removal characteristics.

It is well established in engineering functions such as sandpapering wood, grinding metals and filing hard materials, that coarser abrasive particles remove unwanted material more quickly than fine abrasive particles. The reasons for this become obvious when the material loss effected by covering a surface with coarse scratches is compared with the loss effected by fine scratches (Fig. 18). The above-mentioned functions are two-body abrasive actions whereas toothpaste abrasion of dentine and enamel is a three-body abrasive action. The two-body logic also applies to dentifrice slurries, and is indeed supported by data from tests carried out with abrasive slurries containing particles of different sizes. The data illustrated in Fig. 19 relate to the effect of changing the size of the abrasive particles in a slurry that is brushed against dentine repeatedly, tested in the laboratory.

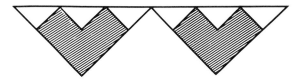

Fig. 18.   A diagrammatic indication of the extra material (shaded) that is removed when the surface of a substrate is covered with deep scratches in place of shallow scratches.

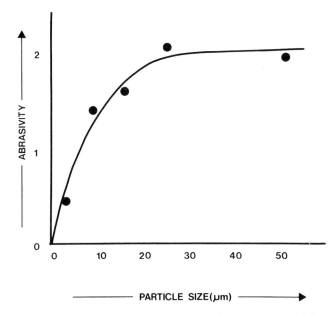

Fig. 19.   The particle size/dentine abrasivity relation for sieved fractions of a calcitic chalk powder. Commercial dentifrices have abrasivities in the range 0–1·5.

Such dentine is not covered with a protective film of pellicle, neither is it likely to be remineralized. Both these possibilities could be in operation under *in vivo* conditions.

F. Concentration

The size/abrasivity relation indicated in Fig. 19 suggests that a plateau is approached. These data refer to abrasive slurries of constant (40% by wt) weight-concentration of abrasive. This means that the number of abrasive particles per unit volume of toothpaste slurry is decreasing as the particle size increases. The levelling off of the relationship indicates the number-concentrations at which the chances of a particle being trapped beneath a toothbrush bristle begins to differ significantly from unity. In the extreme case where the particles become too big to be trapped beneath a toothbrush bristle they are swept aside and are ineffective as an abrasive. The number-concentration of abrasive particles was dealt with by Wright and Stephenson (1967) who showed that as the concentration is increased the abrasive power increases until the chances of particles being trapped approaches unity. Any further particles added are not effective at increasing the rate of abrasion because there are more than enough particles available and the maximum abrasivity level is controlled by the size and hardness of the mineral powders.

XII. POLISH AND PARTICLE SIZE RANGE

Whilst the logic of the effects of particle size and concentration on the abrasive power of slurries is clear the importance of using a powder of narrow particle size *range* is not so obvious. Fig. 20 shows, diagramatically, the abrasive action caused by two types of powder. The uniform powder (narrow size range) will leave scratches, on soft substrates, that are of depth approximately equal to 1/10th of the particle diameter. Repeated applications of such an abrasive will always result in scratches of the same depth being left in the surface.

If a powder of the same weight median diameter, but containing much larger and much smaller particles, is used in the same way; large occasional scratches will occur. If the proportion of large particles permitted is particularly unsuitable; additional deep scratches will be formed before the previous deep scratches have been eliminated by the more general abrasion, with scratches of medium depth. The particle size range factor is of little

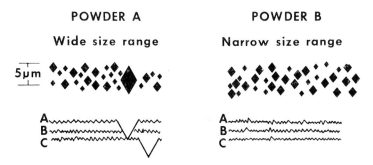

Fig. 20. The polishing powers of powders containing (A) a wide range of particle sizes and (B) a narrow range of particle sizes. As the substrate is progressively abraded to thicknesses A, B and C coarse scratches are not eliminated with the wide size-range abrasive.

consequence to abrasivity as such, but is the controlling factor in the quality of the surface finish.

When fine and coarse powders of the same mineral are blended their abrasivity equals that of a powder of the overall mean particle size but the depth of the scratches produced by the blend is that of the coarsest fraction.

XIII. POLISHING POWER

From the above considerations of particle size and concentration we can see a strong relation developing between particle size/concentration/ abrasivity/surface finish. The surface finish, scratch depth and degree of polish are the expressions for the roughness of a prepared surface. Although the evidence is sparse to support the hypothesis, it is reasonable to suspect that a rough surface on the tooth will be more likely to become contaminated by some form of deposition than a smooth surface. Thus one should strive to preserve a high quality finish after a toothbrushing session.

The degree of polish of a dry surface (i.e. the ability to reflect light without losses by interference from surface asperities) is related to its roughness on a scale in the order of the wave length of visible light, $1/2$ μm. On an atomic scale (in the order of Angstrom units) even highly polished metal surfaces could be considered rough. On a microbiological scale (5 μm is the approximate size of microorganisms encountered in plaque) dull, non-reflective surfaces may be classed as relatively smooth. This latter concept is reinforced if one considers the typical profile of a scratch in dentine. Figure 17 shows that typical dentine scratch has sides that deviate from the general surface contour by an angle of less than 20°. Thus a microorganism in the vicinity of a 1 μm deep scratch on the tooth surface would not consider the scratch as a deep crevice in which it could resist physical disturbance from the toothbrush or tongue. Add to the presence of a fresh, 1 μm deep scratch an acquired pellicle film (which will be more or less continuous within the hour); and it becomes clear that the light reflectivity (i.e. freedom from 1 μm-type asperities) is of little clinical significance. Furthermore, as the teeth are always viewed wet; achieving optical reflectivity, when observed dry, does not enhance their appearance. A suggested order of clinically significant polishing power is listed in Table VI. Defects and scratches as deep as 5 μm may improve the chances of microorganisms resisting the cleansing actions of their environment but such deep scratches are very unlikely to occur on the enamel crown except, perhaps, after the teeth have received a scale and "polish", prophylaxis treatment.

A prophylaxis treatment is carried out to remove calculus for therapeutic reasons and is usually completed by a thorough brushing with a highly abrasive (to enamel) medium. A highly abrasive prophylaxis paste is used for speed and efficiency in the removal of stained pellicle and residual calcified deposits that were not completely removed by the scaler. Brasch *et al.* (1969) showed that the scratches caused by a pumice prophylaxis were not removed by six months of normal dietary attack and regular toothbrushing with a commercial toothpaste. Discounting the disadvantage of losing several microns of well fluoridated enamel; the "polished" surface was not free of light-interfering defects. The enhanced whiteness attributed to prophylaxis is achieved by removing stained pellicle.

IV. ACID EROSION

A study of abrasion is not complete until the relation between abrasion and erosion is discussed. The acid erosion of dentine and enamel might be treated separately from abrasion and polishing. However, acid attack from the dietary intake was observed to upset experiments intended to study abrasion *in situ*. Figure 21 shows the loss of dentine and enamel from an insert in a volunteer's upper central incisor during a seven month period. During this period the diet and toothbrushing habits were controlled. When the diet was generally normal to low in fresh fruit and low pH foodstuffs the dentine was lost more rapidly than enamel regardless of toothbrushing habits. When the diet was changed to include fresh fruits, pickles and low pH beverages the disruption of the surfaces made it difficult to continue measurements, but it was apparent that enamel was lost faster than dentine. Figures 10 and 11 show the effect of changing the diet.

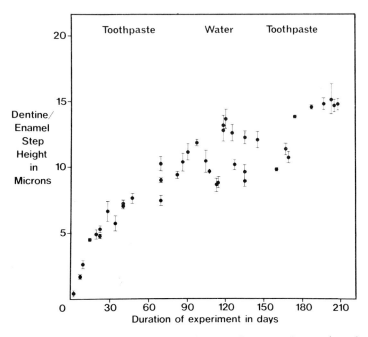

Fig. 21.   The development of height differences between flattened surfaces of human dentine and enamel over a period of 200 days when toothpaste or water are used during toothbrushing. The volunteer was consuming a low fruit diet during this test. (See Figs 10 and 11.)

(Note the apparent preferential attack at the dentine/enamel junction.)

Levine (1972) and Smith (1975) drew attention to the increased rate of fruit juice consumption in recent years, and the difficulties arising when dentists have to diagnose hard tissue losses in the absence of caries. Both these authors stress the importance of the diet and in particular point out the danger of a large, frequent intake of fresh fruits such as oranges and apples.

We now have to question our eating and oral hygiene habits. It is suggested that breakfast starting with fresh fruit juice, followed by well-sugared cereals and finishing with sugared coffee will demineralize enamel by direct acid erosion followed by plaque induced acid formation in inaccessible areas. If such a breakfast is followed by a vigorous tooth-brushing session, with a dentifrice that is highly abrasive to enamel, then enamel loss will be significant, especially if the teeth are not protected by the partial replacement of hydroxyl ions by fluoride ions, as shown by Xhonga and Sognnaes (1973).

Protection of the teeth of the adult population against erosion is, in itself, a strong case for encouraging them to use a properly formulated fluoride toothpaste. In the above consideration of the actions of abrasive particles in dentifrices I hope it becomes obvious that controlling the relevant parameters is important to maintain a physical balance of cleaning, polishing and abrasion. With present day technology we are able to control all the necessary parameters and maintain the chemical stability (and even enhance the activity) of active ingredients. In the near future caries and tooth tissue loss by erosion attack could be reduced to an insignificant level compared with troubles caused by gingival and periodontal diseases. The next generation of research projects aimed at improving current dentifrices will almost certainly be directed towards minimizing such gum disorders.

REFERENCES

Ashmore, H., Van Abbé, N. J. and Wilson, S. J. (1972). The measurement *in vitro* of dentin abrasion by toothpaste. *Brit. Dent. J.* **133**, 60.

Barrett, C. S. (1972). "Structure of Metals". McGraw-Hill Inc., New York, Toronto, London.

Brasch, S. V., Lazarou, J., Van Abbé, N. J. and Forrest, J. O. (1969). The assessment of dentifrice abrasivity *in vivo*. *Brit. Dent. J.* **127**, 119.

Bull, W. M., Callender, R. M., Pugh, B. R. and Wood, G. D. (1968). The abrasion and cleaning properties of dentifrices. *Brit. Dent. J.* **125**, 331.

Cordon, M. (1971). Method for measuring the abrasion of dentine by dentifrices. *J. Dent. Res.* **50**, 497.

Cowell, C. R. (1974). An appliance for the study of tooth tissue *in vivo*. *Brit. Dent. J.* **137**, 61.

Davis, W. B. (1975). Reduction in dentin wear resistance by irradiation and effects of storage in aqueous media. *J. Dent. Res.* **54**, 1078.

Davis, W. B. and Winter, P. J. Measurement *in vitro* of enamel abrasion by dentifrice. *J. Dent. Res.*, **55**, 970.

Davis, W. B. and Rees, D. A. (1975). A parametric test to measure the cleaning power of toothpaste. *J. Soc. Cosmet. Chem.* **26**, 217.

Dean, S. K. and Doyle, E. D. (1975). Significance of Grit morphology in fine abrasion. *Wear* **35**, 123.

Eastoe, J. E. and Miles, A. E. W. (1967). "Structural and Chemical Organisation of Teeth", Vol. II. Academic Press, New York and London.

Eccles, J. D. and Jenkins, W. G. (1974). Dental erosion and diet. *J. Dent.* **2**, 153.

Forward, G. C. (1975). A new technique for enamel solubility reduction (E.S.R.) measurement. *Helv. Odont. Acta.* **17**, 64.

Foulk, M. E. and Pickering, E. (1935). A history of dentifrices. *J. Amer. Pharm. Ass.* **24**, 975.

Grabenstetter, R. J., Broge, R. W., Jackson, F. L. and Radike, A. W. (1958). The measurement of the abrasion of human teeth by dentifrice abrasives: A test utilising radioactive teeth. *J. Dent. Res.* **37**, 1060.

Heath, J. R. and Wilson, H. J. (1971). Classification of toothpaste stiffness by a dynamic method. *Brit. Dent. J.* **130**, 59.

Heath, J. R. and Wilson, H. J. (1974). Forces and rates observed during *in vivo* brushing. *Biomed. Engng.* February, 1961.

Hefferen, J. J. (1974). How abrasive should a toothpaste be? *Pharmacy Times* July, 50–52.

Johnson, N. W. (1971). *Archs. Oral Biol.* **16**, 385.

Larsson, B. T. (1969). Losses of tooth substance and tooth brushing in a national dental service. *Sverige Tandläk. Tidn.* **61**, 58.

Levine, R. S. (1972). Fruit juice erosion—an increasing danger. *J. Dent.* **2**, 85.

Lindhe, J. (1964). Orthogonal cutting of dentine. *Odont. Revy.* **15**, Suppl. 8.

Lobene, R. A. (1968). Effect of dentifrices on tooth stain with controlled brushing. *J. Am. Dent. Ass.* **77**, 849.

Macfarlane, D. W. (1971). The dynamic stiffness of toothbrushes. *J. Periodont. Res.* **6**, 218.

McHugh, W. D. (1970). "Dental Plaque" (Symposium, Dundee 1969). E & S Livingstone Ltd., Edinburgh and London.

Macphee, T. and Cowley, G. (1969). "Essentials of Periodontology and Pedodontics". Blackwell Scientific, Oxford and Edinburgh.

Manly, R. S. (1943). A structureless recurrent deposit on teeth. *J. Dent. Res.* **22**, 479.

Manly, R. S., Wiren, J., Harte, D. B. and Ahern, J. M. (1974). Influence of method of testing on dentifrice abrasiveness. *J. Dent. Res.* **53**, 835.

Manly, R. S., Brown, P. W., Harrington, D. P., Crane, G. L. and Schichting, D. A. (1975). Laser diffusometer for estimation of smoothness of human dental enamel produced by dentifrice abrasives. *Archs. Oral Biol.* **20**, 479.

Manley, J. L., Limongelli, W. A. and Williams, A. C. (1975). The chewing stick: its uses and relationship to oral health. *J. Prev. Dent.* **2**, 7.

Miller, C. H. (1972). Design challenge for toothbrush manufacture. *Chemist Drugg* July, 164.

Padbury, A. D. and Ash, M. M. (1974). Abrasion caused by three methods of toothbrushing. *J. Periodont.* **45**, 434.

Peterson, J., Williamson, L. and Casad, R. (1975). Caries Inhibition with MFP—Calcium Carbonate Dentifrice Fluoridated Area. I.A.D.R. Conference, London.

Pfrengle, O. (1964). Abrasive and cleansing capacity of polishing substances in toothpaste. *Am. Perf. Cosm.* **79**, 43.

Powers, J. M. and Craig, R. G. (1972). Wear of fluorapitite single crystals I, II and III. *J. Dent. Res.* **51**, 168, 605 and 611.

Rees, D. A. and Davis, W. B. (1975). An *in vivo* Method for Assessing Dentine and Enamel Loss. 53rd General Session of I.A.D.R.

Robinson, H. B. G. (1969). Individualising dentifrices: the dentists' responsibility. *JADA.* **79**, 633.

Schiff, T. and Shaver, K. J. (1971). The comparative effect of two commercially available dentifrices on tooth surfaces as determined by a tooth reflectance meter. *J. Oral Med.* **26**, 127.

Scott, J. H. and Symons, N. B. B. (1971). "Introduction to Dental Anatomy", 6th Edn. Livingstone, Edinburgh and London.

Smith, M. L. (1935). The influence of particle size, shape, aggregation and hardness on the abrasiveness of fine powders. *J. Soc. Chem. Ind.* Aug., 269T.

Smith, B. G. N. (1975). Dental erosion, attrition and abrasion. *Practitioner* **214**, 347.

Suomi, J. D. (1971). Prevention and control of periodontal disease. *JADA.* **83**, 1271.

Tainter, M. L., Alford, C. E., Hinckel, E. T., Nachod, F. C. and Priznar M. (1974). A quantitative method for measuring polish produced by dentifrices. *Proc. Toilet Goods Ass.* **7**, 38.

Wilkinson, J. B. and Pugh, B. R. (1970). Toothpastes—cleaning and abrasion. *J. Soc. Cosmet. Chem.* **21**, 595.

Wright, H. N. and Fenske, E. L. (1937). Relative abrasive properties of the more commonly used dentifrice abrasives. *JADA* **24**, 1889.

Wright, K. H. R. and Stevenson, J. I. (1967). The measurement and interpretation of dentifrice abrasiveness. *J. Soc. Cosmet. Chem.* **18**, 387.

Wright, K. H. R. (1969). The abrasive wear resistance of human dental tissues. *Wear* **14**, 263.

Wright, K. H. R. (1969). Designing against wear—1. The basic mechanisms of wear. *Tribology* August, 152.

Wright, K. H. R. (1975). Private communication.

Xhonga, F. A. and Sognnaes, R. F. (1973). Dental erosion: progress of erosion measured clinically after various fluoride applications. *JADA* **87**, 1223.

COSMETIC MARKET AND TECHNOLOGY IN JAPAN

Nobukazu Fukuhara
Shiseido Co. Ltd.,
5–5 Ginza 7 Chome,
Chuo-Ku, Tokyo, Japan

I. MARKET TRENDS

A. Outline of the Japanese Cosmetic Industry

The Japanese cosmetic industry has developed rapidly over the past 20 years, and is still continuing to do so. This has been bolstered by Japan's remarkable economic growth with consequent increase in national income, expanded cultural exchanges with the USA and European countries, and increasingly active consumer buying. Figure 1 illustrates cosmetic shipments, GNP, per capita consumption, disposable incomes, and population. As shown in the figure, the average growth rate registered a phenomenal high of 16·7% during the period 1967–74, as compared to the GNP rate of 17·1%. As is well documented in Table IV cosmetic shipments in 1974 stood at US$1257 million a figure equivalent to 27% of the total shipments by the pharmaceutical industry or 3% of those by the foodstuff industry.

B. The Organization and Activity of the Cosmetic Industry

In Japan, the Japan Cosmetic Industry Association, a national organization has under its jurisdiction the Tokyo Cosmetic Industry Association (TCIA), the Kinki Cosmetic Industry Association (KCIA) and the Aichi Cosmetic Industry Cooperatives (ACIC). Its activities are:

1. to submit collective opinion of the industry to the Government, other agencies etc.
2. to carry out study and make investigation for the improvement of the quality of the cosmetic products, consumer protection and further the knowledge of the consumer concerning cosmetic products so they may select the appropriate products; and appropriate action for consumer complaint.

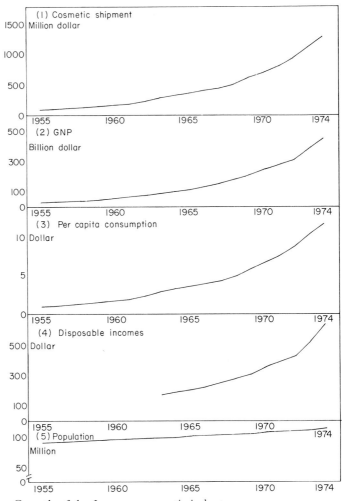

Fig. 1. Growth of the Japanese cosmetic industry.

These three associations are composed of manufacturers, that have their principal premises of business located in east Japan (TCIA), west Japan (KCIA) and Nagoya area (ACIC). The members of each association must be manufacturer of cosmetic products. Today TCIA has 222 members, KCIA (171) and ACIC (24) and accordingly, there should be 417 members in the JCIA; however, since some manufacturers have membership both in the TCIA and KCIA, the total number is slightly less than 417. The organizational structures are:

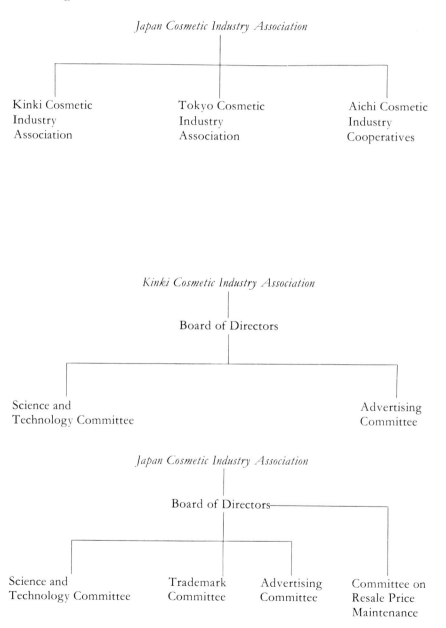

Japan Cosmetic Industry Association

Kinki Cosmetic Industry Association — Tokyo Cosmetic Industry Association — Aichi Cosmetic Industry Cooperatives

Kinki Cosmetic Industry Association

Board of Directors

Science and Technology Committee — Advertising Committee

Japan Cosmetic Industry Association

Board of Directors

Science and Technology Committee — Trademark Committee — Advertising Committee — Committee on Resale Price Maintenance

Tokyo Cosmetic Industry Association

Board of Directors

- Public Relations Committee
- Taxation Committee
- Scientific and Technology Committee
- Consumer Relations Committee
- Budget Committee

- Planning Committee

- Cosmetic Ingredients Standard Committee
- Product Test Method Committee
- Technical Informations Committee
- Color Additive Committee
- Committee on Pharmaceutical Affairs Law
- Committee on Fire Service Law

JCIA discussed and deliberated the following subject matters at the Head Office and also at the Osaka Office during 1975.

1. Plan to establish standard test methods for cosmetics and to make a list of standard ingredients for cosmetic products.
2. Studies on the definition and limit of claims of Quasi-Drugs.
3. Studies on the method to obtain approval for contract manufacturing, repacking and packaging of various items of cosmetics into one composite set.
4. Studies on safety substantiation of cosmetic and cosmetic ingredients and documentation of data.
5. Investigation and studies on coal-tar-colors for cosmetics.
6. Investigation and studies concerning GMP for cosmetics.
7. Studies and investigations on consumer complaint.

Recently, safety substantiation has become a great issue throughout the cosmetic industry. In 1975, TCIA organized various committees staffed by experts under the technical committee to cope with this problem. As there is a strong movement towards regulation, it will be necessary for the industry to expend time, money and effort to cope with this problem.

C. Sales Channels

Distribution routes in the cosmetic industry can be broadly classified as:

(1) Sales Company Route:

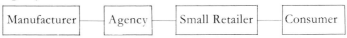

Examples: Shiseido, Kanebo Cosmetics, Kobayashi Kosei, Max Factor, Revlon, Teijin Papilio, etc.

(2) Agency Route:

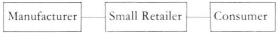

Examples: Kissme Cosmetics, Mandom, Momotani Juntenkan, Yanagiya, Utena, Pias, Cheseborough-Ponds etc.

(3) Direct Sales:

Examples: Helena Rubinstein, Pfizer (Coty), Estée Lauder, Elizabeth Arden, Cosmelt, etc.

(4) Door to Door Sales:

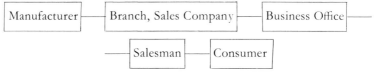

Examples: Pola Cosmetics, Japan Menard Cosmetics, Ryuhodo Pharmaceuticals, Naris Cosmetics, Avon, Shanson Cosmetics, etc.

(1976 *Cosmetic Marketing Strategy*; Nov. 25, 1975)

Major cosmetic manufacturers using Route (1) have grown rapidly through the systematic organization of the retailer and the introduction of the beauty consultant system. Together with the door to door sales method. These two distribution systems typify the Japanese cosmetics industry. The manufacturers using the agency route are experimenting difficulties resulting in decreased market share, although this group is the largest. The direct-sales group is composed of foreign-capital companies, and is characterized by manufacturers who concentrate on expensive products. This method serves their purpose of maintaining prestige by selection of sales outlets.

D. Advertising

The total advertising expenditures of the entire Japanese industry for fiscal year 1974 was $3.898 million. Table I shows the allocations of this sum by media. Newspaper and television advertising made up the greater part, amounting to 67·2% of the total.

Table I
Advertising expenditures by medium

Medium	Advertising expenditures 1974	
	$ million	%
Newspaper	1315	33·7
Magazines	207	5·4
Radio	186	4·7
Television	1306	33·5
Sum of four main media	3014	
Direct mail	164	4·2
Outdoor etc.	632	16·2
Export	88	2·3
Sum excluding four main media	884	
Total advertising expenditure	3898	

From Tokyo Cosmetic Industry Association, 1974 Business Report.

*(US$1 = ¥ 300).

Note: Terms used in Table I are defined as follows:

Newspapers: Advertising and plate-making charges (excluding design charge) of national dailies and industrial newspapers
Magazines: Advertising and plate-making charges (excluding design charge) of national monthly, weekly and specialist magazines

Radio and television: Broadcasting charges of national commercial broadcasting, and production charges (including those of commercial stations, advertising agencies, etc.)
Direct mail: Mailing and dispatch costs (excluding production costs of contents)
Outdoor, etc.: Advertising expenditure for the following 9 items: inserts, matchboxes, ad balloons, films, transport advertising, street posters, exhibitions, neon signs, billboards (including media and production costs for only those media where costs are measurable, and only among these 9 media)
Export: Foreign currency expenditure on advertising, and yen payments within Japan to overseas media (excluding transactions overseas)

Advertising expenditures by the cosmetics industry for fiscal year 1974 totalled $202 million for the four main media (newspapers, magazines, radio and television), ranking fairly high among all industries. (Table I shows the seven industries with the highest advertising expenditures.)

The term "cosmetic industry" refers to manufacture of cosmetics and cleansing foams, including skin and hair cosmetics, cosmetic devices, toothpaste, soap, detergent, soap powder, and household chemical products.

Table II
Advertising expenditures for the four main media: (newspapers, magazines, radio and television) by industry, 1974

	*$ million	%
Medical treatment, education, information etc.	555	18·4
Food and beverages	455	15·1
Housing and building materials	289	9·6
Service and recreation	217	7·2
Cosmetics and detergents	202	6·7
Pharmaceuticals	171	5·7
Wholesale and department stores	169	5·6

From Tokyo Cosmetic Industry Association, 1974 Business Report.
* (US$1 = ¥300).

Many other media besides the main four mentioned above are used for cosmetics advertising; i.e. direct mail, films, neon signs, billboards, posters, etc. All are effective for cosmetics advertising; however, television, which reaches many audience levels covering wide areas, has become the most important. It is highly effective for advertising commodities such as cosmetics which rely heavily on creating an image or mood, and which must be presented to as many consumer levels as possible, in as near their actual form as possible. In particular the recent widespread use of color television has enabled emphasis on color, increasing television's importance even further. In this connection, statistics for 1974 indicate that television accounted for the overwhelming proportion of 74·1% of the advertising revenue of the four main media (Table III).

Table III
Advertising revenue of the four main media

	$ million	%
Television	150	74·1
Magazines	29	14·2
Newspapers	18	9·0
Radio	5	2·7
Total for four media	202	100·0

From Tokyo Cosmetic Industry Association, 1974 Business Report.

The importance of television to the cosmetics industry is also indicated by the fact that quite the opposite situation existed in, for example, the publishing, financial, insurance, wholesale, department store and other business fields, as shown in Fig. 2.

Besides these four media, however, poster advertising is also important. Posters are produced to launch virtually every new product and as PR material for the dissemination of new policy. Significant effect lies in the fact that while cosmetics advertising uses a wide variety of media, it does so, not separately through each, but in an integrated manner to get a better overall result.

E. Sales and Trends

Table IV gives tabulations of the shipments classified by items during the 10-year period 1965–74, which are graphically illustrated in Fig. 3.

These statistics are indicative of some characteristic points, which may be summarized as follows:

In Japan, skin care cosmetics such as beauty washes, creams and milky lotions are used in large quantities, as can be concluded from the market share of these products which constitutes a little over 40%. As regards sales trends during the 10-year period, medicated and make-up cosmetic sales increased somewhat, while hair cosmetics sales decreased, but not to

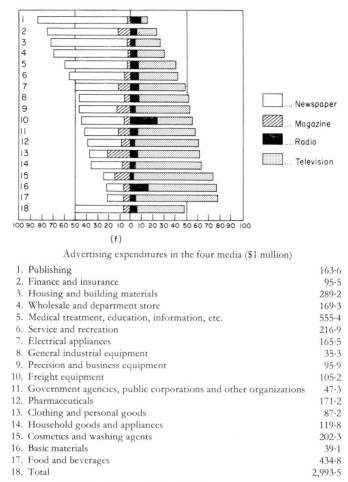

Advertising expenditures in the four media ($1 million)

1. Publishing		163·6
2. Finance and insurance		95·5
3. Housing and building materials		289·2
4. Wholesale and department store		169·3
5. Medical treatment, education, information, etc.		555·4
6. Service and recreation		216·9
7. Electrical appliances		165·5
8. General industrial equipment		35·3
9. Precision and business equipment		95·9
10. Freight equipment		105·2
11. Government agencies, public corporations and other organizations		47·3
12. Pharmaceuticals		171·2
13. Clothing and personal goods		87·2
14. Household goods and appliances		119·8
15. Cosmetics and washing agents		202·3
16. Basic materials		39·1
17. Food and beverages		434·8
18. Total		2,993·5

(Advertising in Japan, 1974) *Dentsu News*, 20 March 1975.

Fig. 2.   Component ratios of use of the four main media by industry (1974).

a large degree. The increase in sales of perfumes and eau de colognes in Japan were relatively low as compared with those of foreign countries and may be explained in several ways. The predominant factor may be attributed to the difference in the Japanese way of thinking and living. Despite the poor showing of fragrances at the present stage, there are all indications that this particular field may develop into one of the most successful lines in the cosmetic business in the future. Cosmetics for men show low rates of increase as hair cosmetics are excluded from the statistics.

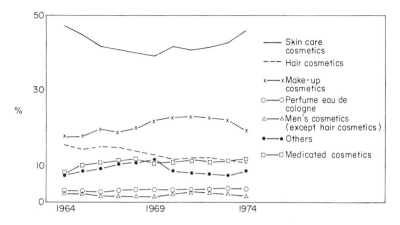

Fig. 3.   Shipments classified by items during period 1965–74.

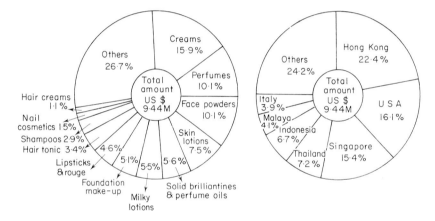

Fig. 4.   Cosmetic exports in 1974. (From the Japan Cosmetic Industry Association Report.)

Judging from the amount of money men are spending for cosmetics, however, there is ample indication that such sales are on the increase.

F. Export/Import Status

As shown in Fig. 4, exports in 1974 registered US$9·44 million with Hong Kong, the USA and Singapore purchasing over 50% of the total. Figure 5 also shows that imports in 1974 were US$26·99 million. Major trade

Table IV
Shipments classified by items (unit: $1000)

No.	Items	1965	Share %	1966	Share %	1967	Share %	1968	Share %
	Skin care cosmetics								
1	Vanishing cream	26 426	17·1	23 036	14·6	22 982	13·7	24 519	13·0
2	Cold cream	31 433	20·3	30 717	19·5	33 111	19·7	34 134	18·1
3	Cleansing cream	12 823	8·3	14 626	9·3	14 670	8·7	16 089	8·5
4	Milky lotion	27 391	17·7	27 007	17·1	28 212	16·8	31 917	16·9
5	Foundation	18 194	11·8	17 669	11·2	25 443	15·1	31 112	16·5
6	Lotion	38 537	24·8	44 558	28·3	43 867	26·0	50 862	27·0
7	Pack								
	Total	154 804	44·6	157 613	41·4	168 285	40·5	188 633	39·6
	Hair cosmetics								
8	Solid brilliantine	14 108	28·9	17 632	31·0	22 548	37·2	25 574	39·4
9	Liquid hair groom								
10	Hair cream	5 003	10·2	6 372	11·2	6 049	10·0	5 470	8·4
11	Hair oil	2 334	4·8	2 044	3·6	1 935	3·2	1 895	2·9
12	Solid brilliantine (stick)	3 958	8·1	4 542	8·0	4 658	7·7	3 975	6·1
13	Hair tonic	8 566	17·5	8 743	15·4	8 864	14·6	10 106	15·6
14	Hair spray	13 179	27·0	15 543	27·4	14 905	24·6	16 065	24·7
15	Set lotion	1 707	3·5	1 922	3·4	1 690	2·7	1 830	2·9
	Total	48 855	14·1	56 798	14·9	60 649	14·6	64 915	13·6
	Make-up cosmetics								
16	Face powder	4 284	7·0	3 645	4·9	3 611	4·6	5 181	5·5
17	Pressed face powder	26 056	42·6	33 082	44·6	34 955	44·8	37 810	40·3
18	Other face powder	1 939	3·2	707	1·0	536	0·7	342	0·4
19	Lipstick	16 142	26·4	19 735	26·6	20 374	26·1	26 080	27·8
20	Rouge	1 154	1·9	2 884	3·9	2 354	3·0	3 103	3·3
21	Eye brow and Eye lash	2 781	4·5	4 851	6·5	6 278	8·0	7 395	7·9
22	Eye make-up	3 699	6·0	4 593	6·2	5 303	6·8	8 621	9·2
23	Nail cosmetics	5 148	8·4	4 641	6·3	4 597	6·0	5 307	5·6
	Total	61 203	17·6	74 138	19·5	78 008	18·8	93 839	19·7
	Perfumes Eau de Cologne								
24	Perfume	5 669	54·9	5 450	50·3	6 212	48·5	6 227	40·1
25	Eau de Cologne	4 649	45·1	5 392	49·7	6 590	51·5	9 287	59·9
	Total	10 318	3·0	10 842	2·8	12 802	3·1	15 514	3·3
	Men's cosmetics (except hair cosmetics)								
26	Men's cream	4 530	53·9	4 365	59·6	4 227	55·0	4 233	49·6
27	Men's milky lotion	536	6·4	475	6·5	622	8·1	1 145	13·4
28	Men's lotion	1 505	17·9	266	17·3	1 371	17·8	1 663	19·5
29	Others	1 827	21·8	200	16·6	1 470	19·1	1 487	17·5
	Total	8 398	2·4	7 326	1·9	7 690	1·9	8 528	1·8
	Others								
30	Others	29 468	8·5	34 361	9·0	42 074	10·1	50 115	10·5
	Medicated cosmetics								
31	Medicated cream	4 825	14·3	6 616	16·7	8 516	18·4	8 136	14·9
32	Medicated lotion	2 190	6·5	1 711	4·3	1 763	3·8	2 326	4·3
33	Hair tonic (medicated)	13 726	40·6	15 768	39·9	16 578	35·9	17 141	31·4
34	Hair color								
35	Others	13 027	38·6	15 458	39·1	19 302	41·9	26 940	49·4
	Total	33 768	9·8	39 553	10·5	46 159	11·0	54 543	11·5
	TOTAL	346 814	100·0	380 631	100·0	415 667	100·0	476 087	100·0

	Year											
1969	Share %	1970	Share %	1971	Share %	1972	Share %	1973	Share %	1974	Share %	No.
26 411 .	11·7	36 663	13·2	38 571	12·3	46 135	12·4	56 764	12·3	77 191	13·5	1
46 846	20·8	51 020	18·4	52 012	16·6	59 961	16·1	75 854	16·4	96 415	16·9	2
18 540	8·2	20 993	7·6	25 448	8·1	32 346	8·7	44 698	9·7	52 671	9·2	3
36 940	16·4	41 302	14·9	47 905	15·3	53 636	14·4	61 201	13·2	77 978	13·7	4
36 906	16·4	40 587	14·7	48 533	15·5	65 561	17·5	78 148	16·9	93 451	16·4	5
59 857	26·5	70 547	25·5	81 755	26·1	94 693	25·4	117 339	25·3	140 301	24·6	6
		15 898	5·7	19 112	6·1	21 053	5·5	29 172	6·2	31 993	5·7	7
225 500	38·8	277 010	41·2	313 336	40·4	373 385	41·1	463 176	42·2	570 000	45·4	
9 570	13·0	8 320	10·8	8 316	9·2	8 150	7·6	8 519	7·0	9 410	7·1	8
16 324	22·3	16 625	21·6	21 672	24·0	25 516	23·9	27 007	22·0	26 787	20·1	9
6 476	8·8	7 167	9·3	8 053	8·9	10 481	9·8	11 190	9·1	13 114	9·9	10
1 785	2·4	2 102	2·7	2 090	2·3	2 294	2·1	2 662	2·2	3 574	2·7	11
4 410	6·0	4 358	5·7	4 089	4·5	3 824	3·6	4 052	3·3	4 416	3·3	12
12 511	12·0	12 907	16·8	15 816	17·5	19 568	18·3	21 861	17·8	25 073	18·8	13
20 063	27·4	22 921	29·8	27 129	30·0	32 147	30·1	40 060	32·7	43 842	32·9	14
2 242	3·1	2 488	3·3	3 195	3·6	4 986	4·6	7 144	5·9	6 922	5·2	15
73 381	12·6	76 888	11·4	90 360	11·7	106 966	11·8	122 495	11·2	133 138	10·6	
4 648	3·7	6 079	4·0	6 821	3·9	8 414	4·1	9 266	3·8	13 399	5·6	16
47 786	37·7	55 117	36·3	65 639	37·3	74 056	36·2	82 929	34·3	79 476	33·1	17
288	0·2	185	0·1	229	0·1	286	0·1	179	0·1	801	0·3	18
29 977	23·7	31 889	21·0	37 250	21·2	52 343	25·6	65 758	27·2	62 620	26·1	19
1 547	1·2	3 729	2·5	5 661	3·2	6 135	3·0	11 992	5·0	13 728	5·7	20
12 645	10·0	13 264	8·7	15 300	8·7	17 752	8·7	20 863	8·6	22 608	9·4	21
19 663	15·5	30 053	19·8	33 979	19·3	32 230	15·7	36 404	15·1	35 002	14·6	22
10 096	8·0	11 617	7·6	10 894	6·3	13 510	6·6	14 085	5·9	12 625	5·2	23
126 650	21·8	151 933	22·6	175 773	22·7	204 726	22·5	241 476	22·0	240 259	19·1	
7 645	38·3	7 717	35·0	7 611	29·5	9 449	29·9	13 083	32·0	14 409	31·6	24
12 321	61·7	14 316	65·0	18 201	70·5	22 131	70·1	27 817	68·0	31 252	68·4	25
19 966	3·4	22 033	3·3	25 812	3·3	31 580	3·5	40 900	3·7	45 661	3·6	
4 455	16·2	5 285	33·0	5 616	24·9	5 612	22·9	6 164	23·7	6 704	36·0	26
1 125	11·7	1 504	9·5	1 970	8·7	2 249	9·2	2 563	9·8	2 753	14·8	27
2 046	21·2	6 335	39·9	11 820	52·4	13 133	53·7	13 083	50·2	4 727	25·4	28
2 077	20·9	2 743	17·3	3 151	14·0	3 473	14·2	4 249	16·3	4 417	23·8	29
9 653	1·6	15 867	2·4	22 557	2·9	24 467	2·7	26 059	2·4	18 601	1·5	
64 968	11·2	56 702	8·4	59 792	7·7	68 575	7·5	81 591	7·4	103 903	8·3	30
10 776	17·4	7 311	10·1	10 705	12·2	11 392	11·6	14 825	12·3	18 867	13·0	31
2 092	3·4	3 230	4·5	6 362	7·3	9 815	10·0	11 266	9·3	12 872	8·9	32
14 358	23·2	13 175	18·3	13 522	15·4	13 457	13·7	14 370	11·9	17 290	11·9	33
21 797	35·3	31 857	44·2	33 902	38·6	35 434	35·9	39 826	32·9	45 277	31·2	34
12 765	20·7	16 467	22·9	23 258	26·5	28 483	28·8	40 644	33·6	50 772	35·0	35
61 788	10·6	72 040	10·7	87 749	11·3	98 581	10·9	120 931	11·1	145 078	11·5	
581 906	100·0	672 473	100·0	775 379	100·0	908 280	100·0	1 096 628	100·0	1 256 639	100·0	

Japan Cosmetic Industry Association's Report (1975).

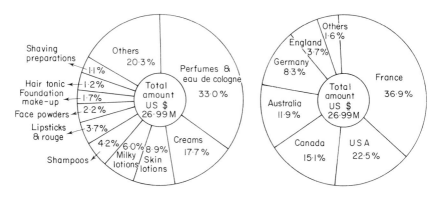

Fig. 5. Cosmetic imports in 1974. (From the Japan Cosmetic Industry Association Report.)

partners, amongst others, were France, the USA and Canada, with perfumes, eau de colognes and creams occupying a substantial portion of the imports.

II. COSMETICS WHICH ARE CHARACTERISTIC OF JAPAN

A. Background

The Japanese archipelago is an area of about 377 000 km² surrounded by sea. Stretching from north lattitude 25°–46°, it is situated in the north temperate zone. As can be seen from the data in Fig. 6, Japan is characterized by relatively high temperatures and humidity and distinct changes in the four seasons. Because of these factors, many seasonal cosmetics must be produced, as can be readily seen in the variety of the cosmetics. In other words, cosmetic manufacturers are required to produce cosmetics conforming to the different seasons. Temperature conditions to which cosmetics are exposed are very extreme and cosmetic manufacturers, therefore, are required to provide quality that can withstand these rigorous conditions.

In Japan, a population of 109·7 million live in an area of 377 000 km². In addition to the high density of population that stands at 291/km² (world average 28/km²), urbanization has progressed considerably in this country. Approximately 65% of women are salaried women (age 20–24) who are expected to use large quantities of cosmetics. In Japan, where means of transportation and mass media such as television, radio, newspapers, and magazines are highly developed, fashions are disseminated quickly; and large quantities of cosmetics are being produced to meet the fast changing

COLOUR PLATE

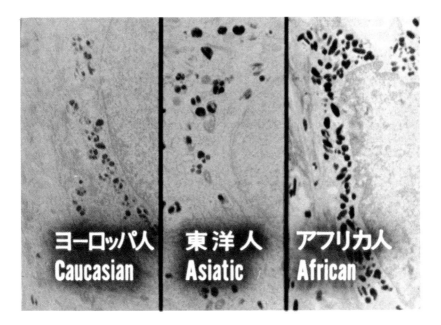

ヨーロッパ人
Caucasian

東洋人
Asiatic

アフリカ人
African

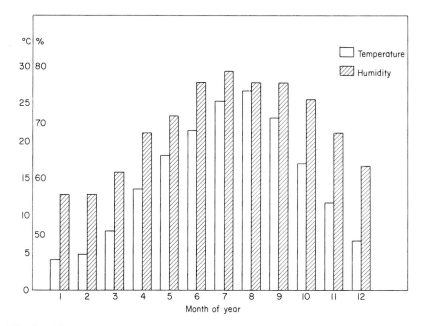

Fig. 6. Temperatures and humidity in Tokyo. The figures are the average during 1941–70. (From the Rika-Nenpto.)

situations. Eating habits, housing situations and life customs in Japan are widely different from those of other countries. These differences are reflected in the preference for fragrance, bath preparations and other cosmetics.

Asiatics including the Japanese, are different from other races in physique, colors of the skin, hair, eyebrows, and features. These differences are reflected in cosmetics. As can be observed in Plate 1, Asiatics are different from other races in size, number and distribution of melanin granules, and have the specific skin color. It is reported that Japanese hair is black in color, round in section and thick. On account of these properties, the Japanese usually bleach their hair before dyeing it, and men's hair dressings are required to be of comparatively high tackiness to keep the hair in place.

B. Skin Care Cosmetics

In skin care cosmetics such as creams, lotions and milky lotions which are segmented according to their function, skin condition and season, it

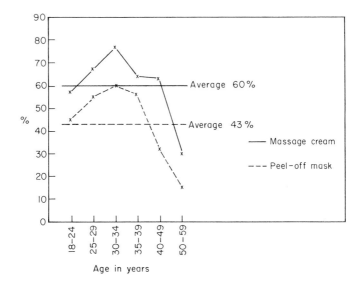

Fig. 7.   Usage rates of massage creams and peel-off masks in Japan. (From the Shiseido Report.)

should be emphasized that a large variety of products with a combination of these factors are placed on the market, and a large quantity of skin care cosmetics are actually used as shown by the sales statistics. In Japan, the practice of skin care has been handed down from times immemorial, and it can be said that the Japanese use of make-up originated from this practice. As shown in Fig. 7 massage creams and peel-off masks are well used in Japan, and this is very characteristic of Japan compared with other countries.

Table V shows examples of model formulations for the creams (cleansing, massage and nourishing creams) presently on the Japanese market.

Technical advances in developing quality goods have progressed remarkably for the past dozen years or so, and are kept secret as technical know-how by each cosmetic manufacturing company, although part of them are open to the public through patent publications or presentations at symposia.

The themes of research presented in recent years are included in the following research fields:

1. Development of surface active agents and emulsification technology
2. Research to improve the quality of raw materials (refining, decolorization and deodorization)

Table V
Formulas for cream (cleansing, massage and nourishing creams)

	Cleansing cream		Massage cream		Nourishing cream		
Formula No.	1	2	3	4	5	6	7
Mineral oil	35·0	51·0	41·0	44·5			
Squalane					33·0	5·0	34·0
Hydrogenated coconut oil					3·0		
Hydrogenated lanolin					5·0	2·0	7·0
Stearyl alcohol					2·0	7·0	
Cetyl alcohol	2·0						
Octyl dodecanol						6·0	
Diisocetyl adipate							10·0
Petrolatum	10·0	8·0	15·0	12.0	6.0		5·0
Microcrystalline wax	11·0	7·0	5·0	10·0	1·0		11·0
Bees wax		10·0	10·0	6·0			4·0
Stearic acid						2·0	
Glyceryl stearate	3·0		2·0		2·5	2·0	
Polysorbate 20			2·0				
Polysorbate 60	3·0				2·5		
Polysorbate 80				0·8			1·0
Sorbitan sesquiolate				3·2			
Cottonseed glyceride							3·0
Glyceryl oleate		1·5					
Celeth 25						3·0	
Propylene glycol stearate		0·5					
Sodium oleate		0·3	0·1	0·3			
Propylene glycol	5·0				5·0	5·0	2·5
Sodium borate		0·7	0·2				
Water	30·5	20·5	24·2	22·7	39·7	67.5	22·0
Perfume	0·5	0·5	0·5	0·5	0·3	0·5	0·5
Preservatives and antioxidants	q.s.	q.s.	q.s.	q.s.	q.s.	q.s.	q.s.

3. Approaches to make products safe and effective on the skin
4. Research on emulsification techniques from the viewpoint of surface chemistry and rheology

Needless to say, the main function of cosmetics should be consumer satisfaction and the Japanese are especially strict in evaluating the quality of the product. It should be added that a large number of tests are conducted to guarantee the quality of products placed on the market which must be stable under varied circumstances of distribution and storage, because visible defects (separation, color fading, etc.) are not acceptable.

C. Make-up Cosmetics

In recent years, Japan has quickly adopted fashions from the USA and Western Europe, so that little noticeable difference is seen in the products and in the way of using make-up at present. Nevertheless, in the application process, the Japanese have achieved a uniquely Japanese effect. Among existing make-up products, there is a cake face powder which is used with a sponge in combination with water, and is favored in the summer when the temperature and humidity are high, for its cooling effect on the skin.

The following is an example of the formulation and manufacturing process of these cosmetics, which originated as stage make-up.

Formula 8

Talc	85·5
Petrolatum or lanolin	5·0
Sorbitan sesquioleate	2·0
Stearic acid	1·5
Triethanolamine	1·0
Water	q.s.
Color	q.s.
Perfume	q.s.

Procedure: There are two procedures employed in the manufacture of cake foundations: dry-molding process and wet-molding process.

As regards the application of make-up, the method of overlapping cosmetics is widely adopted for the purpose of enhancing facial depth, reducing flatness as much as possible, and to lighten the yellow complexion of the Japanese.

Figure 8 shows the color tones in lipstick. The predominant color was once occupied by the pinkish colors, and then the reddish colors gradually increased. Today a wide variety of color tones has appeared including intermediate shades between pink or red and brown, orange etc. Many factors have contributed to such changes mainly the sales promotion programs of cosmetic companies and the spread and diversification of make-up

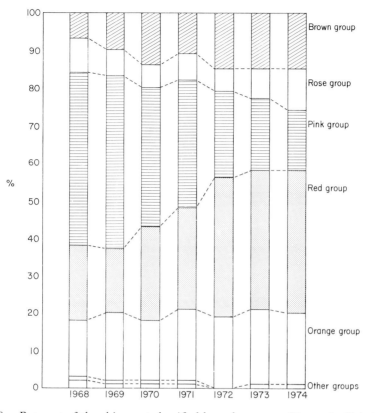

Fig. 8.   Per cent of the shipment classified by colour tone. (From the Shiseido Report.)

products. In Japan, the addition of new lipstick colors is announced mainly in the spring and autumn, each cosmetic company intensifies its sales promotion program and the catch phrases for the season are advertised through various media.

D. Hair Cosmetics

Until the early 1960s, the leading hair cosmetics for men in Japan were vegetable-oil-based solid brilliantines, which suited their relatively coarse textured hair and made possible the styles popular at the time. About 1962, however, liquid and clear gel hair grooms began to appear on the market, and liquid hair grooms have now become by far the most popular. Long hair styles and the widespread use of hair dryers (56·3% in 1973) are recent trends and development in hair fashion, accompanied by the increased use of hair care products among men.

The increasing use of liquid hair grooms can be explained partly by these factors, and partly by improvements of the product quality, to make shampooing the hair easier and to prevent staining clothes and pillows, (both defects of solid brilliantines), and also to give a cooling sensation, all of which have led to wide popular acceptance.

Women are also using hair creams, hair sprays and setting lotions for hair styling. Table VI shows the rate of use.

Table VI
The usage rates of hair cosmetics (women)

	Usage rate (%)
Hair creams	61·9
Hair sprays	54·7
Setting lotions	37·0
Hair oils	11·5

E. Bathing and Bath Preparations

The Japanese people are very fond of hot springs and bathing, not only for the sake of cleanliness but also for health reasons and for sheer enjoyment. Various studies show that the average Japanese takes a bath once every two days, washing outside the tub and warming up in it. In the last few years, sales of bath salts, body shampoos, sponges and bath brushes etc. have grown rapidly.

Japan is one of the fortunate countries in the world endowed with hot springs and mineral springs, and also in having an unusually soft natural water supply throughout the country.

Water hardness:

Tokyo	40– 60 ppm
Europe	50–180 ppm
USA	100–250 ppm

For this reason, ordinary soaps (fatty acids), transparent soaps and body shampoos lather copiously, whereas the use of Syndet Bar is limited and not necessary due to the soft water supply.

F. Cosmetic Raw Materials

In Japan cosmetic raw materials are controlled by the Ministry of Health and Welfare Ordinance. In this way, the standards for properties, purity, and methods of qualitative and quantitative analysis to check raw material quality are established, from the viewpoint of health and hygiene. An example of the form used is shown in Fig. 9.

Japan Wax

Japan Wax is prepared by bleaching the fat obtained from the fruit-rind of *Rhus succedanea* Linné *(Anacardiacca)* .

.Description   Japan Wax occurs as white to light yellowish white mass, having a characteristic odor and taste.

Specific gravity d_{20}^{20}: 0.96 ~ 1.00 (Method 3)

Melting point   50 ~ 53.5 (Method 2)

Acid value   Not more than 25 (5 g)

Saponification value   205 ~ 225

Iodine value   5 ~ 18

Unsaponificable substances   Not more than 1%

Purity   Water   Use the apparatus as illustrated. Place 100 g of Japan Wax in the 500 ml distilling flask A, add 100 ml of xylene and a few pumice stones, and heat the flask A after connecting to the graduated adapter B with the condenser C. Heat the flask A, at the beginning, in order that xylene drops from C at the rate of 2 or 3 drops a second. When the quantity of water in B does not increase any more, make heating strong in order that xylene drops at the rate of 4 drops a second. Stop heating when the distillate becomes clear, and cool naturally. Wash the water drops adhering at the inside of the condenser down into B by a little amount of xylene pouring from the top of C. Then, allow to stand for a while and measure the volume of water: the volume is not more than 0.8 ml.

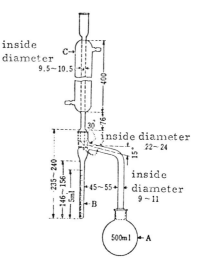

inside diameter 9.5~10.5

inside diameter .22~24

inside diameter 9 ~ 11

500 ml   A

(The figures indicated are in mm)

Fig. 9.   Form used for Japan Wax.

At present, 431 raw materials are listed in the Japanese Standards of Cosmetic Ingredients, and the details may be summarized as Table VII. They can be used in cosmetics and quasi-drugs without the permission of the government.

Table VII
The list of raw materials in the Japanese Standards of Cosmetic Ingredients

	Year			
	1967	1970	1973	Total in 1975
Fats, oils, waxes and derivatives	14	26	32	72
Surfactants	14	4	43	61
Agents	11	—	56	67
High polymers	10	6	12	28
Organic compounds and pigments	14	9	24	47
Inorganic compounds and pigments	26	10	36	72
Fragrance compounds	9	31	—	40
Bacteriostats and preservatives	16	5(-1)	24	44
Total	114	90	227	431

The figures are the number of raw materials

G. Packaging

In the selection of cosmetic container materials, in addition to the obvious considerations of sales appeal and convenience, the important factors of preservation and hygiene, and also ease of production, economy and esthetic acceptability must be satisfied. Plastic, metal and glass containers are frequently used, with the exception of expensive metal compacts and other refill types, and are all disposable.

Plastic containers are used for most liquid cosmetics and shampoos, while for beauty lotions about 90% of the containers are glass. In lipsticks, there has been a recent trend to use plastic elevators instead of metal, and about 80% also have plastic caps.

Table VIII shows the present use of cosmetic packaging materials in Japan.

Table VIII
The final use in Japan (1973)

Use	PVC bottle (%)	PE bottle (%)	Metal bottle (%)	Glass bottle (%)
Cosmetics	26·1	32·8	—	2·0
Foods	68·8	38·0	91·6	90·5
Drugs	—	8·3	—	5·9
Others	Detergents 0·4	Detergents 13·5	Motor oil 2·6	
			Paints 2·7	
	Others 4·7	Others 7·4	Others 3·1	Others 1·6

H. Patents

In 1971 the Japanese Patent Law was partially amended, and the system of laid open application was adopted.

Since most of the applications are published in the Japanese Official Gazette for laid open application before examination, the technical trends can be followed readily by studying them. The laid open applications in the cosmetic industry for 1973 and 1974 are listed in Table IX.

Analysis of the figures shows that cosmetic-related applications made up just over 0·2% of the total, and amongst these the different types of products were fairly evenly represented.

Table IX
The laid open applications in the cos-
metic industry

	Year	
Classification	1973	1974
General	57	71
Skin	54	100
Hair	55	80
Oral	45	61
Fragrance	62	90
Others	6	5

The figures are the number of laid open applications and are total of main class and sub-class in Japanese classification.

III. CONSUMER EXPECTATIONS AND CONSUMER PROTECTION

A. Introduction

In the mid-1950s, Japan entered a period of high-level economic growth accompanied by a mass consumption economy. In the industrial world, the technological revolution brought about mass production, and by aggressive marketing, the products were distributed widely throughout the country and on the initiative of the manufacturers without due consideration of consumer needs was produced and pushed their products by aggressive sales and publicity. On the other hand, consumers began to question the fact that daily-use items being supplied to them were almost entirely determined by the manufacturers' one sided initiatives. In other words, products were being forced on them by the manufacturers: they were given no alternative. Better service began to be demanded of manufacturers: this was the first step towards the consumer movement. Ever since, the movement has been escalating in the midst of a system which increasingly emphasizes social demands towards quality, price, service, environmental control, safety etc.

Simultaneously with this growth of consumer consciousness, both manufacturers and the government were turning their attention to consumer protection. Based on the strong conviction that consumer benefit and safety must be assured, the enterprises undertook improvement at all levels from production to sales, while the government pressed ahead with enactment of necessary laws and regulations. Today, with such laws and regulations in force, the enterprises are undertaking further improvement in all areas to assure maximum product safety and consumer benefit.

What, in fact, are consumers expecting of the product? And what are manufacturers providing? How is the government promoting this? This chapter seeks to answer these questions.

B. Consumer Opinion

1. *Expectations Toward Products*

Consumer expectations toward cosmetics cover quality, safety, and taste. Their expectations of each might be summed up by saying that they are searching for "the real thing", that is, a product they find to be safe, useful and of value. This is true not only of cosmetics but of all consumer products, and this trend has come about with mass production, wide distribution, and the profusion of new products coming on the market each year, consumers have begun exercising their rights to choose and to demand as a matter of course.

What exactly, then, are they demanding of cosmetics, and what form does consumer consciousness of cosmetics take? This may be broadly expressed as follows:

Demand for a product of real value.

A tendency to prefer function over frills, especially among the young.

Own initiative in choosing a product from among many that suits their own taste.

Being safety conscious a demand for adequate safety assurance of the product.

A two-fold trend, of preference for high-class products on the one hand and demand for low-priced products on the other. The latter group prefers practical utility, and regards frills as superfluous as long as the basic function fulfilling their purpose is provided.

A trend that appears with longer experience of using cosmetics is away from mere consciousness of how others see them but towards using cosmetics for personal pleasure and satisfaction.

Thus, consumer expectations of the product may ultimately be defined as: product quality enhancing higher value, taste emphasizing individuality, and the demand for product safety.

2. The Consumer Movement

In the 1960s, Japan entered an intensified mass consumption era. At the same time, new consumer problems arose, which are attributed to the following causes:

Consumer's freedom of choice of appropriate commodities and services were being endangered.

Continual price spiraling acted to hold down the consumption level in spite of increased incomes, widening the gap, and causing growing anxiety over future living standards.

Widespread increase in industrial air and water pollution and by harmful waste resulted in pollution. Also the concentration of population in the cities was a contributing factor to these pollutions and lack of public funds to combat these problems were beginning to draw attention.

All of these problems which were non-made disasters directly affected consumers and their immediate environment and it was from the consciousness of the consumers' right to protect their own interests and safety that the consumer movement arose. Cosmetic manufacturers were greatly affected by these social trends. The "anti-resale" movement which raged from the mid 1960s to the early 1970s, and the intensified campaign for product safety have both rocked the cosmetic industry. As a result of the "anti-resale" movement, the list of applicable items was reduced as of 1 September 1974. Until then, the Resale Price Maintenance Contract System had been applicable to 5153 items (by volume and container) of the following five commodities: cosmetics, pharmaceuticals, toothpaste, household bath-soap, household synthetic detergents (as from the end of December 1973). Of these, toothpaste, soap and detergents were entirely removed from the list, and cosmetics retail-priced over ¥1000 and many pharmaceuticals including sleeping pills, tranquillizers, stimulants, insert repellants, insecticides etc. were also removed. This reduced the number of items on the list to almost over half. At the end of December 1974, a total of 2581 items remained, including 1970 cosmetic items priced at under ¥1000 (37 manufacturers), and 611 pharmaceuticals (32 manufacturers). Also from the safety standpoint, the opposition to production and sale of products not deemed to be safe, or which were definitely unsafe, has been gaining momentum, and legal controls are being tightened. At the same time, strict controls are being self-imposed by the manufacturer within the industry, so as to allow only those products whose safety is adequately substantiated on the market.

For reference: Resale Price Maintenance Contract System. This system (abbreviated to "Resale") was instituted in 1953 by amendment of the Antimonopoly Act, as an exemption from the Act. It consists of vertical contracts between the manufacturer wholesaler retailer, whereby the manufacturer fixes the wholesale and retail prices of a product in advance, and has them retailed at the directed price.

3. *Consumer Protection*

Before discussing consumer protection measures in the cosmetic industry, we shall first look at the present state of these measures in industry as a whole. Japan already had laws and legislations relating to consumer protection which were applied to consumer products in general. The main laws and legislations are: Pharmaceutical Affairs Law; Food Sanitation Act; Electrical Appliance and Material Control Act; Measurements Act; Industrial Standards Act; Anti-Monopoly Act; Misrepresentative Premium Offers and Misrepresentative Labelling Prevention Act; etc. Consumer protection is being enforced by these separate laws and legislations which, however, were not necessarily enacted originally for this purpose.

On the principle that all administrative duties should give precedence to public welfare to achieve true prosperity, that is, the people's living standard should no longer be sacrificed for economic gain, but rather that the economic power should serve to raise the living standard of the people, the Basic Consumer Protection Act was promulgated into law on 24 May 1968 and came into force on the 30 May. The basic concept of this law is not limited to strengthening of consumer protection and promotion of consumer education alone, but lies in permeating the whole of the administration with the basic ideology of precedence of public welfare. Figures 10 and 11 show in outline the system of the Basic Consumer Protection Act and its structural organization.

The Basic Consumer Protection Act is fundamental and comprehensive legislation for consumer protection, consisting of 20 articles, divided as follows:

Chapter 1   General Provisions

Chapter 2   Policies etc., Relating to Consumer Protection

Chapter 3   Administrative Agencies etc.

Chapter 4   Consumer Protection Authorities etc.

The matters to which the policies set forth in Chapter 2 apply, are the existing separate acts (Pharmaceutical Affairs Law; Food Sanitation Act; Electrical Appliance and Materials Control Act etc.), which are specific legislation for individual products, to safeguard and promote consumer interest. Consumer protection with regard to cosmetics is also governed basically by the new Act, while detailed provisions are contained in the Acts listed below. The laws applying to cosmetics are broadly divided into those concerning products and those concerning sales. Those concerning products are:

Pharmaceutical Affairs Law

High-pressure Gas Control Act

Fire Services Act

Fair Competition Statutes

Those concerning sales include:

Law against Private Monopoly and for Maintenance of Fair Trade (Antimonopoly Act)

Misrepresentative Premium Offers and Misrepresentative Labelling Act

Unfair Competition Prevention Act

Resale Price Maintenance Contract System

Of these, the Drugs, Cosmetics, and Medical Devices Act is the representative law affecting cosmetics, directly and comprehensively. It sets forth regu-

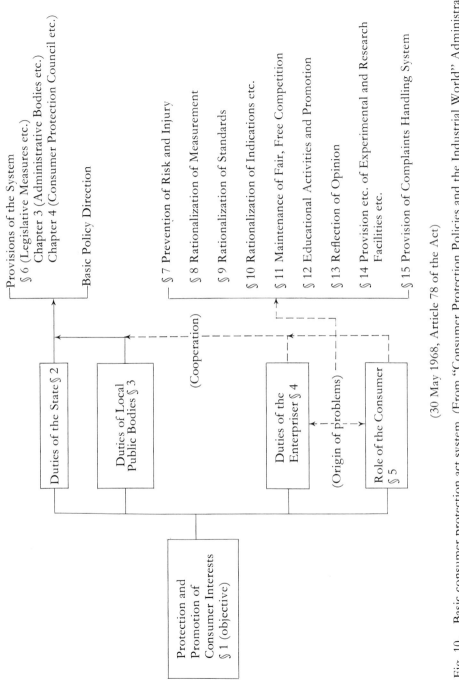

Provisions of the System
§ 6 (Legislative Measures etc.)
Chapter 3 (Administrative Bodies etc.)
Chapter 4 (Consumer Protection Council etc.)

Basic Policy Direction

§ 7 Prevention of Risk and Injury
§ 8 Rationalization of Measurement
§ 9 Rationalization of Standards
§ 10 Rationalization of Indications etc.
§ 11 Maintenance of Fair, Free Competition
§ 12 Educational Activities and Promotion
§ 13 Reflection of Opinion
§ 14 Provision etc. of Experimental and Research Facilities etc.
§ 15 Provision of Complaints Handling System

(30 May 1968, Article 78 of the Act)

Duties of the State § 2

Duties of Local Public Bodies § 3

(Cooperation)

Duties of the Enterpriser § 4

(Origin of problems)

Role of the Consumer § 5

Protection and Promotion of Consumer Interests § 1 (objective)

Fig. 10.   Basic consumer protection act system. (From "Consumer Protection Policies and the Industrial World" Administrative Information Research Sec. 20 Nov. 1975.)

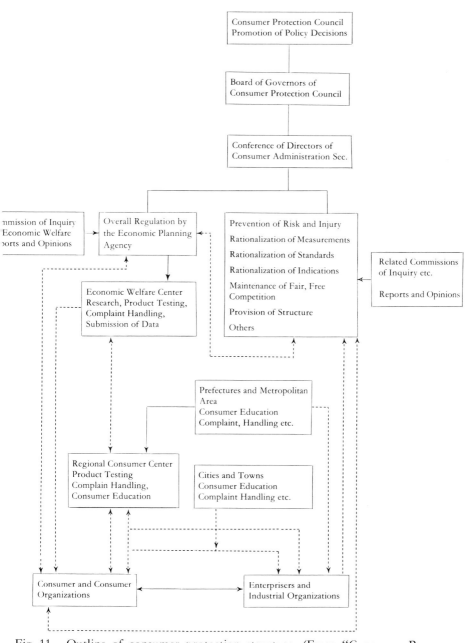

Fig. 11. Outline of consumer protection structure. (From "Consumer Protection Policies and the Industrial World" Administrative Information Research Society.

lations for manufacturers and sale cosmetics, and medical devices, and stipulates that manufacturing import and sale of such products requires authorization by the Ministry of Health and Welfare. Cosmetics are defined in the law as "products for application to the body by applying, spraying, or similar methods, for the purpose of cleansing, beautification, increasing attractiveness, changing the appearance, or maintaining healthy skin or hair, and whose action on the body is mild". The last part of the definition refers particularly to the basic attitude towards efficacy and safety of cosmetics, and sets forth the requirement for safety assurance and prevention of misbranding. The Act also stipulates that manufacture of an individual product shall be commenced only after the approval of the Ministry of Health and Welfare, after prior checking of the formulation manufacturing procedure, efficacy and etc. Furthermore, it contains standards and specifications for labelling, raw materials, e.g. prohibiting products whose contents have changed and does not meet standards, and also products formulated with raw materials which do not meet safety standards. For aerosol products such as hair-sprays, provisions against fire or explosion of the container are stipulated in the High-Pressure Gas Control Act. Products formulated with large quantities of inflammable material, such as alcohol, are regarded as dangerous materials under the Fire Services Act, which prescribes their handling and storage. Thus, from manufacturing to sale, cosmetics are regulated to ensure the safety and protection of the consumer.

C. Quality Assurance

Quality assurance is defined as follows: "a quality product such that the consumer can purchase with confidence and satisfaction, and repeatedly use it over a long period with continued confidence and satisfaction" (Asaka, T. and Ishikawa, H., "Quality Assurance Handbook"). Accordingly, quality assurance is necessary for all stages from product planning to sale including after-service. The same can be said of cosmetics. What does the phrase "good quality" mean for cosmetics? The primary requirement is quality such that anyone can use them with confidence and obtain the desired results. To attain these results, the following are essential:

The product must give the desired effect, that is, it must be a contributing factor in beautifying the user.

Safety of the product

Ease of use

Feeling of satisfaction when applying the product

Satisfaction with the final results

No deterioration of the product, it must have high stability

External appearance of the product must be highly aesthetic

It has always been a trait of the Japanese to seek external beauty, and at the same time a high quality and effective products are in demand. Should the product not have aesthetic appeal, the overall value is lowered. Hence, the manufacturer is concerned with not only the effectiveness of the product, but also with the exterior appearance and the contents, and strives for aesthetic excellence. Recent scientific advances have made prediction of quality possible, so that quality can be sufficiently assured before a product is marketed. In Japan, both manufacturers and consumers have long regarded quality as "life itself", and the search for quality products is a pervading custom. For this reason, manufacturers devote a great deal of effort in producing quality goods. The stages in quality assurance are:

Quality Assurance in Research and Development and in Product Design

1. Raw materials:
   The aim is to develop raw materials of higher safety and performance. Since the raw materials are the most basic and important elements in the composition of a cosmetic, the first step towards creating new properties or increasing safety is upgrading the quality of the raw materials. In Japan, a positive list of 431 cosmetic raw materials are approved for use. On the other hand, use of certain harmful materials is restricted or prohibited. New raw materials, unregistered to the government, must undergo strict safety tests before approval is granted.

2. Human skin physiology:
   As cosmetics are used on the human skin or hair, the structure and physiology of these parts must be thoroughly studied and investigated. Recently manufacturers of cosmetics have been concentrating on the research and development of products compatible with the skin, combined with high safety factors.

3. Formulation techniques:
   Improvement of these techniques is of prime importance. As previously mentioned, both the appearance and safety are of prime importance, with the blending and production techniques. Deterioration, separation, odor change, lowering of satisfaction in use, etc. are very important check-points. Aesthetic appearance also carries great weight. Therefore, products must have resistance to temperature variation over the ranges of $-10°$ to $+50°C$ for certain products, and $-5°$ to $+40°C$ for ordinary

lines without appreciable deterioration in aesthetic appearance. In addition, thermostatically controlled environmental conditions over duplicating climatic conditions are used to carry out tests for stability, preservation, bacterial resistance, etc. Furthermore, the aesthetic values of the product are tested both by sensory tests and instruments.

4. Safety assurance:
   For safety assurance, a variety of tests are conducted on both raw materials and finished products, using animals and humans: patch test, acute toxicity test (oral and percutaneous), subacute toxicity test, maximization test, Draize's test, photopatch test, eye irritation test, and immersion test (in which a guinea pig is actually immersed in the sample solution and the effects on its health are observed), etc. In some cases, teratogenicity, carcinogenicity and metabolism tests are also conducted to maximize the safety level before a product is launched.

5. Performance tests:
   Products are submitted to performance test such as spreading tests, measurements of stickiness, viscoelasticity, hardness (by hardness meter) for creams and related products and breakage tests for lipsticks and related products, and furthermore measurements of particle size, spray pattern, setting strength for hair setting products etc. for aerosols.

6. Field tests:
   At the same time as the scientific tests, field and performance tests are conducted under actual use conditions by a panel of trained specialists. For instance, sunscreens are tested not only in the laboratory but field tested on the beach to confirm the experimental findings. In this way, the expert panel designs tests under conditions of actual use by consumers to predict performance before marketing of the product.

Quality Assurance During the Production Stage
1. Preparation of standard samples and procedures:
   Before the start of production, standard samples of the raw materials and finished product are set up. Furthermore, for efficient production with minimum of rejects, standard operation procedures are set up, thus quality control and production efficiency may be maintained.

2. Acceptance inspection of materials:
   Raw materials are tested by established methods such as properties, purity, presence of harmful substances etc., and only those which comply with the standards are accepted. The same holds true for all other materials.

3. Manufacturing:

The question here is whether the existing plant equipment and operational manual is able to handle the new product line. However for the ordinary products, preplanned operational procedures ensure production of quality product. To this end, countless samplings are taken during production to check that the product meets all quality standards. To meet these ends some of the cosmetic manufacturers have instituted Good Manufacturing Practice. In certain instances, sterilized rooms are provided for the filling and packaging operations. These rooms are manned by operators who have undergone thorough health examination. The Japanese Government is currently studying methods to enact GMP regulations, and as a first step, conducted factory inspections of about twenty companies at the end of 1975. However most manufacturers have already instituted GMP procedures on their own initiative for the sake of higher quality and consumer pretection.

4. Quarantine:

Further quality checks are made while the contents are held in quarantine for quality check before filling into containers. This is one of the aspects of GMP.

5. Filling:

Since it is important at this stage that the net contents per container are accurate, within tolerance and that no contamination by exterior matter, dust, bacteria, etc. should occur, special attention is given to accurate control of the filling machines and hygienic conditions of the surroundings. As mentioned earlier, certain products are filled and packed in sterilized rooms by operators who had undergone thorough cleansing procedures.

6. Inspection:

Hence final tests and inspections are made on the performance, stability, appearance, odor, sterility, usability, etc., of the product actually packed into containers. Since this is the last stage, immediately before dispatch, besides the regular scientific inspection, visual checks are made by trained inspectors who compare each item one by one with standard samples.

Quality Assurance in Marketing

Cosmetics are products which must be readily available to the consumer anywhere at any time. Moreover, the same quality must be supplied throughout the country and for repeat sales, the quality must be within tolerance. There is also a need to furnish consumers with information on correct usage and on the product itself, and to give advice in reply to their inquiries. Provision of a sales network and thorough training of retail staff and beauty consultants answers these needs.

Thus, as previously explained, quality assurance must not be partial, but should be a total function and cover the whole range from research, planning, design, trials, production, purchase, manufacture to sales. Only when full assurance is ensured in each area can overall quality be assured. This is the concept underlying quality assurance as it is practiced in Japan today.

ACKNOWLEDGEMENT

I would like to thank the Japan Cosmetic Industry Association for supplying statistical data regarding sales, advertising etc.

BIBLIOGRAPHY

"Statistics Manual", Research and Statistics Dept., Ministry of International Trade and Industry.
Maruzen, "Rika-nenpyo".
Cosmetic Marketing Strategy, 1976. Nov. 25, 1975.
Advertising in Japan, 1974. *Dentsu News*, Mar. 20, 1975.
Asakura, Kiso Hifukagaku, "Basic Dermatology".
Nanzando. "Cosmetic Science".
Japanese Standards of Cosmetic Ingredients, 1976.
Packaging, Nos. 209 and 215, Packaging Co.
Japanese Official Gazette, Patent Office, Ministry of International Trade and Industry.
Shiseido Report.
Consumer Protection Policies and the Industrial World, Administrative Information Research Soc., 20 Nov. 1975.
Tokyo Cosmetic Industry Association, 1974 Business Report.

PREDICTING SKIN FEEL

E. L. Cussler
Department of Chemical Engineering,
Carnegie-Mellon University,
Pittsburgh, Pennsylvania, USA

I. INTRODUCTION

The acceptance of skin products is strongly influenced by how they feel on the skin. Any creams which make skin feel silky, creamy or soft will certainly be more successful than creams which make skin feel rough, dry or slimy. Likewise, lotions which make skin feel fresh, moist, and natural will be preferred over lotions perceived as harsh, rough, and grainy.

However, in spite of its obvious importance, few scientific studies of skin feel exist. These studies are scattered through fields like psychology, cosmetic chemistry and dermatology. In many ways, this scattering is a symptom of the somewhat silly separation of human effort into physical and social science. Cosmetic scientists, with very real past successes in colloid chemistry and chromatography, often implicitly disparage those in market research and econometrics. The distrust is mutual: men and women planning corporate actions rarely embrace without question the conclusions of "the boys in the lab".

In this paper, we try to connect scientific studies of the physical properties of skin with available subjective measurements of consumer reactions. Because previous work is fragmentary, this paper is more a guide for future progress than a catalog of past success. Recognizing that those who will work in this area have divergent backgrounds, I have kept the mathematical level as simple as possible. I have omitted all mention of formulations and ingredients. I have not discussed changes in skin feel caused by sebum and sweat. I have even restricted the discussion of skin rheology to phenomenological considerations, and have not reviewed the diffusion of water and other materials into skin. With this focus, I can explore in quantitative terms why cosmetics change the feel of skin.

The paper has four key sections. The first briefly reviews physical properties and psychophysical methods important in assessing skin texture. This provides the background for the next two sections, which discuss ways of duplicating skin feel and of improving skin texture. Finally, the vocabulary used to describe cosmetic and skin texture is critically outlined.

II. TOOLS FOR ASSESSING SKIN FEEL

We commonly assess the feel of skin and of cosmetics with our fingers. We rub our hands together, or rub cream into the skin of our arm. Other assessments are more casual: if we rub our knees together and the skin feels funny, we almost always check this feel with our fingers.

This assessment is almost always dynamic. If we move our fingers along the skin, we can tell much more about its texture than if we simply rest our fingers at a single point. As a result, it is important that we have a knowledge of dynamic physical properties if we want to understand the feel of skin. We will need to know the viscosity of cosmetic creams, the elastic modulus measurements of skin, and the coefficient of friction of cosmetic residues on the skin.

The assessment of skin texture is also almost always relative. After a cosmetic is applied, we want our skin to feel better, not just to feel good. As a result, we want to emphasize psychological scaling procedures which emphasize relative assessments. These procedures provide the greatest amount of information, and so will be central to any comparisons between theory and experiment.

Using the physical properties and psychological tools described below, we are already able to predict the size and direction of some subjective changes in skin feel. For example, we can suggest ways of duplicating the consistency of existing products with less expensive, more available ingredients. We can also suggest formulation changes to improve smoothness. However, because our understanding of skin texture is by no means complete, the following paragraphs supply the tools necessary for future research.

A. Important Physical Properties

1. *Viscosity*

Viscosity is a measure of the resistance to flow. High viscosity suggests a large resistance; low viscosity, lesser resistance. Examples are not hard to find: honey has a higher viscosity than water; hand cream has a higher viscosity than milk; motor oil has a higher viscosity than gasoline.

In more exact mathematical terms, the viscosity is the proportionality constant relating the shear stress τ and the velocity gradient

$$\tau = -\eta \frac{dv}{dx} \tag{1}$$

where η is the viscosity, v is the velocity, and x is the direction normal to the flow. Those versed in continuum mechanics will recognize that this equation is a special case of a more general tensorial equation (Bird *et al.*, 1960). Those intimidated by calculus can be reassured by the fact that for a thin film of thickness h

$$\tau = \eta \frac{v}{h} \tag{2}$$

Fluids which obey these simple relations are called Newtonian fluids.

Unfortunately, most cosmetics are not Newtonian fluids, and obey somewhat more complicated relations (Frederickson, 1965). For example, many cosmetics are Bingham fluids, for which

$$\tau = \tau_0 - \eta \frac{dv}{dx} \tag{3}$$

where τ_0 is a yield stress. In physical terms, this means that the fluid must be pushed a bit before it will move. Toothpaste is an excellent example: if you hold the tube upside down, the toothpaste doesn't run out under the force of gravity. On the other hand, once you get toothpaste moving, you can make it move faster without much difficulty. This means that for toothpaste, τ_0 in Eq. (3) is nonzero and η is not especially large.

Another group of cosmetics behave as power-low fluids, for which

$$\tau = -m \left(\frac{dv}{dx} \right)^n \tag{4}$$

where m and n are adjustable parameters. In many cases, n is less than one; for many cosmetics, n varies between 0·3 and 0·6. This means that doubling the velocity of the fingers won't double the shear stress.

The differences between these descriptions of viscosity are summarized in Fig. 1. Newtonian fluids are linear in Cartesian coordinates, and show a slope of one in logarithmic coordinates. Bingham fluids are linear in Cartesian coordinates, but not in logarithmic coordinates. Power law fluids are curved in Cartesian coordinates but linear in logarithmic coordinates. Although there are many more elaborate ways of describing viscosity, these three simple ones are sufficient for this article.

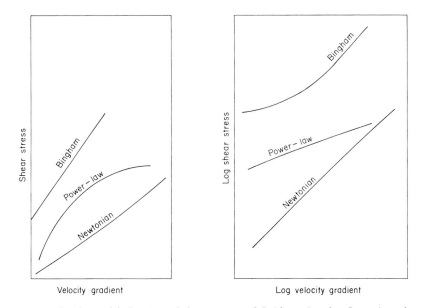

Fig. 1. Rheological behavior of three types of fluids. On the Cartesian plot, the slope is the apparent viscosity, and is independent of velocity gradient only for Newtonian fluids. On the log–log plot, the Newtonian fluid has a slope of one, but the power law fluid has a slope less than one.

2. *Coefficients of Friction*

When the cosmetic layer on the finger is thick, viscosity successfully describes the relation between the force exerted by the fingers and the velocity at which they move. When this layer is very thin, viscosity is no longer applicable, and must be replaced by the concepts of friction described next (Tabor, 1959; Boden and Tabor, 1964).

Like viscous force, shear stress τ caused by friction is described by a simple equation

$$\tau = \mu W \tag{5}$$

where W is the normal force, more commonly called the load; and μ is the coefficient of friction, analogous to the viscosity. Like the viscosity, the coefficient of friction is a linear approximation and is often not constant. In some cases, it can vary with the load, just as the viscosity can vary with the velocity or more exactly, the velocity gradient. However, unlike viscosity, experimental measurements of coefficients of friction are scattered and less well defined.

Three special cases need to be discussed. The first, applicable to rigid solids like metals, begins with the assumption that

$$\tau = sa \tag{6}$$

where s is the shear strength of any contacts between solids, and a is the actual contact area per total projected area. The quantity a is almost always considerably less than one because of surface roughness. However, this area depends linearly on load W:

$$a = \frac{W}{p} \tag{7}$$

where p is the yield pressure of the solid surfaces. As a result,

$$\mu = \frac{s}{p} \tag{8}$$

One implicit implication of this derivation is that the number of contacts can change as the load increases.

The implications of this first case are shown in Fig. 2. The shear force varies linearly with the load, and the coefficient of friction, i.e. the slope, is independent of load. For clean metal surfaces, the shear strength s is about equal to the yield pressure p, so μ equals about one (curve (a)). For lubricated surfaces, where the surface is covered with cosmetic, the shear strength is sharply altered by the lubricant layer but the yield pressure is relatively unchanged. As a result, the coefficient of friction is smaller but still constant, as shown by curve (b).

The second special case for frictional forces is applicable to elastic materials like rubber and skin. For these materials, the shear force is again proportional to contact area a, in Eq. (6). However, this area depends on load in a very different way:

$$a = \left[\frac{Wd}{4E}\right]^{2/3} \tag{9}$$

where d is the effective diameter of a bump on the surface, and E is Young's modulus of the elastic material. As a result,

$$\mu = s\left[\frac{d^2}{16\,E^2\,W}\right]^{1/3} \tag{10}$$

This analysis implicitly assumes that the number of contacts does not change as the area is increased, but that the area of each contact is altered (Archard, 1953).

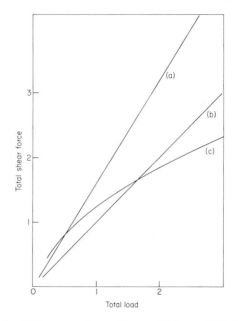

Fig. 2.   Friction for different surfaces. The coefficient of friction is the slope of these plots. Curve (a) is for unlubricated solid surfaces, and has a slope close to one. Curve (b) is for lubricated solid surfaces. Curve (c) is for elastic surfaces like skin.

One characteristic of this case is that shear force is nonlinear in load, as shown by curve (c) in Fig. 2. As a result, the coefficient of friction is not independent of load. Because skin is elastic, this case will be important in the analysis which follows.

The third special case involves the variation of the coefficient of friction with the velocity. This variation, which is responsible for the difference between "standing" and "sliding" friction measured in every introductory physics lab, is qualitatively illustrated in Fig. 3. At vanishingly small velocities, the coefficient of friction reaches the values given in Eqs (8) or (10). At larger velocities, it drops sharply to a minimum and then increases linearly with velocity. While the coefficient is dropping, motion is irregular, characterized by sticking and slipping (Haykin *et al.*, 1940; Fort, 1962). When the coefficient is rising, the force becomes

$$\tau = \eta \left(\frac{v}{b} \right) \tag{11}$$

where h is again the thickness of the fluid layer on the skin. In many cases, this thickness is a function of the specific situation and can only be determined by experiment.

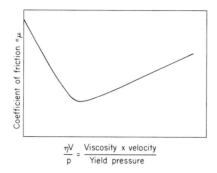

Fig. 3. Variation of the coefficient of friction. The values of velocities below the minimum refers to contact lubrication; the values at velocities above the minimum represent hydrodynamic or boundary lubrication. The drop to the minimum is characterized by unsteady motion, i.e. by sticking and slipping.

3. *Elasticity*

As mentioned above, the feel of skin is most often assessed dynamically, by sliding the fingers over the skin. This sliding is a strong function of viscosity and friction. However, some subjective attributes are assessed by smaller finger motions which deform the skin. Softness, for example, is sometimes assessed by pressing the skin or by gently pulling it back and forth. Thus, the key parameter assessed is elasticity.

Like viscosity and friction, elasticity is described by a simple equation:

$$\tau = E\gamma \tag{12}$$

where E is Young's modulus and γ is the strain. In uncomplicated cases, this strain is the fractional elongation of the sample. For example, if skin is stretched 30%, its strain is 0·30. Like the initial approximations for viscosity and friction, Eq. (12) is a limiting case, defining a "Hookian spring". Such a spring is completely analogous to the Newtonian fluid described by Eq. (1). However, because we will not use more complex concepts of elasticity (Middleman, 1968), we will not discuss them here.

4. *Special Characteristics of Cosmetics and Skin*

The discussion above is basic and is repeated again and again in many textbooks. In fact, the study of the rheology both of cosmetics and of skin is quite extensive.

Whether these more elaborate rheological studies are important to skin texture depends on the research objective. For a complete and exact understanding, we probably need more information than even the extensive measurements made to date. However, in the approximate descriptions of texture developed at the present time, we need no more than the rough outline given above.

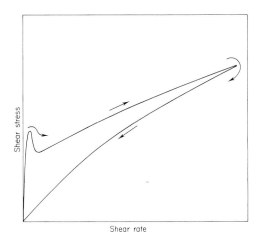

Fig. 4.   Stress and shear rate while assessing cosmetic consistency. The stress and shear change as the cream is removed from its container and rubbed on the skin. The arrows give the variation with increasing time.

Nevertheless, two aspects of these detailed rheological studies are well worth discussing. The first concerns the stresses and velocities actually involved, for example, in taking cold cream out of a jar and spreading it on the skin (Barry and Grace, 1972). Some of these stresses are shown schematically in Fig. 4. Just before the assessment begins, both stress and shear rate are zero. Stress then rises abruptly, especially for a Bingham fluid. Both stress and shear rate (i.e., finger velocity) then increase and decrease in a periodic fashion. However, because the rheological characteristics of the cream can change as water evaporates, the stress-shear rate curve can show hysteresis. Finally, the fingers are again stationary.

The result of this spreading is that a rheological test covers a surprising range of stresses. In other words, the fingers have made a more complete and complex study than we get from measurements with a capillary viscometer and a Brookfield viscometer. The subjective reactions to cosmetic texture must involve unknown averages of the stresses on the fingers.

The second interesting aspect of the detailed rheological studies is the skin itself. Skin is viscoelastic. In other words, it will be elastic when it is quickly stretched a small amount, but it may flow slightly if it is greatly deformed for a long time. These characteristics are commonly summarized by the "springs" and "dashpots" shown in Fig. 5. The springs represent the elastic response of skin; the dashpots, easily imagined as automobile shock absorbers, model the viscous response.

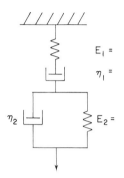

Fig. 5. A viscoelastic model for skin. The values for the springs (E_1 and E_2) and dashpots (η_1 and η_2) are estimated under various conditions by Tregear (1969).

The physical properties of the springs and dashpots have been measured as a function of a wide variety of physical parameters. Probably the most important is humidity (Idson, 1973). Increasing the humidity makes the skin considerably more elastic. This increase can be tempered by using salt or alcohol solutions, which effectively alter the chemical potential of the water and hence its absorption (Park and Baddiel, 1972). These properties and the other aspects of skin rheology provide a fascinating picture of the detailed operation of this largest of body organs.

B. Psychophysical Methods

1. *Panels*

Psychophysical measurements are most commonly made by a panel of perhaps five to twenty subjects. Frequently, these panels are trained by forcing them to define closely the meaning of subjective attributes like smoothness or dryness. They are then asked to evaluate samples for these subjective attributes. Training these panels requires experienced and subtle psychological manipulation (Yoshida, 1968; Marks, 1974a; Marnell,

1974; Stevens, 1975). It also requires that panel members be periodically available for new evaluations. Clearly, trained test panels are expensive.

Such trained panels are essential if the objective is to duplicate skin texture. Panel members can accurately reproduce assessments. They learn to detect minor changes in product formulation, changes which may be difficult to measure with objective instruments. If the research objective is quality control or duplication of an existing product, these expensive panels are an excellent idea.

Trained panels are less necessary if the objective is to predict skin texture. In this case, we want to study textures which vary as widely as possible. For example, for skin dryness, we want to assess skin samples which range from some which are very moist to those which are chapped and blistered. Moreover, we are interested in knowing how consumers evaluate skin dryness without having been carefully forced to define what they mean. Untrained consumers are customers. As a result, I am somewhat sceptical of using trained panels to suggest product improvements.

These two cases are illustrated in more detail by the hypothetical example in Fig. 6. Imagine that we want to determine skin oiliness after application of a cosmetic cream. If our goal is to duplicate the oiliness of an existing preparation, we may want to evaluate many very similar preparations of similar viscosity. Differences between these preparations, which are shown in Fig. 6. by the letter A, will best be evaluated by a trained panel capable of precise distinctions.

On the other hand, if we want to determine how oiliness is affected by cream viscosity, we will want to test widely different preparations. "Vis-

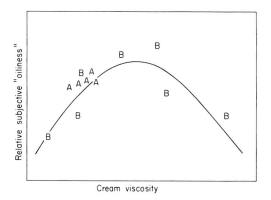

Fig. 6. A hypothetical experiment for evaluating "oiliness". If the samples have the similar physical properties shown by the A's, a trained test panel will give better results. If these samples have the widely varying properties shown by the B's, a trained panel is less important.

cosity" in this case can be measured under arbitrary conditions. Differences between these preparations, shown in Fig. 6 by the letter B, are easily perceived by untrained subjects. Thus, whether a trained test panel is necessary depends on the research objective.

2. Scales

The common method of measuring subjective reactions is to give subjects a selection of samples and ask for their responses. The average responses then become the appropriate psychological measurements. However, the choice of samples and the type of response requested can sharply affect the quality of the information received.

The four types of scales used commonly to assess skin texture are shown in Table I. This classification, roughly based on that suggested by Stevens (1960, 1975) and Marks (1974a), is best illustrated by specific examples. Nominal scales aim at identifying samples of equal texture. Subjects are presented with a small number of similar samples, often six or less. They are then asked which two samples feel most alike. In most cases, the samples are chosen so that at least two feel identical. This method is used to construct the "universal curves" used to duplicate texture, and is more completely discussed in Section III.B.

With nominal scales, we can try to duplicate existing products. Such scales are simple to use because people know what you want. However, these scales do have one major disadvantage, implicit in the use of equality. Imagine that people are given felt, cotton broadcloth, wool suiting, and raw silk, and asked which feel the same. They don't know what to answer. Even samples of some wools and synthetic wool substitutes feel very

Table I
Psychophysical scales for skin feel

Type scale	Basic operation	Average response	Examples
Nominal	Determine equality	Number of cases	Year cars made; "universal curves" of cosmetic consistency
Ordinal	Determine greater or less	Median; percentiles	Cooler cream; smoother skin
Interval	Assign scores from a list	Mean; standard deviation	Student grades; "skin feel index"
Ratio	Determine relative reaction	Geometric mean; percent variation	Relative viscosity; relative smoothness

different. As a result, nominal scaling is restricted to very similar groups of samples.

The common alternative, called ordinal scaling, is to present the samples and ask which have the greatest subjective attribute. Such scaling produces a relative rank for each sample. For example, Prall (1973) presented subjects with five different skin samples and asked which was roughest, whch was next roughest, and so forth. Such straightforward tests can isolate the chief physical factor responsible for subjective attributes like roughness.

The disadvantage of ordinal scales is that they depend on the samples chosen. The roughest sample in one study will not automatically be the roughest sample in a second study using different samples. Thus ordinal scales do not produce information which allows comparison of different sets of samples. This ambiguity can compromise the value of this second method.

The third method, interval scales, involves assigning numbers characteristic of a subjective attribute or quality. Student grades are one example of this method: in a very smart class, all students may earn excellent grades; in an average class, students will earn both excellent grades and poor ones; but in a dumb group, all students may fail.

In spite of its considerable value, this method is not widely used for cosmetics. One intriguing exception is the skin feel index suggested by Goldemberg and de la Rosa (1971). These authors asked subjects to classify skin according to a variety of adjectives. For example, for smoothness, they asked subjects to use the following numbers:

$$1 = \text{poor}; \qquad 4 = \text{smooth};$$
$$2 = \text{fair}; \qquad 5 = \text{velvety rich}.$$
$$3 = \text{good};$$

They used several other attributes and then arbitrarily added scores to try to achieve an overall reaction. While their choice of attributes and descriptive adjectives may not be perfect, their overall idea is impressive. Although interval scales certainly have significant psychological disadvantages, they deserve more frequent consideration in cosmetic science.

The fourth method, ratio scaling, both produces the most information and is the most difficult to use. In this method, subjects are asked to choose one sample as a standard and to grade other samples relative to it. As an example, imagine that we want to study the smoothness of ten skin samples. We choose one sample as a standard, and assign to it the number ten. The second sample feels twice as smooth, so its score is twenty. The third is only one fifth as smooth, so it is assigned the number two. Thus this method combines the inequality of ordinal scales and the spacing of interval scales to produce a very powerful tool (Marks, 1974b).

Ratio scales provide so much more information than the other types that they should be used whenever feasible. Indeed, their power and success has inspired advocates who argue that no other scales should ever be used. Unfortunately, when test panels use ratio scaling on very similar samples, they become confused, and can give erratic results. In spite of this, ratio scaling is invaluable in efforts to predict subjective skin attributes *a priori*.

3. *Psychophysical Laws*

We now want to correlate the psychophysical information obtained using the test panels and scales described in the previous paragraphs. Such correlations can indicate the relationship between two subjective attributes, or between one subjective attribute and the objective stimulus responsible for it. Correlation coefficients are the easiest way to search for such relationships. However, although these are very useful as an initial screening method, they often are of little aid in duplicating or predicting cosmetic and skin texture.

An approach of considerably more potential is to use one of two psychophysical laws (Marks, 1974a; Stevens, 1975). These laws can often quantify consumer reactions. The first, proposed by Fechner, suggests that

$$\left(\begin{array}{c}\text{subjective}\\\text{assessment}\end{array}\right) \propto \log \left(\begin{array}{c}\text{objective}\\\text{stimulus}\end{array}\right) \tag{13}$$

In other words, doubling the stimulus always increases the assessment by about 30%. The second, urged by Stevens, states that

$$\left(\begin{array}{c}\text{subjective}\\\text{assessment}\end{array}\right) \propto \left(\begin{array}{c}\text{objective}\\\text{stimulus}\end{array}\right)^k \tag{14}$$

The effect of doubling the stimulus now depends on the value of the experimentally measured exponent k. For length, the exponent is one; doubling the physical length doubles the assessed length. For electric shock, the exponent is 3·5; doubling the current increases the assessment about ten times.

Stevens' law, often superior to that of Fechner, can describe responses to a surprising variety of physical stimuli. Some of the experimentally determined exponents are shown in Table II. The success of Stevens' law may not have anything to do with fundamental principles; it may work better only because it has two adjustable parameters and Fechner's law has one. Nevertheless, there is no question that it is frequently successful.

In spite of these successes, both Stevens' and Fechner's laws are difficult to apply to cosmetics, because the appropriate objective stimulus is not

Table II
Stevens' Law Exponents*

Subjective assessment	How assessed	Objective variable	Average exponent	Remarks
Warmth	Sun lamp on back or forehead	Watts in sun lamp	1.0	Exponent varies from 1·3 to 0·7 as area exposed varies
Coolness	Metal contact on arm	Temperature of contact	1·0	—
Smoothness	Fingers feel samples of sandpaper	Grit diameter	−1·5	Roughness is inversely proportional to smoothness
Hardness	Squeezing rubber samples	Modulus of elasticity	0·8	Inversely related to softness
Viscosity	Fingers feel Newtonian liquids	Newtonian viscosity	0·4	Stirring gives similar values
Spreadability	Fingers feel Newtonian liquids	Newtonian viscosity	−0·5	Also possible for non-Newtonian liquids
Taste	Sugars in non-Newtonian liquids	Viscosity	−0·5	Viscosity was arbitrary measurement with Brookfield viscometer
	Sucrose in mouth	Concentration	1·3	Data scattered
	Salt in mouth	Concentration	1·4	Significant temporal effects
	Acids in mouth	Concentration	0·8	Different substances give slightly different exponents
Odor	Heptane vapor	Concentration	0·6	Again, different substances can give different exponents
Electric shock	Current through fingers	Current	3·5	Voltage dependence unknown

*Values from Stevens (1975); Marks (1974); Arcelus and Cussler (1975); Moskovitz (1971).

known. This is most easily illustrated by the subjective assessment of viscosity. Newtonian fluids are easily and successfully analyzed by Stevens' law: subjectively assessed viscosity is plotted vs. Newtonian viscosity. Non-Newtonian cosmetics cannot be analyzed in a similar way because we don't know which combination of non-Newtonian properties correspond to the objective stimulus. To discover this combination, we must develop a physical model like those in Section IV. Without such models, we cannot achieve the real understanding of skin texture which psychophysical laws promise.

III. DUPLICATING SKIN FEEL

The physical and psychophysical tools described above allow some aspects of skin feel to be predicted and duplicated. How duplication is achieved is the subject of this section.

The obvious way to duplicate the consumer's reactions to a given cosmetic is to duplicate all the physical properties of that product. The substitute product would be made of identical or very similar materials, combined in a similar way; it would have the same viscosity, the same thermal conductivity, the same surface wetting. It would have an identical color and perfume.

This attempted duplication is often impractical or expensive. Raw materials may be difficult to obtain. Cheaper substitutes for some ingredients may be readily available but produce products having altered rheology. Increased product demand may require making more in larger mixers; these larger mixers rarely produce an identical product, especially an identical emulsion.

Duplicating consumer reactions can now be greatly facilitated by using the so-called "universal curves". These curves, which essentially are generalizations of empirical experience, allow ingredient substitution on a large scale. They show that the physical properties of the product being duplicated do not have to be exactly duplicated under all conditions, but only under extremely specialized ones. As such, they provide an important route for producing different products which "feel" the same.

While the ideas presented below are relatively recent, they seem surprisingly complete. This does not mean that a universal curve is available for every situation that is encountered; indeed, the curves available refer only to a specific part of subjective assessment. However, the curves already published clearly show how others can be developed.

A. How to Use a Universal Curve

Three universal curves reported for the subjective spreadability of different types of cosmetic materials are shown in Figs 7–9 (Barry and Grace, 1972; Barry and Meyer, 1973). These curves include, as a shaded region, estimates of the experimental error involved in their use. Each is shown as a function of shear stress and shear rate over the ranges studied experimentally. These curves do *not* contain rheological information, but rather summarize psychological determinations of identical feel.

The significance of these curves is easy to state, but was for me initially hard to understand: "A universal curve for a specific subjective attribute represents the locus of the intersections of the stress–strain curves for cosmetic materials which feel identical." This significance is best illustrated by a hypothetical example.

Imagine that we want to duplicate the consistency of the cosmetic cream whose rheological properties are shown by curve A in Fig. 7. Since curve A is a straight line with a slope of one, this cream is a Newtonian

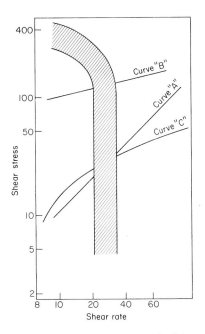

Fig. 7.   A universal curve for the consistency of oil-in-water emulsions. The shaded area gives the experimental error. The fluids represented by curves "A" and "C" feel the same, different than that represented by curve "B".

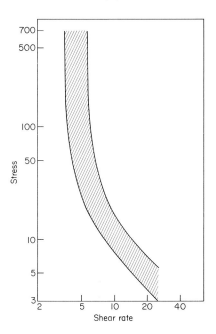

Fig. 8. A universal curve for the consistency of lipophillic creams. The shaded area represents the experimental variation.

fluid of fixed viscosity (cf. Fig. 1). We have made two non-Newtonian creams as possible substitutes for this original product; these are shown by curves B and C in Fig. 7. Both these creams are made with cheaper ingredients, but neither is a Newtonian fluid. Since curve B is a straight line with a slope less than one, it can be described as a power law fluid (cf. Fig. 1). Since curve C is not a straight line, its rheological behavior is more complex than the models described previously.

Because curves A and C intersect at the universal curve, they will feel identical. As a result, the inexpensive cream represented by curve C can be substituted for that described by curve A. Because curves A and B do not intersect, they do not feel identical. The material illustrated by curve B will not have the same consistency as that shown by curve A.

One important corollary of these curves is that no two Newtonian fluids of differing viscosity can feel the same. Such fluids would all be parallel to curve A in Fig. 7 and hence intersect the universal curve in different regions. As a result, they will have a different subjective "consistency". On the other hand, a particular Newtonian fluid can feel the same as a large collection of non-Newtonian fluids if all intersect the universal curve at the same point.

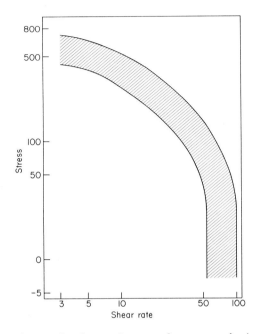

Fig. 9.   A universal curve for the consistency of aqueous gels. Again, the shaded area represents the experimental error.

B. How to Construct a Universal Curve

Clearly, each universal curve must be based on experimental evidence garnered for a particular class of materials and for a specific type of assessment. For example, the curve in Fig. 8 is based on the subjective consistency of lipophillic creams. For other situations than those already studied, experiments are necessary to develop a new curve.

These experiments, which are based on ideas of Wood (1968), involve presenting members of a test panel with samples of varying physical properties and simply asking which samples have the same subjective attribute. This subjective attribute should be as specifically defined as possible, either in writing or by discussion with the test panel.

The physical properties of the samples presented should commonly go well beyond the range expected in the product. This wide range will accurately define any trend in the curve. If a smaller range is used, the inevitable experimental errors will obscure any trend, and make the curve less reliable. If all samples already seem subjectively as close as possible to the product to be duplicated, there is no reason to construct the curve.

Once samples of very similar feel have been identified, their rheology should be measured as a function of stress and strain rate. A single measurement with a capillary or Brookfield viscometer is *not* sufficient; more complete measurements are essential. However, because the largest errors in constructing these curves are subjective, the rheological properties need not be determined to a high degree of accuracy.

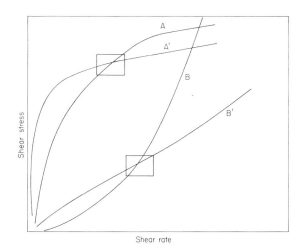

Fig. 10. The construction of a universal curve. The fluids represented by curves A and A′ feel alike so their intersection becomes part of the universal curve. The fluids represented by curves B and B′ feel alike, so their intersection is another part. However, the fluids represented by curves A and B feel different, so that their intersection is not used here.

The next step is to plot the rheological information, and determine the intersection of the stress–strain rate curves of identical fluids. The intersections of the various groups of fluids form the locus of the universal curve. This is qualitatively shown in Fig. 10. The two curves labeled A and A′ represent materials which feel the same; thus their intersection becomes one point on the universal curve. The curves B and B′ are a second, similar example. The resulting universal curve can then be used as a guide for modifying existing products.

C. Other Characteristics of the Universal Curves

Curves like those described above should facilitate quality control and shelf-like studies. They identify the stress and shear rate important in duplicating skin texture. As a result, the stress and shear rate chosen for experiments should be those on the universal curves, and not values picked for convenience.

All three universal curves shown above suggest that the choice of stress is much more important than the choice of shear rate. For example, the stress in Fig. 7 varies one hundred times, while the shear rate varies about two times. However, this may not always be the case: the universal curve for liquid and semi-solid foods, shown in Fig. 11 (Sherman, 1975), shows that whether stress or shear rate is more important depends on the region studied.

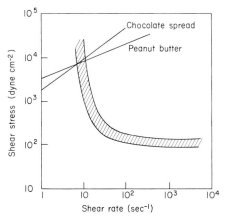

Fig. 11.   A universal curve for liquid and semi-solid foods. Since peanut butter and chocolate spread have stress-shear rate curves which intersect at the universal curve, they have the same consistency.

In spite of these known exceptions, it is still tempting to conclude that the shear rate in Figs 7–9 is that used by the fingers. In other words, the universal curves are saying that the fingers use approximately constant shear rate to assess a wide range of stress. The extent to which this is true is discussed in the next section.

IV. IMPROVING SKIN FEEL

The universal curves in the previous section allow duplication of skin feel under a variety of circumstances. They will become an invaluable aid in cosmetic formulation, especially as a guide for ingredient substitution. They seem a major, secure accomplishment. However, the universal curves give no guide for product improvement. They give no indication of how cosmetic rheology should be changed to make skin feel smoother, or softer, or creamier.

To predict product improvements, we must understand more completely the nature of perception. We need to understand which physical effects on the fingers correspond to specific subjective attributes. For example, in the cases discussed below, we will find that spreadability closely corresponds to the shear force on the fingers, that warmth is perceived as skin temperature, and that skin smoothness is proportional to the coefficient of friction. Once we have this understanding, we can predict the exact changes in rheology which will double the spreadability or triple the smoothness.

At the same time, we must emphasize that the ideas below are fragmentary and incomplete. They should not be used without careful checks. Nevertheless, their major promise for predicting product improvements justifies their careful consideration.

A. Predicting Subjective Viscosity (de Martine and Cussler, 1975)

The way in which subjective improvements can be effected is illustrated by three special cases. The first case is the assessment of subjective viscosity. When water is rubbed between the fingers of one hand and honey is rubbed between the fingers of the other, the fingers of both hands move at the same speed; but the water and the honey feel very different. Clearly, this feeling is not based on velocity differences. What is it based on?

One possibility is that this difference in feeling depends on the force used to push the finger. By experiment, we found that honey and water were both assessed with a constant normal force, so that the difference in feeling must come from differences in the shear force. Thus, when we say that "honey is more viscous than water", we may mean that the shear force of honey on the fingers is greater than that of water.

To test this possibility, both psychophysics and rheology are used. We first recognize that the thickness of the fluid on the fingers is much less than the thickness of the fingers themselves. As a result, we approximate the fingers as the parallel plates. From Eq. (2), we see

$$\begin{matrix} \text{subjective} \\ \text{viscosity} \end{matrix} \propto \begin{matrix} \text{shear} \\ \text{stress} \end{matrix} = \text{viscosity} \left(\frac{\text{velocity}}{\text{thickness}} \right) \qquad (15)$$

Although the velocity is constant, the thickness is not. For Newtonian fluids (Stefan, 1874),

$$\text{thickness} \propto \sqrt{(\text{viscosity})} \qquad (16)$$

When we combine these equations, we find

$$\frac{\text{subjective}}{\text{viscosity}} \propto \text{viscosity} \cdot \frac{\text{velocity}}{\sqrt{\text{viscosity}}}$$

$$\propto \sqrt{\text{viscosity}} \tag{17}$$

In other words, to double the subjective viscosity, we must increase the actual Newtonian viscosity four times.

The variation suggested by Eq. (17) is consistent both with earlier experimental work (Stevens and Guirao, 1964) and with our own experiments, shown as circles in Fig. 12. The liquids used were silicone oils whose Newtonian viscosities covered a 100 000 fold range. The exponents in both the literature and our work are 0·44 and 0·40, in good agreement with the value of 0·50 predicted by Eq. (17). Such underestimation is a common psychophysical phenomenon, and is discussed in considerable detail elsewhere (Marks, 1974a).

A second related experiment, shown as triangles in Fig. 12, also supported the guess that subjective "viscosity" is, in fact, a measure of shear force. In this experiment, we attached small sleds to the fingers which prevented the fluid film from thinning. From Eq. (15), we would expect subjective "viscosity" to vary with the 1·00 power of the physical viscosity; in fact, it varies with the 0·89 power, again in reasonable agreement with the prediction.

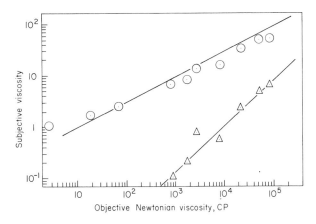

Fig. 12. Predictions of subjective viscosity. The circles correspond to measurements between the fingers, where the liquid film on the fingers was thinned by rubbing. The squares are results where the liquid film was kept constant. The solid lines are not best fits of the data, but predictions of Eqs (17) and (15).

Even for non-Newtonian fluids, the subjective attributes of "viscosity" and "spreadability" are perceived as shear force on the fingers, as shown in Figs 13–14. The non-Newtonian liquids, shown as squares, were all shear thinning, including aqueous solutions of hydroxypropylmethylcellulose

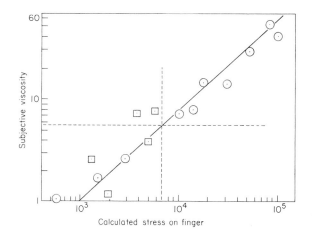

Fig. 13. Predictions of subjective viscosity including non-Newtonian fluids. The circles are Newtonian fluids and the squares are non-Newtonian. The correlation coefficient between the subjective and predicted values is 0·95.

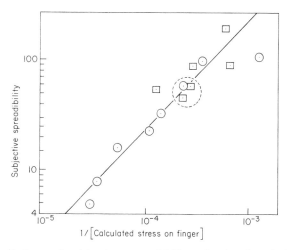

Fig. 14. Predictions of subjective spreadability. Again, the circles represent Newtonian fluids; the squares are non-Newtonian ones, and the solid line is a theoretical prediction. The three fluids within the dashed circle feel the same but have radically different rheological properties.

and of polyacrylamide. In predicting the stress on the fingers, we have assumed that subjective viscosity is assessed by rubbing the fingers back and forth, and that spreadability is assessed by a smooth spreading motion.

These results explain the important corollary of the universal curves which states thàt no two Newtonian liquids of different viscosity can feel alike, but that a large number of non-Newtonian fluids can have the same feel as one Newtonian fluid. Any fluids which produce the same force on the fingers will feel the same. For example, the three fluids within the dotted circle in Fig. 14 have very similar spreadabilities, but very different rheological properties. They are a silicone oil of viscosity 70 cp, a 2% solution of hydroxypropylmethylcellulose ($m = 630$; $n = 0.32$); and an 8% solution of polyacrylamide ($m = 390$; $n = 0.47$). All these fluids produce a similar force on the fingers; therefore, all have a similar spreadability.

B. Predicting Subjective Smoothness (Cussler, Zlotnick and Shaw, 1977)

As in viscosity and spreadability, subjective smoothness can be predicted *a priori* from physical theory. For subjective viscosity and spreadability, the physical theory used fluid mechanics, and the key physical variable was the scientifically defined viscosity. For smoothness, the physical theory involves friction, and the key physical properties will include the coefficient of friction on the skin.

To assess skin smoothness, most people move their fingers lightly across a characteristic skin area. Pressing the skin hard seems to reduce sensitivity. This light motion is not completely steady, but involves some sticking and slipping across the skin.

One possibility is that smoothness is perceived as inversely proportional to the force required to have the finger slip across the skin. To test this hypothesis, we assume that each slip results from a bump on the surface. These bumps have an effective diameter d, and are evenly separated by some distance l. By combining Eqs (6) and (9) we obtain

$$\text{smoothness} \propto \left[\frac{\text{force}}{\text{bump}} \right]^{-1}$$

$$\propto \frac{1}{s} \frac{4E}{wd}^{2/3} \tag{18}$$

where the load per site w is

$$w = \frac{W}{A/l^2} \tag{19}$$

The prediction of relative smoothness now requires knowledge of the shear strength s, the Young's modulus of the skin E, and the size d and spacing l of the stimulus-inducing spheres.

Unfortunately, few studies of skin texture contain enough detail to allow a definitive test of the prediction in Eq. (18). Some useful results have been obtained by Stevens and Harris (1962) for the subjective texture of sandpaper. To test our prediction, we assume that the spacing l is proportional to the size d. This assumption will be exact if the grains of sand are packed closely together on the sandpaper surface. By experimental measurement, we found that the load is proportional $d^{-0.3}$. As a result

$$\text{smoothness} \propto d^{-1.8} \qquad (20)$$

This prediction is in good agreement with the data in Fig. 15.

However, skin is very different from sandpaper. To test the predictions of Eqs (18–20) for skin itself, we next turn to the results of Prall (1973), who measured subjective skin smoothness as a function of scratch resistance, friction on the skin, and surface topography. It is unclear how Prall's measurements of friction are related to more fundamental properties, but they are clearly a function of both the size and spacing of bumps on the skin. Any use of these measurements will be approximate.

To test the predictions of Eq. (4), we assume that Young's modulus E is proportional to scratch resistance; that the spacing of bumps is proportional to their size; and that the bump size d is inversely proportional

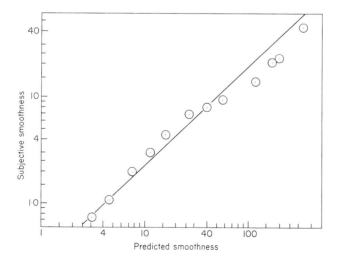

Fig. 15.   Predictions of sandpaper smoothness. The data, taken from Stevens and Harris (1962), agree closely with the solid line predicted with Eqs (18–20).

to the topography. The first assumption is a common approximation in mechanical engineering, and the second was successfully used in the prediction of sandpaper smoothness. The third assumption, that unevenness is inversely proportional to topography, is partially justified in Fig. 16.

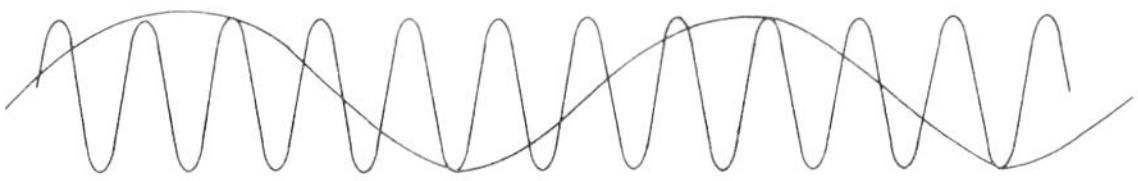

Fig. 16.   Schematic surface profiles for skin. The curve with the large period represents a skin surface of low topography, i.e. low surface length per linear length. The curve with the short period represents a smoother skin surface of high topography.

Without detailing the line integrals involved, the surface with the smaller bumps will involve a longer surface profile, and hence a larger topography.
    Using these approximations, we find from Eqns (18–19) that

$$\text{smoothness} \propto [\text{scratch resistance}]^{2/3} [\text{topography}]^2 \qquad (21)$$

This equation is tested in Fig. 17. The upper part of this figure gives the results for actual samples of skin, while the lower part represents data for skin models. Prall did not report the relative smoothness, but rather the rank of smoothness: for five samples, the smoothest is assigned the number five; the second smoothest is called number four etc. The predicted rank of skin smoothness in Fig. 17 does agree reasonably well with the rank observed experimentally. These predictions contain no adjustable experimental parameters, and are based on measurements of scratch resistance and surface topography.
    These results form an interesting contrast with the analysis of Prall, who used the data at the bottom of Fig. 17 to derive a five-parameter empirical equation:

$$\text{smoothness} = 9 \cdot 4 - 0 \cdot 0014 \text{ (scratch resistance)} - 0 \cdot 0786 \text{ (topography)}$$
$$- 0 \cdot 0029 \text{ (friction)} + 0 \cdot 00002 \text{ (scratch resistance)} \times \text{ (friction)} \qquad (22)$$

The units of scratch resistance, friction, and topography must be those specified. Prall then used this empirical equation to predict the ranks shown as squares at the top of Fig. 17.
    The two approaches symbolized by Eq. (21) and Eq. (22) are complimentary. The empirical approach of Eq. (22) is possibly more accurate over the range studied, since it involves five adjustable parameters compared with none in Eq. (21). However, Eq. (22) cannot be confidently extrapolated or applied to different types of skin surfaces. It would not predict

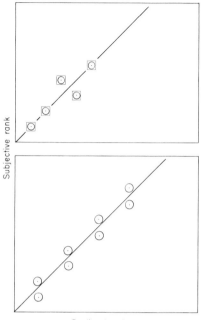

Fig. 17. Predictions of skin smoothness. The data, from Prall (1973), consist of the relative rank of skin smoothness. The predictions shown by circles result from Eq. (21). The predictions shown as squares in the upper graph are those calculated from Prall's empirical result, Eq. (22). This result was obtained from the data in the lower graph.

the relative smoothness of surfaces of equal topography but different sizes and spacings of surface roughness. Because Eq. (21) depends on a definite physical model, it includes a more exact characterization of the surface. It can be extrapolated and applied to new situations with greater confidence.

C. Predicting Warmth and Coolness

This final discussion illustrates how theories of heat transfer can produce results like those found from fluid mechanics used in the first two topics. Parallel derivations can use theories of mass transfer to explain some aspects of odor and flavor.

When one bare foot rests on the bathroom floor and one rests on the bathmat, the foot on the floor feels colder, in spite of the fact that both floor and mat are at the same initial temperature. The obvious hypothesis is that more heat is conducted away from the floor than from the mat, reducing the skin temperature. To test this hypothesis, we measured the skin temperature during subjective assessment of the warmth of heated slabs of metal, wood, and glass. The skin temperature was measured using a small thermocouple pressed into the skin. As shown in Fig. 18, these skin temperatures do correlate well with the relative warmth of the slabs. Other research is consistent with these conclusions (Stevens and Marks, 1971).

Skin temperature can often be calculated from the physical properties of the materials in contact with the skin. Two special cases illustrate these calculations. The first is the "windchill factor" commonly given on winter weather reports. For example, the report will say, "The temperature outside is 24°F. However, because of a 15 mph wind, it feels like 0°F." These statements, based on Antarctic experiments which do not include a psychological component (Siple and Passel, 1945; Court, 1948; Arkin, 1974), essentially calculate the bare skin temperature in the wind relative to the values in a 4 mph wind, which is assumed to be characteristic of a brisk walk.

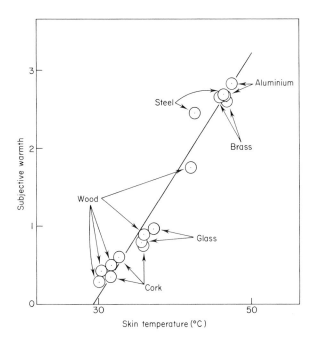

Fig. 18.   Warmth vs. skin temperature. Again, the solid line is that expected theoretically.

The second example recognizes that for thin layers of cosmetic, the skin temperature is proportional to the thermal conductivity of the cosmetic divided by the thickness of the cosmetic layer (Bird *et al.*, 1960). Most common cosmetic materials, except water, have similar thermal conductivities. For an emulsion, the thermal conductivity is dominated by the continuous phase, i.e. for an o/w emulsion, by water; and for a w/o emulsion, by oil. This suggests that the abrupt consumer reactions near a colloid inversion may be associated with an abrupt change in thermal conductivity and hence of subjective warmth.

These ideas suggest how subjective warmth can depend on the physical properties of cosmetics. They are clearly a limited attempt; for example, they do not include any effects of evaporative cooling or astringency. Nevertheless, when they are combined with ideas describing viscosity, spreadability, and smoothness, they provide a strategy for predicting subjective reactions and improving cosmetic products.

V. DEFINING A BETTER VOCABULARY

The above sections show how universal curves can be used to duplicate skin feel, and how physical models can predict skin feel. However, both methods assume a cosmetic vocabulary which has not been carefully defined.

Specific cases vividly illustrate this shortcoming. For example, the universal curves are for equal "consistency." The concept of "consistency" makes good sense when one scoops cream out of a jar and starts spreading it on the skin. The same idea does not apply at all after the cream is rubbed in. As a second example, a predictive theory for "thinness" does not differ significantly from that for "spreadability." To avoid these limitations, we must define more carefully the words used to describe skin feel.

A. Texture Profiles

The most direct way to sharpen the description of skin is to use a "texture profile," a classification of the words used to describe skin. Such classifications are often used in the food industry to improve the effectiveness of test panels (Szczesniak, 1963; Sherman, 1969). Their chief function may well be to force these panels to use common definitions of subjective words.

A possible texture profile for cosmetics is shown in Table III. This profile is a composite of the fragmentary studies reported in the literature

(Prall, 1973; Goldemberg and de la Rosa, 1971). I am not confident of the accuracy of this profile; it is an initial try, subject to revision.

The profile in Table III does have important features which should be retained after revision. One of these is the particular choice of key words. Wherever possible, these words have been chosen as independent and closely related to a known physical property. They are not chosen as the most important cosmetic attributes which are both interdependent and functions of several physical properties.

Table III
A tentative texture profile for skin

Probable physical property	Key word	Secondary words
Vision	Evenness of color	Blemished, hairy, flaky, dry, chapped, raw, cracked, flushed, rough
Viscosity	Thin	Viscous, spreadable, wet, equal consistency, creamy, thick, oily, rich, slippery
Coefficient of friction	Smooth	Rough, tacky, velvety rich, dry, waxy, tense, soft, draggy
Skin temperature	Warm	Cool, hot, cold, dry, sweaty

Several examples illustrate this choice. Smoothness is not a function of thinness or of warmth. It is a strong function of the coefficient of friction, but varies significantly with viscosity only at high viscosity. It is not a strong function of temperature, and varies only slightly with color. As a result, it is a good key word.

The softness of cosmetic creams varies closely with smoothness. Softness is also largely independent of color, thinness, and warmth. Within our present knowledge, we could use softness as a substitute for smoothness. However, as our experiments continue, we may find softness is more commonly assessed by pressing the skin and not by rubbing it. If so, it may be more closely connected with the elastic modulus than the coefficient of friction.

In contrast, creaminess, a very important subjective attribute, depends on both thinness and smoothness. Correspondingly, it varies strongly with the viscosity and with the coefficient of friction. Indeed, in some cases, it seems possible to change both of these physical properties and still retain the same creaminess. As a result, creaminess seems a bad choice for a key word in the texture profile, although its importance makes it an excellent choice for panel tests.

A second important feature of the proposed texture profile is its obvious redundancy. This takes two forms. First, some words like "dry" and "rough" appear at several points because they can apparently be assessed in several different ways. It may be reasonable to avoid these attributes in panel tests.

The second type of redundancy is the use of synonyms and antonyms. Table III contains many examples of this: smooth skin is not rough; warm skin is not cool; spreadable cream is not highly viscous. The results in the next section illustrate how this type of interrelation is removed.

B. A Minimum Vocabulary

To reduce the vocabulary in Table III to the minimum number of words required, we gave a test panel of 24 untrained adults a selection of 14 cosmetics, oils, and foods. We asked them to evaluate by ratio scaling a set of 10 subjective attributes, including spreadability, softness, smoothness, and coolness. We then ran a simple log-linear regression to determine the relations between the various words. Such a regression is consistent with Stevens' law, discussed in Section II.B.

Three of the words can successfully predict the seven other words which we studied. Since several trios give roughly equivalent results, we chose thinness, smoothness, and warmth for further study. Our predictions use the equation

$$\log \left(\begin{matrix} \text{relative assessment} \\ \text{for a specific word} \end{matrix} \right) = a \log (\text{smoothness}) + b \log (\text{smoothness})$$

$$+ c \log (\text{warmth}) \qquad (23)$$

where a, b, and c are the experimentally measured parameters shown in Table IV. At first glance, this analysis seems to use an inordinate number of parameters; however, on closer inspection, one realizes that many of the parameters are probably one, zero, or minus one within experimental error. For example, Fig. 19 shows that softness correlates with smoothness without any reference to thinness or warmth.

Another way of illustrating the interdependence of the cosmetic attributes studied is given in Fig. 20. In this figure, the Cartesian axes correspond to the three key words of thinness, smoothness, and warmth. The fact that these attributes become the principal axes suggest that they are a type of verbal eigenvectors for the cosmetic vocabulary. The other attributes are

Table IV
Relations between words
The coefficients below should be used in the equation:
log (attribute) = a log (smoothness) + b log (thinness) + c log (warmth)

Attribute	a	b	c
Softness	0·8	0·2	0·0
Creaminess	2·2	−0·9	−0·1
Thickness	1·1	−1·6	−0·0
Spreadability	0·1	1·2	0·0
Hardness	0·4	−1·2	−0·2
Dryness	0·5	−0·8	0·2
Coolness	0·2	−0·0	−0·8

shown as vectors. The angle of each vector indicates its relation to the three key attributes, while its length gives the sensitivity of the panel to this particular attribute.

Several examples illustrate this. Softness and smoothness are almost parallel, indicating that they are often used interchangeably. Thinness and spreadability show similar behavior. Coolness is in almost the opposite direction to warmth, showing that these words are antonyms. Dryness is a very short vector, indicating that it did not vary significantly for the cosmetics used.

One large and interesting vector is creaminess. This attribute varies strongly with both thinness and smoothness, or in terms of the physical attributes in Table III, with viscosity and with coefficient of friction. It is the only attribute studied to do so. This characteristic behavior may be the reason why creaminess is often chosen as the single attribute for careful study. This behavior, and indeed all the information in Table IV, exemplifies the major returns possible from straightforward investigations of the cosmetic vocabulary.

VI. CONCLUSIONS

At the beginning of this paper I pointed out that it would not be a conventional review, but rather a primer for future development. As I reread the above, I realize that this is more true than I had hoped. As a result, any conclusions must be tentative.

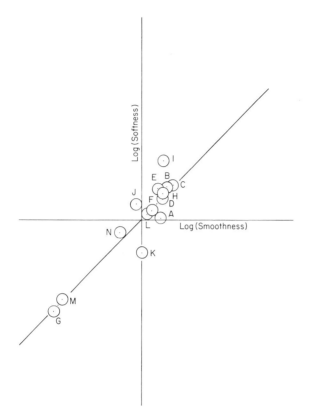

Fig. 19. Softness vs. smoothness. These data were obtained by ratio scaling. The correlation between softness and smoothness is 0·9.

Five prospectives do seem clear:

(1) *Rheology*. We currently have more complete rheological methods than we can effectively use. No elaborate rheological study should be started without carefully identifying the connection with the feel of skin and cosmetics.

(2) *Psychophysics*. Psychological testing is of sufficient sophistication not to limit our progress. Whenever feasible, we should use interval and ratio scales, rather than paired comparison tests.

(3) *Universal Curves*. These curves are a solid, effective technique for duplicating cosmetic consistency. Although each curve may have a narrow range of applicability, they should prove useful for duplicating existing products.

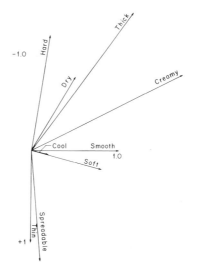

Fig. 20.   The interdependence of the various attributes. Each attribute can be represented as a vector in a three-dimensional orthogonal space where smooth, thin, and warm represent principal axes. The projection of this space on the smooth-thin plane is shown.

(4) *Subjective Predictions*. These predictions do offer the real prospect of providing the intellectual framework for understanding perception. This can help initial product development, but may be too crude for changes in detailed formulations.

(5) *Vocabulary*. Additional studies which narrow the vocabulary used in cosmetics are urgently needed. These should reduce the vague descriptions of cosmetics and skin to a much more exact picture, and thus facilitate better predictions.

With these prospectives, we can work to put the feel of skin on a more scientific basis.

ACKNOWLEDGEMENTS

Susan J. Zlotnick helped to prepare this paper. The work was partly supported by the National Science Foundation Grant GK-32313, and the National Institute of Arthritis, Metabolic, and Digestive Diseases Grant 1-RO1-AM-16143. The author is supported by the National Institutes of Health Research Career Development Award 1K04-AM-70461.

REFERENCES

Archard, J. F. (1953). *Nature* **172**, 918.

Arkin, M. A. (1974). Wind Chill, Environmental Information Summaries C-3, National Oceanic and Atmospheric Administration.

Barry, B. W. and Grace, A. J. (1972). Sensory testing of spreadability: investigations of rheological conditions operative during application of topical preparations, *J. Pharm. Sci.* **61**, 335.

Barry, B. W. and Meyer, M. C. (1973). Sensory assessment of spreadability of hydrophilic topical preparations. *J. Pharm. Sci.* **62**, 1349.

Bird, R. B., Stewart, W. E. and Lightfoot, E. N. (1960). "Transport Phenomena". Wiley-Interscience, New York.

Bowden, F. B. and Tabor, D. (1964). "The Friction and Lubrication of Solids, Clarendon, Oxford.

Court, A. (1948). *Bull. Amer. Meteor. Soc.* 487.

Cussler, E. L., Zlotnick, S. J. and Shaw, M. C. (1977). Texture perceived with the fingers. *Perception and Psychophysics* **21**, 504. *J. Soc. Cosmet. Chem.*

de Martine, M. L. and Cussler, E. L. (1971). Predicting subjective spreadability, viscosity and stickiness. *J. Soc. Cosmet. Chem.* **22**, 635.

Fort, T. (1962). *J. Phys. Chem.* **66**, 1136.

Fredrickson, A. G. (1965). "Principles and Applications of Rheology", Prentice-Hall, Englewood Cliffs.

Goldemberg, R. L. and de la Rosa, C. P. (1975). Correlation of skin feel of emollients to their chemical structure. *J. Pharm. Sci.* **64**, 976.

Haykin, S., Lissovsky, L. and Solomonovich, A. (1940). *J. Phys.* **2** (3), 253.

Idson, B. (1973). Water and the skin. *J. Soc. Cosmet. Chem.* **24**, 197.

Marks, L. E. (1974a). "Sensory Processes", Academic Press, New York.

Marks, L. E. (1974b). On scales of sensation. *Perception and Psychophysics* **16**, 358.

Marnell, G. M. (1974). "Scaling, A Sourcebook for Behavioral Scientists", Aldine Pub. Co., Chicago.

Maskovitz, H. R. (1971). *Perception and Psychophysics* **9**, 371.

Midelleman, S. (1968). "The Flow of High Polymers", Wiley-Interscience, New York.

Park, A. C. and Baddiel, C. B. (1972). Rheology of the stratum corneum II. A physico-chemical investigation of factors influencing water content in the corneum. *J. Soc. Cosmet. Chem.* **23**, 13.

Prall, J. K. (1973). Instrumental evaluation of the effects of cosmetic products on skin surfaces with particular reference to smoothness. *J. Soc. Cosmet. Chem.* **24**, 693.

Rabinowicz, E. (1965). "Friction and Wear of Materials", Wiley-Interscience, New York.

Sherman, P. (1969). *J. Food Science* **34**, 458.

Sherman, P. (1975). "Factors influencing the instrumental and sensory evaluation of food emulsions." *In* "Theory, Determination and Control of Physical Properties of Food Materials", (Ed. C. K. Rha), Reidel, Boston, 256.

Siple, P. A. and Passel, C. F. (1945). *Proc. Amer. Philo. Soc.* **89**, 177.

Stefan, J. (1874). *Akad. Wiss. Wien., Math. Natur. K1. Abt.* **11**, 713.

Stevens, J. C. and Marks, L. E. (1971). *Perception and Psychophysics* **9**, 391.

Stevens, S. S. (1961). *In* "Sensory Perception", (Ed. W. Rosenblith), MIT Press, Boston.

Stevens, S. S. and Harris, J. R. (1962). *J. Exptl. Psychol.* **64**, 489.

Stevens, S. S. and Guirao, M. (1964). *Science* **144**, 1157.

Stevens, S. S. (1975). "Psychophysics". Wiley-Interscience, New York.

Szczesniak, A. S. (1963). *J. Food Sci.* **28**, 385.

Tabor, D. (1959). "General Mechanism of Friction." *In* "Friction in Textiles", (Eds H. G. Howell *et al*.) Textile Book Publishers, New York.

Tregear, R. T. (1969). *J. Soc. Cosmet. Chem.* **20**, 467.

Wood, F. W. (1968). *Soc. Chem. Ind.* monograph **27**, London, England. 40.

Yoshida, M. (1968). *Japanese Psychol. Res.* **10**, 1.

CURRENTLY USED SUNSCREEN MATERIALS— FORMULATION AND TESTING

F. Greiter, S. Doskoczil and P. Bilek
*Forschungsabteilung (Research Department) Greiter AG,
A-3400 Klosterneuburg-Weidling, Austria*

I. INTRODUCTION

The VIIth International Congress on Photobiology, held in Rome, featured the slogan "LUX VITA EST".

The majority of presentations, however, rather left a feeling of "LUX MORS EST".

How did this come about?

(i) The impressive data given by the dermatologists describe an increase of chronic and actinic skin damage induced by irradiation and – as secondary processes – of precancerous and malignant lesions of the skin (Ippen, 1976; Wiskemann, 1976; *HEW News.* 1976).

(ii) This does not only result from unreasonable exposure to sun, but also from physical inactivity, internal and external exposure to chemicals, and all ranges of irradiation which reach man through all kinds of lamps, radio and TV sets (Greiter, 1975).

This means that an organism – often in poor condition anyway and accordingly capable of reduced resistance only – is exposed to an increasing irradiation energy from non-natural sources.

(iii) The assumption will be correct that on account of recent leisure time activities and the present trend towards sun worshipping, the sum total of all irradiation effects from non-natural sources over the past 50 years will become apparent.

Our clothes, which are often made of translucent, synthetic fabrics, will be worthy of consideration as well.

Table I
Some ultraviolet filters currently in use

Chemical name	Trade name	Generally used maximum concentration (%)
p-Amino-benzoic acid	Pabanol	7
Ethyl-p-aminobenzoate, ethoxylated	SC 9155	6
Ethyl-p-aminobenzoate, N-propoxylated	Amerscreen P	2
p-Dimethylamino-amyl-benzoate	Escalol 506	2
2-Ethylhexyl-salicylate	Ingredient of "Sonnelan"	10
Triethanolamine-salicylate	Synarome W	10
Trimethyl-cyclohexyl-N-acetylanthranilate	Ingredient of "Parsol Ultra"	10
Octyl-cinnamate	Prosolal S 8	1
p-Isopropyl-ethyl-cinnamate	Ingredient of "Neo-Heliopan"	6
p-Methoxy-isoamyl-cinnamate		6
p-Methoxy-2-ethoxyethyl-cinnamate	GIV-TAN F	3·5
p-Methoxy-2-ethylhexyl-cinnamate	Parson MCX, and ingredient of "Neo-Heliopan"	7·5
p-Methoxy-cyclohexyl-cinnamate	Ingredient of "Parsol Ultra"	8
p-Methoxy cinnamatic acid and salts	Solprotex II	4
α-Cyano-β-phenyl-2-ethylhexyl-cinnamate	Uvinul MS 40	3
2-Hydroxy-4-methoxy-benzophenone	Eusolex 4360, Uvinul M 40	4
4′ Phenyl-benzophenone-2-ethylhexyl-2-carbonate	Eusolex 3573	5
2,2′-Dihydroxy-4-methoxy-benzophenone	Cyasorb UV 24	4
2,2′ Dihydroxy-4,4′-dimethoxy-benzophenone	Uvinul DS 49	3
2,4-Dihydroxy-benzophenone	Uvinul 400	3
2-Phenylbenzimidazole-5-sulfonic acid	Eusolex 232	7

Table I—*continued*

Chemical name	Trade name	Generally used maximum concentration (%)
3,4-Dimethoxyphenyl-glyoxylic sodium salt	Eusolex 161	4
2-Phenyl-5-methyl-benzoxazole	Witisol	6
Benzalazin (Dibenzalhydratin)	Eusolex 6653	2
Dianisoylmethane	Antisolaire DAM	5
5-(3,3-Dimethyl-2-norbornylidene)-3-penten-2-one	Prosolal S 9	3·5
3-(4-Methyl-benzylidene)-D,L-camphor	Eusolex 6300	6
3-Benzylidene-D,L-camphor	Ultren bk	8
Guanine		2

We are therefore justified to ask which possibilities for protection exist, and which contribution can be afforded by the cosmetics industry in particular.

II. ESTABLISHED MATERIALS AND METHODS

(i) If we disregard the disputed method of systemic protection by means of beta-carotene and protection by more or less ultraviolet-blocking (UVB) textiles (Wittels, 1973; Ippen and Goerz, 1973), we are left with cosmetic agents, available as various systems of mixtures, gels, and solutions, into which predominantly UVB light absorbing filters are incorporated.

Substantial differences exist between the USA and Europe insofar as the establishment of the concept of "Sonnenschutzfaktor" (Sun Protection Factor, subsequently called SPF) has emphasized sun protection in Europe, whereas in the USA a large number of products promise a "tan" in the first place, and in general prefer low to medium sun protection.

(ii) Concerning the filter vehicles used there are different opinions, too:

In the USA oil in water (O/W) emulsion systems or alcoholic solutions are preferred.

In Europe – particularly in Central Europe – water in oil (W/O) emulsion systems are frequently used and are available in tubes and jars. Comparative trials have shown that these products have a better substantivity (Fitz-patrick *et al.*, 1975; Cripps, 1976).

Ultraviolet filters, which are currently used, are manifold; a list, drawn up from Germany, part of which is given in Table I, illustrates this fact IKW, 1976).

(iii) The effectiveness is tested by spectroscopic investigation and SPF determinations on human skin.

(iv) After the introduction of the SPF the following problems have arisen:

(a) Some manufacturers think that the highest SPF is always the best. This attitude led to a contest for the highest SPF.

The quantities of filter substances needed for this objective often exceed physiological tolerance.

Table II
Water in oil system—solid

Ingredients	(%)	Comments and action
Mixture of cetylic and stearylic alcohol	1·00	Emulsifier. Lipid providing substance
Beeswax	3·00	Mixture of esters from the C_{18}–C_{36}–acid and the C_{24}–C_{36}–alcohol. Temperature and emulsion stabilizer
Lanolin, puriss.	14·00	Mixture of various fatty acid esters. Approved "lipid substance" with emulsifying properties
Fatty acid ester	9·00	Facilitates spreading on top layer of skin
Liquid hydrocarbon	9·00	Mixture. Produces lipid providing surface film and stabilizes emulsion
Saturated hydrocarbons	18·00	Mixture. Produces resistant, lipid surface film, and stabilizes emulsion
Cinnamate	4·00	UVB filter for oily phase
Benzophenone	3·00	UVA and UVB filter for oily phase
Distilled water	32·30	Solvent. Swells upper layers of skin
Phenylbenzimidazole	3·00	UVB filter for aqueous phase (even an emulsion which has broken down should contain enough UV filter in each phase to ensure that adequate UV protection is given!)
Propylene glycol	3·00	Moisturizer and solvent for preservative
Magnesium sulfate	0·30	Stabilizes structure
PHB ester	0·20	Preservative against microbial contamination
Perfume	0·20	Should not include any photoreactive components!

(b) The clinical determination of the SPF meant a boom for some investigators, at times affecting the accuracy of the results.

The method of a single trial with 10–20 volunteers under artificial sunlight does not do justice to natural sun conditions. As a consequence of test areas which are too small (8×5 mm) and a non-defined thickness of product layer the end results are not significant with regard to practical usage.

Again and again we have learned that clinical trials under artificial light only yield approximate values. Hence it is mandatory to carry out field tests under solar radiation, employing a clearly defined method and quantity of application.

III. NEWER MATERIALS AND METHODS

A. Suitable Bases for Sunscreens

As already stated above (II, para i), the W/O emulsion system and certain oily solutions are to be preferred on account of their superior resistance to water. The following examples – more or less varied – have proved to be useful for many years.

Table III
Water in oil system—liquid

Ingredient	(%)	Comments and action
Fatty acid ester	6·00	Emulsifier
Liquid hydrocarbon	12·00	Mixture. Functions as lipid surface film and stabilizes emulsion
Cinnamate	4·50	UVB filter for oily phase
Isopropyl-iso-stearate	7·30	Facilitates spreading on top layer of skin
PHB ester	0·25	Preservative against microbial contamination
Propylene glycol	4·30	Moisturizer and solvent for preservative
Magnesium sulfate	0·80	Stabilizes structure
Distilled water	64·55	Solvent. Swells upper skin layers
Perfume	0·20	Should not include any photoreactive components

The formulas in Tables II and III will have the following properties:

sufficiently thermostable,
easy to spread due to low viscosity,

penetrate well into upper skin layer (since lipophile and hydrophile),
high protection against ultraviolet,
resistance to environmental pollution,
good skin and eye tolerance (pH = 6·5),
good water-resistance,
limited protection against cold,
do not impair the skin's natural function.

Table IV
Oily-alcoholic system

Ingredients	(%)	Comments and action
Camphor derivative	4·70	UVB filter for oily phase
Benzophenone	2·80	UVA and UVB filter for oily phase; increases protection against UVA range
Fatty acid esters	38·00	Facilitate spreading in top layer of skin. Protects the skin. Increase substantivity
Liquid lanolin	4·00	Emollient
Alcohol	50·20	Solvent
Perfume	0·30	Should not include any photoreactive components

This formula will yield:

agreeable application properties,
thermostability,
easy penetration into stratum corneum,
good water-resistance,
high protection against ultraviolet,
no impairment of the skin's natural function.

B.   Ultraviolet Filters

Since every foreign substance may at some time or other become dis-
agreeable for the human organism, the basic rule in processing filter
substances must be to use "as little as possible".

The most effective filter is that which is incorporated in low concentration into a base with good skin tolerance and will be present as long as
possible on the skin.

With the filters taken from the list in Table I, and given in detail in
Table V, we have had long experience in their use (Doskoczil and Greiter,
1974).

Table V
Details of ultraviolet filters taken from Table I

Chemical name	Optimum solubility (weight) in cosmetic solvents (%)	Transmittance in terms of % at wave length (in nm) of *								Skin compatibility	Stability in water as a function of the system of the base	Comments
		280	290	295	300	305	310	330	340			
1. Ethylhexyl-p-methoxy-cinnamate	14	33	20	18	17	15	15	53	90	good	In alcohol-aqueous solution: above 70% alcohol—good; below 70% alcohol-less satisfactory; in oily-alcoholic solution—good; in W/O—good; in O/W—less satisfactory.	According to manufacturer no pharmacological effect
2. Diethanolamine salt of p-methoxycinnamic acid	8	18	21	23	26	29	37	100	100	good		Depends on the pH
3. 3-(4-Methyl-benzylidene)-camphor	5	18	9.5	9	9.5	10	13	78	98	good		According to manufacturer no toxicologic effect, not even as a pure substance
4. Triethanolamine salt of 2-phenyl benzimidazole-5-sulfonic acid	10	51	35	33	31	38	49	100	100	good		Depends on the pH
5. 2-Hydroxy-4-methoxy-benzophenone	4	25	24	30	36	41	41	38	45	good		UVA filter
6. p-Amino-benzoic acid (PABA)†	8	4	5	7	12	22	45	100	100			

*1 mg of substance in 100 ml solvent. Thickness of layer: 1 cm.
†The esters of p-amino-benzoic acid (PABA), which have recently been very popular in the USA, are more and more subject to controversies. Phototoxic properties have been described in the literature (Greiter and Doskoczil, 1976; Hodges et al., 1976).

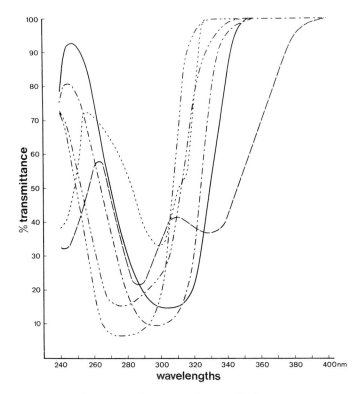

Fig. 1.   Curves of ultraviolet absorbing filters. All filter curves are measured at identical conditions. One mg of substance weighed into 100 ml solvent. Thickness of layer 1 cm. Narrow slit. Range of 240–400 nm. Beckmann DB Spectralphotometer.

See Table V: 1. ——————— 3. —·—·—·—·—·—5. - - - - - - - - - - - -
         2. —··—··—· 4.———————— 6. —·--—·--—

1. *Comparison of Curves* (Figs 1–3)

A comparison of the curves in Fig. 1, shows that filters which, in lower concentration have good absorption values in the UVB and UVA range, do far better than filters which do not have these properties.

For a practical utilization of these values, and taking the range of formulation mentioned under Tables II–IV as a basis, the following rule results.

The maximum permissible transmittance at a wavelength of 310 or 340 nm respectively must be determined. When 25 mg of a sunscreen preparation are weighed into 100 ml solvent (other measuring conditions see Fig. 1) the following maximum permissible transmittances should result:

For SPF 3
appr 20–25%
at 310 nm

For SPF 4
appr. 15–20%
at 310 nm

For SPF 6
appr. 3–10% at 310 nm
appr. 40–50% at 340 nm

The entire range of absorption of sunscreen agents with SPF 3, 4 and 6 is illustrated by the three absorption curves in Fig. 2.

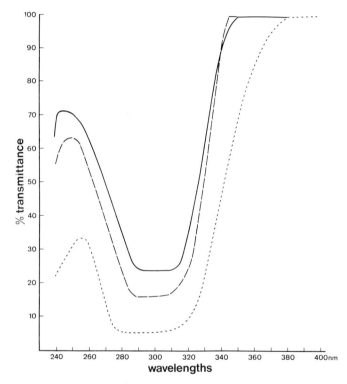

Fig. 2.   Ultraviolet absorption curves of sunscreen agents.

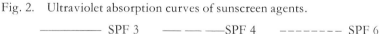

——————— SPF 3   — — ——SPF 4   ———————— SPF 6

Provided the same filters and bases are used, proportionate alterations of the filter concentrations will permit valid conclusions to what extent already known and approved SPF values may need modification.

The ideal absorption curve for a preparation containing an ultraviolet wideband filter (Doskoczil and Greiter, 1974; Greiter and Doskoczil, 1976) results from an optimal combination of those filters which are currently approved and generally used in Europe.

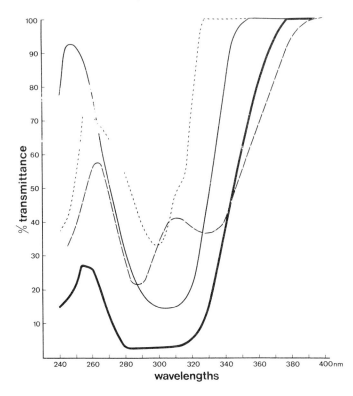

Fig. 3.　Absorption curves of a sun protective agent containing wideband filter, resulting from 3 ultraviolet filters. Sun protective agent containing wideband filter: 25 mg weighed into 100 ml solvent; all individual ultraviolet filters: 1 mg weighed into 100 ml solvent. Other measuring conditions see Fig. 1.

──────── Sun protective agent containing wideband filter
─ ── ── Benzophenone
─ ── ── ── Benzimidazole
──────── Cinnamate

Such preparations will not only absorb erythemogenic UVB light, but also part of the photoactive, non-erythemic UVA light. This seems of special importance, because on account of the present environmental situation—as already stated under I, para. 2—more and more agents causing photoreactions affect the human organism. A growing number of phototoxic and photoallergic reactions is the result.

2. Solar Radiation

Here again it should be emphasized that not only the ultraviolet range, but also visible and infrared light will definitely need more investigation (Greiter, 1975).

Although the energy emitted by photones of these wavelengths does not suffice for the development of primary photochemical lesions to the same extent as that of ultraviolet radiation, the arising heat should not be neglected. If one is aware of the fact that temperature is an important factor in secondary photochemical lesions (dark reactions), late effects can by no means be excluded. The complex influence of long-wave radiation is still largely unknown, and it is hard to understand why to date these wave ranges have not received greater attention.

It is in this context that the "heretic question" should be considered whether or not dealing with solar radiation in terms of multiple mono-chromatic bands, which is more or less common practice, can be meaningful for the various experimental studies in the field of photobiology.

In our opinion, the entire spectrum of solar radiation should attract attention to arrive at a more correct evaluation of the effects of sunlight.

With a view to biological protection the only relevant question is how much of the entire spectrum is to be kept off from man in order to avoid as far as possible any kind of damage by radiation.

3. Skin Care

In addition to the ultraviolet filters the base is of special importance. It should be almost neutral, well compatible with the skin, and resistant against all influences.

Oil of almonds, cocoa butter, emulsifiers, preservatives, and perfumes can, *per se* or after contamination, become photosensitizing agents. They should only be used upon careful consideration. If any doubt arises, such substances should be avoided.

Some manufacturers still think that complicated formulas are "more valuable" and specific active components for skin care offer advantages for the consumer.

This attitude may—particularly with respect to sun protective agents—give rise to quite a number of intolerance reactions.

We recommend the use of simple formulations, employing substances that have been found safe regarding skin tolerance.

4. Skin Compatibility Tests

Skin compatibility testing is of special importance for sun protective agents.

Products which are offered for sensitive skin and/or extreme radiation shall be examined repeatedly according to the Shelanski Patch Test. If there is any doubt, especially when new substances are being used, the substance itself and the entire product are to be analysed.

5. Eye Compatibility Tests
Eye compatibility testing is just as important. This holds particularly true for O/W emulsion systems, aqueous-alcoholic, and oily-alcoholic solutions.

6. Perfumes
In choosing perfumes and preservatives special care is mandatory.

For very or extremely sensitive skin bases should be chosen which do not require such substances.

7. Sun Protective Agents
The use of photoactive substances, such as Bergapten, in o.t.c. sun protective agents must be rejected, because the amount necessary for the achievement of an increased tan has been reported to exceed 1% of Bergapten (Lane-Brown, 1976).

Apart from the problem of an uneven application, resulting in uneven tanning, phototraumatic and phototoxic reactions are likely.

We are therefore justified to expect that legislation will stop such practices and the industry will refrain from using such substances in o.t.c. sunscreens.

8. Pigments
The addition of pigments, which absorb not only parts of ultraviolet radiation, but also of visible light, may become increasingly desirable.

This is particularly true for conditions of extreme irradiation and for patients suffering from actinodermatoses, who at times should not be exposed to daylight at all.

The addition of beta-carotene improves the filtering properties, too. However, it is a bit difficult to stabilize this sensitive substance.

9. Testing
Spectroscopic testing of ultraviolet filters yields useful data for a suitable dosage and combination of the filters.

Laboratory testing under artificial sunlight is an essential prerequisite for practical usage under natural sunlight.

10. Test Methods
Accurate test methods are required.

A recommendation to this end was drafted at the VIIth International Congress on Photobiology.

Different views as to the necessity of field tests (see also III.9), the technique of test area determination and product application, and the testing of product substantivity will have to be overcome.

Our method how to standardize test area size and thickness of product layer is largely unknown and will be illustrated by the following three pictures (Figs 4–6).

(a) *Laboratory tests*   In these we use opaque adhesive tapes with circular, punched out test sites. There have been found suitable for smaller test areas, since this shape allows for application of the entire product quantity without leaving any residue (see Fig. 4).

Size of test areas for determining the effect of sun protective agents = 7·1 cm². Size of test areas for determining the skin's inherent protection time = 3·1 cm².

(b) *Field tests*   In field testing rectangular areas of equal size are used (see Fig. 5).

Size of test areas for determining the effect of sun protective agents = 30 cm². Size of test areas for determining the skin's inherent protection time = 10 cm². Size of untreated control areas = 12 cm².

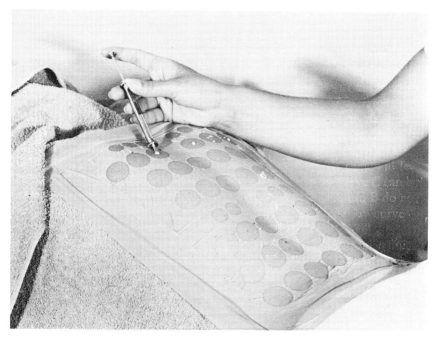

Fig. 4.   Laboratory testing; suitable for smaller test areas.

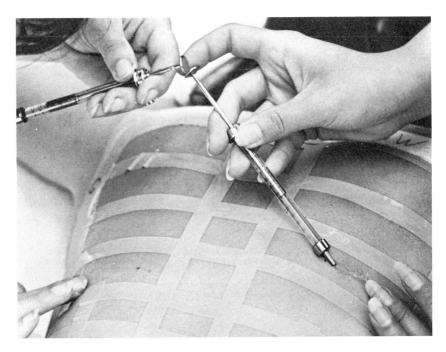

Fig. 5. Field testing of rectangular areas of equal size.

(c) *Product quantity for the tests* Exact product quantities are applied by means of a syringe and distributed with the finger (see Figs 4 and 5). This method offers the following advantages:

test area size more meaningful with a view to practical application, accurately defined thickness of layer in cm = 3

$$= \frac{\text{product quantity applied per test area in cm}^3 \ (= \text{ml})}{\text{size of test area in cm}^2}$$

clearly recognizable skin reactions,

the resulting SPF values are confirmed by practical usage.

An investigation of the various layer thicknesses actually applied in practice—depending on the preparation system used—resulted in values between 6·3 and 20·0 μm (Doskoczil and Bilek, 1973–6). In laboratory testing the application of layer thicknesses lower than 28 μm has so far failed, because no adequate instruments are available.

(d) *Water-resistance tests* Testing the water-resistance of sun protective agents in praxi is best performed by the Fitzpatrick and Pathak method.

Other methods have been described by Ippen and Goerz (1973), Tronnier *et al.* (1973) and Pathak *et al.* (1973).

According to our method, which is based upon the Fitzpatrick and Pathak procedure, the volunteers have to swim during the time of exposure (skin's inherent protection time x SPF) for altogether 15 mins under natural sunlight.

These tests are conducted in sea-water as well as in standardized pool water (pH 7·2; 0·6 mg Cl/1).

(Incidentally, sun protective agents are removed to a greater extent from pool-water than from sea-water.)

(e) *Test results*   A specific problem is to read the test results. In our experience this is best done by visual evaluation by three trained experts (dermatologist, physiologist, biochemist).

Parallel to this reflectometric measurements are performed (see Fig. 6).

These results have not been satisfactory.

A new, interesting procedure is described by Kölmel (1976). It employs an instrument which measures erythema without contact and can thus also be used for smaller test areas; it is especially useful for differentiating the various degrees of redness.

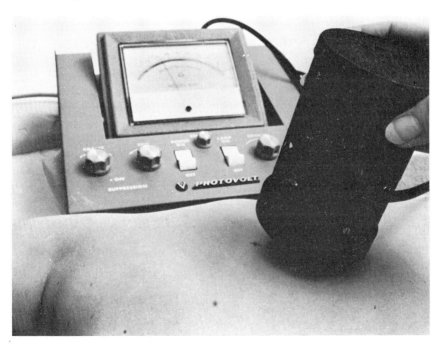

Fig. 6.   Reflectometric measuring equipment.

(f) *Test evaluation* The statistically correct evaluation of a SPF-test is the necessary conclusion of every test procedure.

The methods existing at present either permit a statistically correct evaluation (Hoppe *et al.*, 1974) or allow for a safe realization in practical testing (Greiter, 1974).

A method taking into account both requirements has not been developed so far.

IV. RESULTS

A. Ultraviolet Filters

With the ultraviolet filters listed in Table V, we have had a long, positive experience.

From all inquiries made and from an evaluation of all complaints received from 1970 to 1975 the following result was obtained:

Table VI
Evaluation of complaints from 1970 to 1975

System of preparation	Total production in test region (pcs.)	Number of complaints		Consulted physician and invited to hospital for objectivation‡	Actual clinical tests	Hospital findings
		Total	Skin and eye intolerance			
W/O	8 187·806	126	39	14	3	Hyper-sensitivity*
O/W	12 161·614	200	36	14	2	Acute eye damage†
Aqueous alcoholic	520·224	5	5	1		
Oily	2 227·702	4	3	2		
Aerosols	730·258	9	1	1		

*To certain substances, once to 2-phenyl-5-methyl-benzoxazole.
†Which had been caused by other foreign bodies.
‡The apparently low interest to go to hospital at manufacturer's expense leaves some doubt whether the original diagnosis of the physician had been correct.

B. Approved Materials and Methods

The methods explained under III have been approved and are increasingly utilized in Europe. This means that the light absorbing or reflecting filters must not be seen out of context of the whole preparation, and that a correct evaluation of the effectiveness of a sun protective agent can only be made by adequate testing, based on the requirements of practical usage.

C. Protection Times

The determination of the skin's inherent protection time is occasionally difficult, because there may be substantial differences, depending on the type of skin, the general condition of the test person at the time of the test, and the intensity of irradiation.

The following irradiation times and the corresponding SPFs have proven reliable for healthy skin for almost all conditions:

10 mins: sensitive skin	SPF 6
15 mins: skin of average sensitivity	SPF 4
20 mins: skin of little sensitivity	SPF 3

V. CONCLUSION

The growing importance of a highly natural, physiological sun protection is emphasized.

Established and newer methods of sunscreen testing are reported. Our own experience is described and special attention is focused on the ultraviolet filters and bases most commonly employed in Europe.

ACKNOWLEDGEMENTS

Thanks are due to Mrs Rauscher for translating and typing the manuscript and Mrs David for the graphical work involved.

REFERENCES

Cripps, D. J. (1976). VIIth International Congress on Photobiology, Rome, *Symp. Abstr.* 220 and Round Table Discussion on Topical Photoprotection of Normal Skin.

Doskoczil, S. and Bilek, P. (1973–6). Untersuchungen am ÖISM Wien (Studies Carried Out in the Austrian Institute of Sports Medicine). Unpublished.

Doskoczil, S. and Greiter, F. (1974). UV-Filter für Sonnenschutzmittel (Ultraviolet Filters for Sun Protective Products). *Öst. Chem. Z.., Heft* 2.

Fitzpatrick, T. B. and Pathak, M. A. (1975). Sunlight and Man, Ch. 49, 765. University of Tokyo.

Greiter, F. (1974). Sonnenschutzfaktor—Entstehung, Methodik (Sun protection factor—development, methods). *Parfüm. Kosmet.* **55**, 70–75.

Greiter, F. (1975). Spektralphotometrische Messungen zur Beurteilung von UV-Filtern für Sonnenschutzmittel, Fensterglas, Glas- und Plastikmaterial für Sonnenschutzgläser sowie Suntex-Material für UV-durchlässige Badebekleidung (Spectrophotometric measurements in evaluating the effectiveness of ultraviolet filters in sun protective glasses made of glass and plastics, and of UV-through bathing clothes made of suntex fabrics). *Parfüm. Kosmet.* **56**, 129–132.

Greiter, F. and Doskoczil, S. (1976). Die Problematik photodynamischer Substanzen für die Kosmetik (Difficulties with photodynamic substances in cosmetics). *Parfüm. Kosmet.* **57**, 149–156.

HEW News (1976). US Department of Health, Education, and Welfare, 9/76.

Hodges, N. D. M., Moss, S. H. and Davies, D. J. G. VIIth International Congress on Photobiology, Rome, *Symp. Abstr.* 156.

Hoppe, U., Kopplow, H. J. and Wiskemann, A. (1974). Statistische Auswertung des Lichtschutzfaktors (Statistical evaluation of the light protection factor). Society of Cosmetic Chemists of Great Britain.

IKW-Inquiry (1976). Industrieverband Körperpflege- und Waschmittel (Manufacturers' Association Personal Hygiene Products and Detergents), BRD-6000 Frankfurt, Karlstraße, 21.

Ippen, H. (1976). VIIth International Congress on Photobiology, Rome. *Symp. Abstr.* 39.

Ippen, H. and Goerz, G. (1973). Photodermatosen und Porphyrien (Photodermatoses and prophyria). Self-published, 93–94 Düsseldorf.

Kölmel, K. (1976). *Ärztl. Kosmetol.* **6**, 135–139.

Lane-Brown, M. M. (1976). VIIth International Congress of Photobiology, Rome. *Symp. Abstr.* 289.

Pathak, M. A., Fitzpatrick, T. B. and Parrish, J. A. (1973). Final Report Piz Buin, Harvard Department of Dermatology, (October).

Tronnier, H., Mayerus, M. F. *et al.* (1973). Ergebnisse eines praktischen Lichtschutztests I. Vergleichsuntersuchungen zur Lichtempfindlichkeit und Lichtschutzwirkung (Report on a practical light protection test I. Comparative studies on sensitivity against light and effectiveness of light protection). *Parfüm. Kosmet.* **54**, 140–146.

Wiskemann, A. (1976). VIIth International Congress on Photobiology, Rome. *Symp. Abstr.* 47.

Wittels, W. (1973). Die klinische Prüfung von Kosmetika, Sonnenschutzpräparaten und UV-durchlässigen Textilien (Clinical investigation of cosmetics, sun protective products, and ultraviolet transmitting textiles). *Parfüm. Kosmet.* **54**, 74–77.

COLOUR IN COSMETICS

I. D. Rattee
Department of Colour Chemistry,
University of Leeds, Leeds, England

I. INTRODUCTION

Although colour has an objective origin it is a completely subjective experience. The physicist will define colour as that part of the visible spectrum remaining after reflection or transmission from an object of light consisting of the whole or part of the visible spectrum. However the words "visible spectrum" encompass a phenomenon which depends upon subjective experience. While colour and light may be discussed in terms of energy, wavelength etc. the fact remains that as Newton (1730) pointed out, "For the rays to speak properly are not coloured. In them there is nothing else than a certain power and disposition to stir up a sensation of this or that colour".

Colour is the language we employ to describe our subjective experience when there is an interaction between an absorbing material or surface, a perceptible (visible) light emission and our eyes. Any variation in any one of these three factors will change the interaction and hence what is called the colour. Although eyes may be replaced by photoelectric measuring instruments the final arbiter of colour is the human viewer. What the viewer sees can only be described by the reaction to the colour stimulus and the language used to describe the experience. Here we find another component in the interaction which is culturally based. Linguistic limitations in the description of colour are known to be accompanied by limitations in colour discrimination. In other words differences in colour which are not important enough to be described in words are not regarded as being subjectively significant even if seen.

The topic of cosmetic colouration is most conveniently discussed in terms of the factors underlying the interactions shown schematically in Fig. 1.

The first interaction (1) results in colour reflection or transmission and involves the incidence of the emitted light energy upon the object with its absorbing colouring matter. It is thus that part of the light reflected or transmitted. It is determined by the chemical structure of the colouring matters and the nature of the light source. The former are most conveniently considered in terms of their specific applications e.g. hair dyeing, skin colourants etc. and this is done in Section V. Colour reflection or transmission can be detected only by a sensor such as the eye or a photoelectric device and it is the interaction of the reflected or transmitted light with the

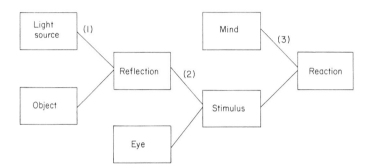

Fig. 1.   Interaction sequence leading to a subjective colour reaction.

sensor (2), that provides the colour stimulus. This depends upon both the nature of the light and the properties of the sensor. The process provides a signal which at its simplest is a metre reading or a digital print out. When the sensor is the human eye, however, the signal is interpreted by the brain thus providing a further interpretive interaction, the colour reaction (3). It can be seen that the process is a consequential selective process the final product of which is what is called colour. Each stage is important in the consideration and is considered separately.

II. COLOUR REFLECTION, COLOUR MEASUREMENT AND METAMERISM

Visible light is a small part of the electronic energy spectrum which ranges from longwave radio transmission to X-rays in energy. The energy of the radiation is governed by the well known equation, $E = h\nu$, where E is the energy, h is Planck's constant and ν is the frequency or reciprocal wavelength of the radiation. The wavelength of visible light lies between the approximate limits of 380 and 750 nm. Yellow light, or rather what human beings react to as yellow light, has a wavelength between 560 and 590 nm.; blue light has a wavelength of less than 480 nm.; red light has a wavelength of more than 630 nm. It can be seen that as we proceed through the familiar rainbow spectrum from red to blue the energy of the radiation increases.

Light sources such as the sun, fluorescent tubes, incandescent filaments etc. emit characteristic spectra which are received in general terms as white light but which contain different proportions of the different energy levels. The properties of a light source may be defined in terms of a *spectral energy distribution curve* which is characteristic and of great importance in relation to the production of the colour stimulus as will be seen.

When electronic radiation interacts with a chemical compound many consequences can follow the absorption of the incident radiation. Organic colouring matters, for example, possess their colour due to an extensive population of delocalized electons which are very easily excited, i.e. they are raised to a higher state of energy by radiation of quite low energy such as visible light. This process involves the absorption of the light energy. Depending upon the characteristics of the chemical structure involved, quanta of different energies are absorbed leading to a filtering effect. Thus, objects described as red absorb visible light energy of shorter wavelengths than 630 nm. while blue objects absorb light energy of longer wavelengths than 480 nm. and so on. This process can be characterized for any coloured surface or solution by the proportion of the incident light quanta which is reflected or transmitted. For simplicity discussion will be confined to reflection. The coloured surface can be described by a *spectral reflectance curve* which relates the relative reflectance to the wavelength of the radiation.

Thus the two interacting components producing the colour stimulus may be characterized by a spectral energy distribution curve and a spectral reflectance curve. Since the coloured object can only reflect light that is received, the actual reflectance at any particular wavelength will be the product of the relative reflectance and the relative energy of the source at that wavelength. For the moment such factors as scattering and refraction which also occur will be ignored. From the interaction of the two components it can be seen that the colour stimulus produced will have a *stimulus curve*. In Fig. 2 the process is shown. Figure 2a shows two typical spectral energy distribution curves. Curve (i) is typical of sunlight while curve (ii) typifies a tungsten filament lamp. Figure 2b shows the spectral reflectance curve for a grey surface. Figure 2c shows the actual reflectance or stimulus curves which arise when the light from the two sources falls on the surface. Clearly the colour stimuli in the two cases differ very considerably and, indeed, it is doubtful whether what will appear as a grey surface in the sunlight will appear grey at all in the tungsten light.

The spectral reflectance curve of a light absorbing surface, being characteristic of its colour producing potential provides the kind of absolute property, independent of either the light source or the observer,

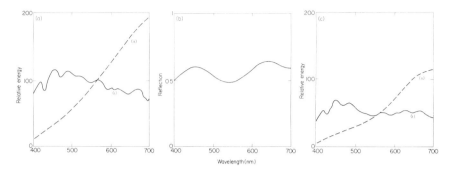

Fig. 2. The interaction of spectral energy distribution and spectral reflectance curves to produce a colour stimulus curve.

which can be used for comparative and computational purposes. Using appropriate equations (Beasley *et al.*, 1965; Kubelka and Munk, 1931; Kubelka, 1948, 1954) the reflectance can be related to the concentration of the colourant. In such computations the ability of most colourants to scatter as well as absorb light is taken into account and many of the equations become so complex that their ready solution is only possible using a computer. The use of the spectral reflectance curve enables the colour to be expressed in terms of three carefully selected standard primary colours established by the Commission International de l'Eclairage (CIE). Using the three CIE coordinates, colours may be given precise specification and removed from the area of subjective judgment. Standardized acceptable colour differences can be established and an element of control imposed over the colour using industries so that, for example, a lipstick produced in Scotland with a particular shade is matched by the same product produced in another factory thousands of miles away. Colours of unlike objects can be matched also, e.g. lipsticks and nail lacquer, although they may be produced in different places. The whole subject of colour measurement and computation is very extensive and its full treatment is well beyond the scope of the present contribution. Excellent descriptions are readily available elsewhere (Billmeyer and Saltzmann, 1968; Colour 73, 1973; Judd and Wyszecki, 1963). The use of the instrumental approach to colour assessment in the cosmetics industry has been rather uneven. The Yardley company has been particularly active (Wheeler *et al.*, 1975) and the subject has been reviewed (Fujiwara *et al.*, 1973).

It can be seen from Fig. 2 that in the two different lights the actual stimulus curves from the grey object depend very strongly on the spectral composition of the light source thus giving rise to the sensation of different colours. This phenomenon is a very general one and is known as *metamerism*. It is particularly important in colour matching as what may prove a match in one light may not be a match in another. Thus two kinds of metamerism are important. The first is that arising simply from the reflectance characteristics of the surface in different lights. The colours produced can be acceptable or not according to circumstances. A carton which is green in daylight and grey in tungsten light may be acceptable if both shades are attractive. Care has to be taken with actual cosmetics however as they may be purchased to blend with particular articles of apparel or accessories. The second manifestation of metamerism arises from the fact that what may be small acceptable differences in colour in one light become unacceptable in another. Sometimes because of the nature of the objects to be coloured the colouring matters used may vary from one object to another although they are required to be the same shade. For example it may be desired to produce ceramic bathroom tiles and acrylic baths of the same shade but using different colouring matters; a lipstick may be required to match a nail varnish; a sweater may need to match a shirt. The forms of the problem affect many industries. Due to small differences in the individual spectral reflectance curves the actual colour stimulus curves may be the same in one light but not another. Such effects are readily calculable using instrumental/computational methods otherwise different formulations have to be checked for acceptability of the degree of metarism.

A simple form of shade specification which is often used is the standard shade card or in its fully developed form the colour dictionary. The use of standard shades for reference rather than spectral reflectance curves or CIE tristimulus values clearly requires account to be taken of the metameric phenomenon since both the shade and reference standard are likely to show the effect. A useful piece of equipment for this kind of rudimentary shade control is a "viewing box" which provides the possibility of inspection under a variety of selected light sources.

III. THE COLOUR STIMULUS: OBSERVER METAMERISM AND COLOUR BLINDNESS

The reflectance resulting from the light/surface interaction cannot be detected, of course, without a light sensitive sensor which may be a photomultiplier, a photographic film or the human eye. The colour stimulus is the reaction of the sensor to the reflected light and depends upon its spectral sensitivity or response curve. The common terms ultraviolet and infra red refer to the fact that the spectral sensitivity of the human eye is zero below and above certain wavelengths. Such terms have no meaning in relation to sensors with other characteristics. The spectral sensitivity of the sensor represents a further process in the selection of signals which are ultimately recorded. The characteristics of the light source determine what light is available for reflection and the characteristics of the sensor determine what components are detected. Thus the colour experience is quite subjective for all sensors whether they be chemical, electronic or human. Two observers may see a given object under a particular illumination quite differently. This is known as observer metamerism.

As adults grow older the corneal lens yellows producing a filtering effect which diminishes the proportion of reflected blue light reaching the retina. Thus the tendency for older people to see red is physical as well as metaphorical. In an individual the eyes may differ giving rise to observer metamerism between the two. Photomultiplier tubes used in spectrophotometers vary in their characteristics so that absolute values are impossible to achieve in any precise sense although by careful selection and the use of controls the highest quality spectrometers currently available show a satisfactory degree of instrument to instrument comparability. In Fig. 3 the different stimulus curves produced by slightly differing sensors are shown. The degree of difference shown between the sensors actually corresponds with the shift in spectral sensitivity in the human eye which occurs when the eye is adapted to low and high light intensity (the Purkinje shift). It can be seen that the more red sensitive vision sees the colour as weaker and redder than the more blue sensitive (dark adapted) vision.

Observer metamerism clearly adds further effects to the metamerism of the reflecting surface so that individuals vary greatly in their assessment of such effects. Great improvements have been brought about in the textile industry in this regard by the use of instrumental control and colour

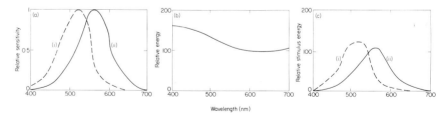

Fig. 3.   Observer metamerism: differences in the stimulus curve produced by changes in the spectral sensitivity of the sensor. (i) Dark adapted human vision. (ii) Light adapted human vision. (a) Spectral sensitivity curves for two sensors. (b) Spectral reflectance curve of observed surface. (c) Different spectral stimulus curves resulting from differences in the sensors.

computation. Colour formulations of minimal metamerism are readily computed in instrumental shade match prediction systems. The use of instruments raises the question of their use of colour specification and control. Observer metamerism through variations in the characteristics of photomultiplier tubes and light sources is largely avoided in single instruments by the use of split beam comparative methods and a single photomultiplier tube. Cross comparison between instruments still presents difficulties and it is necessary to select detectors and sources using calibrated control panels as references.

Carried to its extreme observer metamerism becomes colour blindness and normally relates to the inability to distinguish between red or green light and grey light i.e. so called red or green blindness. Only a small percentage of women are colour blind but about 10% of males are so affected. The sale of cosmetics predominantly to women has made colour blindness of no importance to the cosmetics industry. However the growing effort to create a male market may make it advisable to take into account this deficiency.

IV. REACTIONS TO COLOUR: PSYCHOLOGICAL AND PARAPHYSICAL FACTORS

The colours used in cosmetic materials have two purposes. There is the direct function of colouration as in the case of nail lacquers, hair dyes, eye shadows or lipsticks and there is the indirect function where the colour is present purely to enhance sales appeal or pleasure in use. The indirect function may be extended to include packaging or promotional material so there are few products which utilize colour only for direct colouration.

Clearly the indirect function is based on some interpretation of psychological factors. However direct colouration is not immune to such considerations. The successful marketing of a cosmetic colouring product depends upon an accurate anticipation of the colours which will find a favourable response from contemporary opinion or taste either spontaneously or as a result of appropriate promotion. At the present time there are no real guide lines available to assist the prediction of a popular shade. For example, nail varnishes were at one time exclusively red or colourless but the shade gamut has now widened to include blues, greens, black and even multicoloured effects. Although lipsticks still are largely confined to red shades the available gamut has been considerably extended. The middle nineteen seventies have seen a very considerable expansion in available eye shadow shades. Population movement, immigration and integration are also creating a wider range of cosmetic problems and solutions none of which necessarily stay conveniently compartmented. The application of the very broad correlations between colour and psychological reaction which have been put forward by some psychologists is, under these circumstances fraught with uncertainty. Such correlations have always lacked predictive power and have in any case depended greatly on the context of the interaction between colour and subject.

In the international market some useful conclusions of a very general kind can be drawn about national or regional factors. Reference has been made to the significance of the ability of people to describe colour in words for their ability to discriminate between colours. An extreme variety of this effect is provided by some Bantu whose language encompasses only black, white and red in relation to colours. Thus only lightness and darkness or redness have any significance and although there must be a capability of discriminating between green, blue, and purple etc. the evident differences are not regarded as being worth mentioning. Indeed, without the linguistic tools they cannot be mentioned. These are some indications that the kind of extreme importance put on certain colours by some Africans is at least marginally evident in other peoples. The tendency for a liking for green shades in Muslim countries, a significant preference for purple among older jews, the great significance of pink among Hindus represent choices originating from some deep rooted cultural source. However, the greater degree of international movement and the influence of the news and entertainment media must inevitably erode such distinctions.

Colour associations are of considerable importance and derive from the human capacity to transfer properties. It is well known that lemon and orange flavoured sweets may vary only in their colour. The flavour difference is produced by an interpretation of the taste sensation conditioned by memories of lemons and oranges. In the cosmetic field such associations are also common. Blueness and coolness, greenness and freshness, redness and antiseptic properties are all common connotations. They do depend, however, upon the product so that the mental structuring of the association may be complex. Green and hence mint flavoured toothpaste is difficult to connect with green and hence somewhat mysterious eyeshadow. Associations can be affected by the form of sales promotion but it is clearly better for the sales argument to complement rather than contradict the instructive reactions of the purchaser. This is particularly important where the colour has an indirect function, so that its purpose is to assist in creating some image in the minds of consumers. Red aftershave lotion, or soap giving a grey lather are clearly non-starters in the market place. An interesting study by Austrian, Van Bommel and Schwarz (1964) showed that in the promotion of perfume colour associations played a very significant part. Consumers asked to rate perfumes spotted onto differently coloured papers were found to be little influenced by the colour but when asked to rate perfumes associated with coloured promotional material i.e. displays, packages etc. in the absence of the fragrance, marked effects were noted. Qualities such as sweetness, sharpness, sensuality and expensiveness were used as parameters. Magenta was found to have strong associations with expensiveness. Golden yellow gave an excellent association of ratings which suggested its value as a "perfume" associated colour.

Another very important aspect of human reaction to colour relates to paraphysical phenomena. These do not arise from psychological factors but fall into the same category as optical illusions. Some paraphysical effects arise from persistence of vision effects while others appear to arise from other mechanisms causing a distortion of the neural message between eye and brain. Of particular relevance in the present context is the way in which background colour and relative areas of different colours affect the observer. Very marked differences can be observed in some cases (Albers, 1973). One such effect is known as the Bezold effect and arises when extreme intensity contrasts are juxtaposed e.g. black or white adjacent to a coloured area. The effect is used to good effect in film cartoons and was originally employed to increase carpet design possibilities. Paraphysical factors are of considerable importance in relation to design and colour selection in cosmetics where the interaction of differently coloured areas may have to be taken into account.

V. COLOURING MATTERS AND COLOURATION

A. General

The basis of cosmetic usage is the desire to change personal appearance to produce social, sexual or magical effects in accordance with the cultural interests of the society in which one lives. At different times the same form of self decoration may create quite different social reactions. In D. W. Griffith's classic film of the French revolution "Orphans of the Storm" an aristocratic rake pauses to adjust his lip rouge before plunging into the bushes after a dairy maid. Historically accurate, this image produces laughter in a contemporary audience. Similarly, the clean chinned crew cut hero of the Second World War resembles the skinhead of the 1970s. At one stage the changes in cultural taste followed complex and little understood social changes but today they have become increasingly modified by what has been called "psychomarketing" (Bassin, 1975). However there has been little change over the centuries in the location of the decoration. What has varied, of course, has been the colours and combinations employed. Materials have also changed as natural products have been displaced by synthetic materials. In addition an increasing knowledge of medicine and interest in health has resulted in some traditional cosmetic colouring materials being dropped. It is true that the adoption of clothing led to a decline in body colouration and a concentration on the exposed extremities. Even this change is less one of attitude than visibility and the continual concern of light skinned people outside of South Africa to acquire as dark a sun tan as possible has provided the basis for a continuation of even this form of decoration in modern times. Thus cosmetic colouration may be resolved into the three areas of interest skin, nail and hair colouring and colourants.

Cosmetic colouration using henna or indigo in hair dyeing, kohl as an eye shadow and betel to enhance the redness of the lips has been known to be carried out since well before the fifth century B.C. The materials sold were to a large measure subject to individual control and modification. In the Far East today the bespoke perfumer and powder blender can still be met. The twentieth century has seen the introduction of the cosmetic product promoted by the promise of an identical allure to all who purchase it. There are some who may regret this but it should be recognized that with the product has also come, by and large, a freedom from risks of poisoning and dermatitis.

B. Skin Colouration

There are three main areas of interest here each introducing a different aspect of cosmetic colouration technology. These relate to eye shadows, powders and lipsticks.

In ancient times Kohl was the eye shadow generally used by the semitic people, the Persians and the Greeks. Composed of lead or antimony sulphide it is toxic and unacceptable as a cosmetic product in the more industrial countries which provide the bulk of the cosmetic market. The modern eye shadow or powder is carefully screened for skin sensitization and toxic properties leaving a limited range of colours from the wide range available. Colouring matters found to be satisfactory on the basis of long experience are naturally abandoned reluctantly in favour of unknown products. It is not proposed in this chapter to enter into a discussion of the constantly changing regulations regarding the use of different colouring matters in cosmetics in different countries. The literature is contradictory in many cases as to whether a particular colourant is a safe compound or a potential allergen. For example carmine which is the aluminium lake of the natural product cochineal has been quoted by Hardy (1973) as a potential allergen following work by Calman (1967) while it is listed as a suitable product by Schlossmann and Feldman (1971). Part of the problem of regulation of the use of colours lies in the term "safe". In the United States a Supreme Court decision in 1958 defined the term as implying safe in any concentration i.e. regardless of the quantity actually used in the coloured product. Thus the Food and Drug Administration has moved against many well established compounds. However it must be said that the Supreme Court decision apart, the Food and Drug Administration listing of "delisted" products reveals some alarming traditional inclusions such as iron blue (ferric ferrocyanide) and manganese violet (ammonium manganese phosphate).

Powders and rouges are by tradition red in colour but contemporary fashion has introduced a much wider shade range to include yellows and violets. Eye shadow has in the past spanned a fairly wide range of shades but again the trend is towards a wider range and more intense colouration.

Inorganic pigments have been extensively used because of their stability and general lack of sensitization. A white base of purified titanium dioxide, zinc oxide, alumina hydrate or blanc fixe is normally employed.

Iron oxides are frequently encountered for the production of a wide range of yellow, orange, red and brown shades. The standards of purity demanded by the cosmetics industry are higher than those normally applicable to iron oxides. Thus the standard procedure of dissolution of scrap iron in acid followed by precipitation is unsuitable due to arsenic and lead contamination. Normally pure ferrous sulphate is used, treatment with alkali in the presence of air producing hydrated ferric oxide in the presence of air and which is then the starting point for the various end products.

The shades produced are products of the conditions employed. Thus precipitation of hydrated ferric oxide with alkali, followed by treatment with oxygen produces the ferric oxide monohydrate, $Fe_2O_3.H_2O$. By varying conditions of precipitation and oxidation, shades from lemon yellow to orange can be obtained. If the ferric oxide monohydrate is calcined then a range of red iron oxides results. Again using controlled conditions of precipitation, black iron oxide which is a mixture of ferrous and ferric oxides is obtained.

Carbon black is extensively used. This is prepared by controlled combustion of natural gas in order to achieve the desired purity and freedom from carcinogens.

Ultramarine has also been used extensively in cosmetics although the number of manufacturers is now very few. The ultramarine pigments are complex products resulting from the high temperature (850°C) treatment of appropriate mixtures of sodium carbonate, china clay, sulphur and an organic reducing agent such as charcoal pitch or rosin. The use of china clay makes it necessary for a purification process to remove lead and arsenic. Variation of the formulation produces a range of shades but generally the bulk of manufacture is the familiar Capis lazuli shade.

Pure chromium oxide, Cr_2O_3, is also used as a cosmetic pigment. A variety of green pigments based on chromium are known e.g. Arnandan's Green made by heating ammonium phosphate with potassium dichromate or Dingler's Green which is a mixture of chromic and calcium phosphates. However the general range of "chrome greens" is not suitable for cosmetic use. The product employed is the chromium sesquioxide (C.I. Pigment Green 17) produced to meet rigorous specifications with regard to lead and arsenic content.

Among organic colouring matters employed in powders, the most important group consists of the lithol reds which are either the sodium salts of sulphonated dyes of sparing solubility or the virtually insoluble salts of other permitted metals. Typical of these compounds is the series based on the dye produced by diazotizing Tobias acid and coupling with β-naphthol (I).

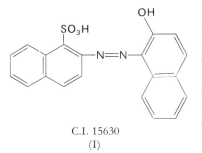

C.I. 15630
(I)

D and C Red 10   sodium salt (orange red)

D and C Red 11   calcium salt (deep red)

D and C Red 12   barium salt (medium red)

D and C Red 13   strontium salt (medium red)

Other examples are given by (II) and (III) below,

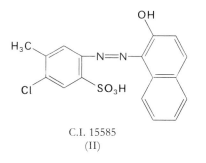

C.I. 15585
(II)

D and C Red 9   barium salt.

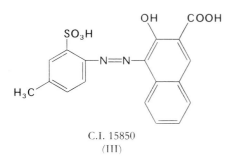

C.I. 15850
(III)

D and C Red 7   calcium salt

with other more soluble dyes it is possible using permitted precipitants to prepare an adequate lake for cosmetic purposes. Tartrazine (IV) has been used for this purpose.

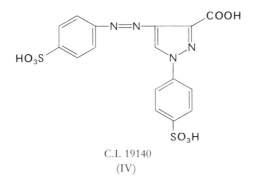

C.I. 19140
(IV)

Indigo has a venerable record as a cosmetic being one of the oldest skin decorative colours. In an appropriately pure form indigo (V) is still used.

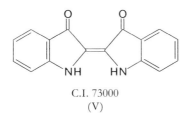

C.I. 73000
(V)

Natural colouring matters are virtually displaced entirely by synthetic colouring matters in cosmetics as well as most other applications. Carmine still finds some use. It is the aluminium lake of Cochineal (VI) which is extracted from the dried bodies of the female *Coccus cacti* insects.

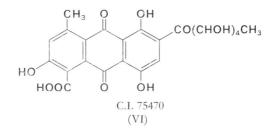

C.I. 75470
(VI)

When incorporated in a powder the effectiveness of a colouring matter depends considerably on its particle size distribution and surface area. These properties affect not only the colour value as Alex (1975) has pointed out but also coverage, tinting strength, smoothness etc. When used in an oily medium as in lipsticks agglomeration characteristics and oil absorption are additional important factors affected by the physical properties of the colourant particles.

Lip stains have been employed for centuries. On the Indian subcontinent betel was used to produce a red stain and vermillion or other pigment colours in a wax medium were used as caste marks (Gloag, 1927). The modern lipstick as a device for the convenient application of lip colourants appeared in 1915 (Wall, 1974). The safety aspects of lipstick colourants clearly cover the possibility of internal effects as well as skin sensitization. Nevertheless, lipstick colourants and media are relatively rarely the source of cosmetic injury complaints (Weissler, 1974). In a survey over the years 1970 and 1971, Weissler showed that only 2·2% and 1·9% of cosmetic injuries were ascribable to lipsticks in the respective years. Further there is no indication that the colourants used were the only basis of complaint. The colourants used in lipsticks must be compatible with the oily base of these products. Both pigments and oil soluble stains are used as varying degrees of permanence are desired by the consumer. However great care has to be taken in the selection of oil soluble colourants due to the loose correlation between oil solubility and carcinogenic activity in aromatic compounds.

The main oil soluble component employed is C.I. 26100 (VII) prepared by diazotizing p-phenylazoaniline and coupling with β-naphthol.

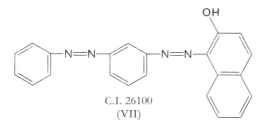

D and C Red 17

C.I. 26100
(VII)

Among the pigments used D and C Reds 10, 11 and 12 derived from C.I. 15630 (I) are of particular importance. The lakes of a number of xanthene dyes are also used. These are prepared by precipitating the dyes with alumina on to permitted substrates such as aluminium benzoate or alumina hydrate. The xanthene dyes used are classic colouring matters i.e. erythrosine, eosine and rhodamine exemplified by (VIII) and (IX) below.

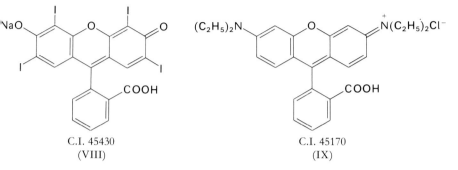

C.I. 45430   C.I. 45170
(VIII)   (IX)

The tetrabromo analogue of (VIII) is Eosine (D and C Red 21 lake—C.I. 45380). According to Calman (1967), Eosine is the main cause of allergic reactions but the use of highly purified versions reduces the incidence drastically.

C. Nail Lacquers or Varnishes

The use of coloured nail lacquers dates from relatively recent times since the necessary or suitable products were not available to the ancients. Thus, nail painting is probably the only unique contribution to cosmetic arts in the field of colouration technology which has appeared during this century. In 1916 Peggy Sage introduced nail varnish (Wall, 1974) and the market has expanded from that point on.

Nail varnishes are different from other cosmetic colouring systems in that they are applied to a relatively robust part of the anatomy permitting the use of substances which would cause considerable discomfort if used elsewhere on the body. Thus the normal nail varnish consists of a pigment or stain in a solvent solution of a suitable film former. This may be cellulose acetate or more usually in modern times a synthetic resin system with somewhat better performance. The resin system has to be chosen with some care as allergic reactions to products such as the arylsulphonamide formaldehyde resins which can be used are known (Cronin, 1967).

The normal colourants used are the lithol red pigments already described. Irridescent effects with the production of interference colours have also been explored (Greenstein and Bolomey, 1971). White inorganic pigments are also used as reducers and also in their own right. In the recent period there has been some departure from the traditional red shades to blacks, browns, greens and blues. Again standard pigments prepared to satisfactory purity levels are employed.

D. Hair Colourants and Colouration

1. *Introduction*

The hair occupies a peculiarly important position in cosmetics. This reflects its very significant cultural standing. Many religions demand that it must not be cut while others insist upon its removal. The arrangement of the hair is universally a matter of human preoccupation. A change in hair decoration fashion among the young may be expected, without fail, to produce apoplexy among the old. Short hair and long hair have both within the past two decades provided cultural distraction of this kind in the western world. The hair as a virility (or femininity) symbol has meant that its loss due to age or illness has been a matter for concern to many. The accidental loss of hair has been regarded as a serious matter by the courts in compensation cases despite its relative lack of useful function. It is not surprising that within this context hair colour and colouration provide the basis for an extensive literature and commercial activity.

The reasons for the colouring of hair vary from a desire to disguise an apparent ageing due to greyness or for many other reasons. From the point of view of the cosmetic colourist it is the most deeply studied colouration problem. This may arise from the fact that most cosmetic colouring is a very temporary affair i.e. eye shadow, lipstick etc. whereas even the most impermanent of hair colourations require a durability to quite severe mechanical abrasion processes such as combing and brushing. The problems posed to the chemist are consequently more challenging and the response has been the provision of many varied solutions to the problems.

2. *The Colour of Human Hair*

Unlike almost all other chosen substrates for colouration human hair is generally strongly coloured. Shades range from very pale yellow or albino hair to very dark black. Due to the fact that the colour will vary in different parts of the scalp precise description of a given head of hair is not possible. However, some kind of classification is desirable for the guidance of salon workers and also for identification purposes in, for example, forensic work. Porter and Fouweather (1975) consider that, in view of the variations of colour over an individual scalp, hair colour can be classified by nine selected colours produced by nylon tufts. They prefer the use of tufts over the Munsell chips suggested by Garn (1948) because of the greater ease of comparison. The nine colours selected by Porter and Fouweather range from black through browns to white/grey but do not include (somewhat oddly) any red hair shade. This is perhaps less serious in the United Kingdom where the tuft system was tested than it might have been in other parts of the world where red hair is more common. Taking a sample of 200 individuals the shade distribution shown in Table I was found.

Table I
Distribution of hair shades in a UK sample (Porter and Fouweather, 1975)

Tuft number	1	2	3	4	5	6	7	8	9
Shade	Black	V. dark brown	Dark brown	Mid brown			Blond		White/ grey
Sample: female (%)	0	28	20	9	14	7	6	4	12
Sample: male (%)	0	43	16	12	9	1	0	0	19

While the nine shades selected as a basis for the classification system might be criticized because of their failure to discriminate in the largest single group, the system is in principle acceptable. While it is clearly imprecise and in any case omits the red hair shades it offers the virtues of simplicity and cheapness. Its operation moreover requires little skill. A much more precise but correspondingly more complicated method has been put forward by Denbeste and Moyer (1968) who advocate instrumental methods. This offers greater discrimination and can be carried to a considerable level of sophistication such as might be needed in forensic work by the measurement of the spectrophotometric absorption curve of a single hair using a microspectrophotometer such as that described by Patterson and Blacker (1969).

The colour of different hairs is produced by the presence of either or both of two melanin pigments. These are the more common eumelanin which is present in black, brown and even blond hair and phaeomelanin which is present in so called red hair. Variations in shade are produced by variations in the concentrations of the pigments in the particle size and distribution of particle sizes in the hair shaft. In addition shade variations can be produced by differences in the level of photooxidation or bleaching of the melanin particles as well as by metabolic changes due, for example, to ageing.

The eumelanins are irregular cross linked polymers which are mainly based on 5:6 dihydroxy indole (XIII) units and conjugated with protein.

Our knowledge of the final stages of the formation of this polymeric pigment is still somewhat scant. The early stages of melanogenesis have, on the other hand, been described in detail by Raper (1927), Duliere and Raper (1930) and Head and Raper (1933). The starting point is the amino acid tyrosine (X) which is successively oxidized to the red pigment dopachrome (XII). The sequence of reactions is initiated by the enzyme tyrosinase and continued by the action of other enzymes. The sequence of reactions is shown below.

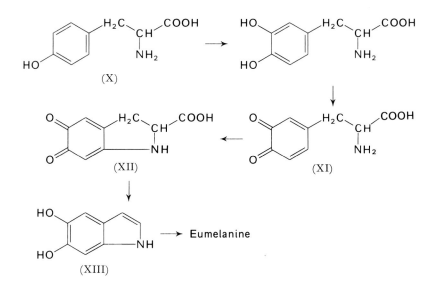

The phaeomelanins arise from a branching reaction in the above sequence in which cysteine reacts with (XI). The reaction scheme is shown below and derives from the work of the Naples school (Prota, 1972; Fattorusso *et al.*, 1970; Prota and Nicolaus, 1967; Nicolaus *et al.*, 1969).

It can be seen that the formation of the phaeomelanins occurs after the formation of the dopaquinone (XI) and depends purely on the presence of cysteine in the melanocytes. The chemistry of the transformation of the dihydrobenzothiazine derivative (XIV) to the phaeomelanins remains obscure. However, oxidative polymerization is almost certainly involved. Thomson (1974) has described the indirect evidence which relates the known components of red hair with the chemical reactions of the initial stages of the process.

The colouring of hair by any kind of dyeing process is capable only of producing darker shades than the original colour of the hair. Since for most of mankind the original colour is a dark shade, this leaves little room

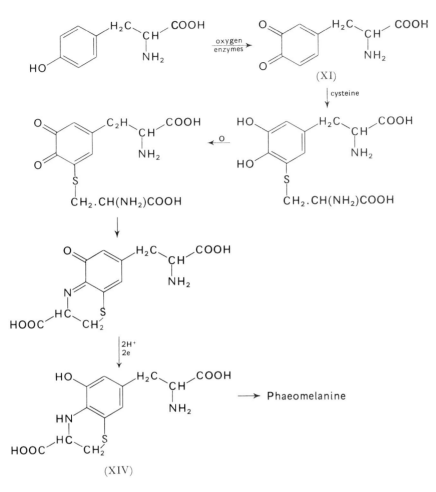

(XI)

(XIV)

for manœuvre. Consequently hair is generally bleached before dyeing. Sidi and Zviak (1966) have commented that while melanin (presumably eumelanin) is fairly readily bleached, hair contains also a "diffuse red pigment" (presumably phaeomelanin) which is difficult to bleach. Certainly red hair resists bleaching and red shades are often apparent in the course of bleaching dark coloured hair. Bleaching is generally carried out with hydrogen peroxide, its use having been demonstrated at the Paris Exposition in 1867. Hydrogen peroxide has the property probably unique among hair bleaching agents, of solubilizing the melanin granules in the hair prior to the bleaching reaction (Wolfram *et al.*, 1970). This probably involves attack by the peroxide anion or some complex of it on the quinonoid ring of the indolequinone. Bleaching is also a feature of hair redyeing since the normal practice is to bleach out an initial dyeing when redyeing to colour new growth since this avoids repeated colouration of already dyed hair.

3. *Physical Chemical Aspects of Hair Colouration*

In general terms the physical chemical aspects of dyeing hair are not greatly different from those of wool dyeing and around which an extensive literature is to be found (Rattee and Breuer, 1975; Peters, 1976). However, the conditions under which hair has to be dyed in the salon without causing excessive discomfort to its owner highlight certain special features of hair colouration and have tended to direct research into the physical chemistry of the process towards certain special problems.

Although it is not possible to define a "normal" hair due to the wide variations in the characteristics of hairs even over the scalp of a single individual (Hunter and Wall, 1974), it is possible to make a general comparison between hair and wool and to make reasonable generalizations about the relative dyeing characteristics of the two fibres.

Medullation is more extensive in hair than it is in wool and the cuticle layer is very much thicker. In wool the cuticle layer is 1–2 scales thick whereas on hair it covers 7–10 overlapping scales (Wolfram and Lindemann, 1971) and is very highly cross linked due to the presence of an abnormal proportion of cysteine in its constituent amino acids. In addition, the hair in its virgin state carries an outer "sheath" which differs from the epicuticle seen on wool (Wolfram, 1968). Thus the very marked affects of the fibre surface on dyeing rates which are apparent in wool dyeing are even more so in the dyeing of hair. Many years ago Speakman and Smith (1936) showed that with a typical acid dye the time of half dyeing (i.e. the time required to achieve 50% of the equilibrium exhaustion of the dyebath) at 60°C was 2 hours with a typical wool sample but 50 hours with the hair sample examined. The problems of penetration of hair under the imposed mild conditions of colouration present three kinds of solution.

  (i) the use of small dye or dye forming molecules which may diffuse sufficiently rapidly;
 (ii) the use of swelling agents to increase the intrinsic diffusion characteristics of the hair;
(iii) the use of solvent assisted systems to change both the hydrodynamics of the system and the diffusion behaviour of solutes.

In general, it is the first option which has received the most attention since long before the nature of the problem of dyeing hair was understood successful systems had been found even as early as the time of the ancient

Egyptians (Wall, 1974) and it is natural enough that research investigations should build upon success.

Wilmsmann (1961) and Holmes (1964) have both reported that the penetrability of human hair to solute molecules is virtually zero when the diffusant molecules exceed 0·6 nm in effective diameter. This is not an absolute limitation but refers to significant penetration of hairs during periods of time which are reasonable in view of the circumstances under which hair is dyed in the salon i.e. at temperatures not exceeding 40°C and for times between 15 and 45 minutes. Thus the search for hair colourants has either involved a limitation to chromogens or chromogen forming compounds of low molecular weight in comparison with textile dyes or some means whereby larger molecules could be assisted to diffuse into the hair. The problem may be put in these terms because the colour yield or extinction of the colourant is closely linked with the extent of its structure and its capacity to adsorb energy in the visible region of the spectrum. The need for colour yield creates a pressure towards maximization of the molecular size particularly as desirable hair shades tend to be dark and this is in opposition to the requirements for easy dyeing. Satisfactory resolution of this contradiction has been found among a relatively limited range of substances as is discussed later.

It has been realized for some years that if some additive such as a swelling agent or a promoter of diffusion could be found which could be used in conjunction with the dye, then larger colourant molecules could be used for hair dyeing thus making the problem of finding alternative colourants more simple. Two aspects have to be considered in this context, namely the circumstances in the dyeing liquor and those in the fibre. The dyebath situation may be represented schematically as in Fig. 4.

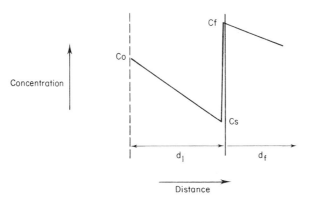

Fig. 4.   A schematic of concentration relationships in an unstirred dyebath.

If the concentration of the adsorbate in the dyebath at the outermost limit is taken as C_o, then the concentration at the fibre surface is C_s where $C_s < C_o$ because of rapid surface adsorption by the hair. Thus the surface concentration in the fibre surface is C_f. The adsorbate will thus diffuse

(i) through the liquor at a rate dependent on the diffusion coefficient in the liquor (D_s) and the concentration gradient which is $(C_o - C_s)/d_1$ assuming that there is no mechanical circulation of the liquor increasing the transport of the adsorbate;

(ii) through the fibre at a rate dependent upon the appropriate diffusion coefficient (D_f) and the concentration gradient which assuming simple slab geometry and incomplete penetration is $(C_f)/d_f$ where d_f is half the thickness of the fibre.

Thus the two fluxes are:

$$J_1 = D_s \frac{(C_o - C_s)}{d_1} \quad \text{and} \quad J_f = \frac{D_f(C_f)}{d_f} \tag{1}$$

But the relationship between C_f and C_s is fixed by the affinity of the adsorbate under the dyeing conditions and consequently

$$\frac{C_f}{C_s} = K \text{ for all times} \tag{2}$$

It can be seen that under these circumstances there are two rate controlling possibilities. Either dye at the surface is replenished at the rate of depletion by the fibre so that the diffusion rate in the fibre controls the situation or diffusion in the liquor phase is so slow that dye at the surface is replenished at a rate less rapid than the fibre is capable of depleting it. In both cases, of course a steady state is set up. In unstirred systems control by both liquor or fibre phases is observed according to circumstances (Rattee and Breuer, 1975). Since hair colouring solutions are generally highly viscous due to the incorporation of surfactants and foaming during application diffusion to the hair surface is inevitably slow. If the liquor diffusion rate was rate determining then significant variation in dyeing rates would be observed with different rates of agitation on the scalp by the operative. There has been no study to determine such effects but salon experience suggests that the effects would be small in most cases showing that the diffusion rate in the fibre is so slow as to give a relative insensitivity to agitation even in a system of this kind. This situation is quite different from that with textile fibres and emphasizes the problem of slow diffusion in the fibre. From the salon operations point of view it is perhaps fortunate as one cause of operator variable is removed.

Just over 20 years ago Peters and Stevens discovered that with certain dyes the rate of adsorption by wool and hair was greatly enhanced by the presence of certain solvents dissolved in the aqueous dyebath (Peters and Stevens, 1956, 1956a, 1957a, 1958). The effect was most pronounced at the point where the aqueous dyebath became just saturated with the solvent. Suitable solvents included butanol, cyclohexanol, benzyl alcohol and thymol. It was found that the dyes giving the most impressive results were those which in a partition experiment between the solvent and water favoured the former. Very rapid dyeing was observed in many cases using quite large molecules and consequently the method of dyeing possessed many features of interest to the hair colourist and patents rapidly followed (Peters and Speakman, 1957; L'Oreal, 1957).

The mode of action of the solvent assisted dyeing process remains in some doubt and it seems probable that a variety of factors may operate with different relative importance in different instances. The appropriate solvents for solvent assisted processes are in all cases alcohols and these are known to have marked effects on internal bonding in proteins. n-Butanol is known to considerably increase the ease of extension of wool (Atkinson, Filson and Speakman, 1959). Other alcohols have been shown to have the same effect (Zahn and Blankenberg, 1964). Denaturation of soluble proteins by alcohols has also been reported (Schrier *et al.*, 1965). Alcohols and phenols have a marked disaggregating effect on dyes in aqueous solution due, presumably, to their lessening of hydrophobic interaction effects. Medley and Ramsden have reported that dyes diffuse more rapidly in an alcohol–water environment than in pure water (Medley and Ramsden, 1960). Microscopic studies suggest that in keeping with a lessening of aggregation in solution, the tendency for dye-fibre binding interactions is also reduced (Karrholm, 1960) thus leading to an increase in diffusion rates inside the fibre. One idea much favoured to account for the effect of the added solvents suggested that the solvent formed a separate solvent rich phase inside the fibre into which the dye was preferentially partitioned (Karrholm, 1956; Peters and Stevens, 1958). However, this view has been shown to be thermodynamically incorrect (Cassie, 1960). In certain cases it has been shown (Butcher and Cussler, 1972) that the solvent reduces the static boundary layer effect at the fibre surface assisting the process of transport across the interface. Cussler and Breuer have demonstrated that one important general effect is the acceleration of diffusion resulting from the coupling of diffusion fluxes between the dye and the solvent (Cussler and Breuer, 1972, 1972a).

There has always been a strong body of opinion among students of solvent assisted dyeing processes that partition of the dye into a solvent rich phase was an important factor in the observed effects. However, the effect of the added solvent is generally to be seen before the water becomes saturated with the solvent and there are many solvents which work extremely effectively well below the saturation level e.g. cresols. It has been shown that one important factor due to phenolic solvents is their effect on swelling or disorienting the cysteine rich surface layers on wool thus promoting dye penetration (Hampton, 1976). However there is no doubt that the partition effect, whatever else might happen, promotes rapid dyebath exhaustion and methods have been proposed to promote the partition. Acid dyes may be complexed with added cationic surfactants to assist in hair dyeing in the presence of solvent assistants (Rapidol, 1959). Added salts have also been claimed to be effective (Gillette, 1964) as have other miscellaneous additives such as benzoic acid, phenyl urea etc. (Unilever, 1965). In most cases the explanation for the enhanced dyeing rates in the presence of these additives is little understood. Simply studying dyebath exhaustion is often extremely deceptive as many solvent assisted systems merely deposit dye on the fibre surface. Where no fastness is sought this may be unimportant in a purely technical sense but it is clearly unwise to develop theoretical ideas on an unreliable experimental basis.

An important general difficulty associated with accelerating the adsorption of dyes by hair using solvents and similar additives is that such agents also tend to promote dye uptake by the skin. Normally the skin remains unstained in hair dyeing by virtue of its grease content which provides an adequate resistance over the duration of the dyeing treatment. However degreasing solvents change this situation and can in some instances lead to sensitization. An alternative approach based on the selective break down of the cross linked cuticle layer by controlled cysteine hydrolysis or reduction appears to be a better approach currently under investigation.

4. *Methods of Colouring Hair*

The desire to change the colour of hair goes back to ancient times. The invention of hair dyeing has been ascribed to the ancient Egyptians (Cooley, 1868). The daily dyeing of the beard was a common practice in ancient Persia (Montseygur, 1915). The products employed in those times and indeed up to the end of the last century were of natural origin. Extracts from henna, camomile flowers, and dye woods were much used, these containing appropriate active ingredients e.g.

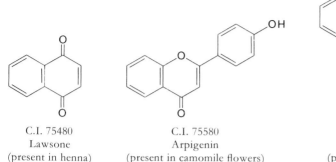

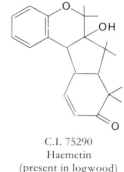

C.I. 75480	C.I. 75580	C.I. 75290
Lawsone	Arpigenin	Haemetin
(present in henna)	(present in camomile flowers)	(present in logwood)

Dyeing methods were tedious. In the reign of Queen Elizabeth I for example hair was dyed to a golden red shade by soaking the hair in warm alum and then in an extract of rhubarb, turmeric and the bark of the barberry (Wall, 1974). The use of pre-coloured wigs was naturally favoured. There has been some attempt in the recent period to market hair colouring preparations based on natural colouring matters following the suggestion that some synthetic hair colourants may be carcinogenic. This has been based on the tendency of the general public to accept "natural" as being synonymous with "safe" notwithstanding the hazards of "natural" blue asbestos, deadly nightshade, toadstools, etc. The question of carcinogenic effects is discussed later but that question apart there seems little likelihood that natural colouring matters will replace the synthetic materials which completely dominate the situation today.

The first use of synthetic colouring materials for human hair was based on Hofmann's observation that p-phenylenediamine gives rise to a brown colouring matter on oxidation (Hofmann, 1863). This was put to use by Monnet (1883) who patented the use of p-phenylenediamine and other compounds for the production of brown shades on hair in an oxidative dyeing process. The process was based on treatment of the hair with a solution of the diamine and hydrogen peroxide. This remains the basis of the majority of hair dyeing treatments but there have been continual attempts to find a more straightforward or "direct dyeing" process using colouring matters instead of colour formers.

The contemporary market for hair colouring and hair colourants shows some sophistication and the mode of colouring which is favoured depends upon the end use of occasion. There are basically three systems:

(a) *Permanent colouration*   This is clearly a relative term since the growth of the hair continually presents undyed new hair. However, permanent in this context means the need to redye every 3–4 months. The colour is fast to shampooing and is particularly favoured by the 35+ age group to cover greyness etc. The shades are normally close to the natural hair colours i.e. browns and blacks and oxidative dyeing is used exclusively.

(b) *Semi-permanent colouration*   A wider age group of consumers employ this approach which meets the demand for a process which colours the hair for 6–8 weeks and may then be removed or changed. The colouration has some resistance to shampooing but will not stand repeated wet treatment. The colourants used are not the pigment forming system used in permanent colouration but direct dyeing dyes.

(c) *Temporary colouration*   This is not expected to be more durable than most other cosmetic colouration. The colour has to be readily applied and readily removed. Frequently it is applied in an aerosol spray. Consequently purely surface colouration is desired although it has to be fast to rubbing, combing or perspiration. Selected textile dyes are often used and some special non-penetrating hair colouring polymers have been described.

The three systems involve different aspects of dye chemistry and will be considered separately

5. *Oxidative Hair Colourants*

(a) *General*   The general principle of oxidative hair colouration has been indicated already in outline i.e. the oxidation of a diamine to form a colouring matter. The procedure has however been raised to a high level of sophistication by the use of a variety of amines, oxidizing agents and also additives which participate in the reactions to modify the main colour produced. Thus the process involves three components the primary intermediate (i.e. the diamine providing the main basis for colour development) the colour coupler (i.e. an additive able to react with products of the diamine reaction to produce alternative shading components) and the oxidizing agent. Commercial products based on these components contain also a number of other agents designed to assist marketing, or facilitate the process of colouration but such additives may be regarded as having effects which are not relevant to the topic under discussion.

Normally the oxidizing agent is hydrogen peroxide. Many others have been proposed such as persulphate, (Erdmann and Erdmann, 1888) potassium dichromate, (Corbett, 1971), chloramines etc. (Bandrowski, 1894) but have not succeeded in displacing the use of the hydrogen peroxide used by Hofmann in the original experiments (Hofmann, 1863).

The original hair colouration processes employed straight primary intermediates. Monnet's use of *p*-phenylenediamine (Monnet, 1883) was soon extended by the Erdmanns to cover aminophenols, *N*-substituted derivatives of *p*-phenylene diamine and of, aminophenols, and naphthalene derivatives (Erdmann and Erdmann, 1888). By 1911 Gaston Bondon was able to market a range of standardized hair dyes under the name—"Inecto". However, in much of the early work inadequate attention was paid to the problems of dermatitis and skin sensitization. The dyeing of human hair on the scalp was not always understood to require a slightly different approach as compared with the dyeing of fur. In the 1920s research conducted by the suppliers of the Inecto hair dyes showed *p*-phenylenediamine to be one cause of trouble and "notox" hair dyes were introduced containing no *p*-phenylenediamine. The search for more satisfactory products and the introduction of reliable testing have further improved the situation. Just over 10 years ago a new class of heterocyclic bases was introduced (Corbett, 1971) with reported weaker sensitization. The two classes of primary intermediates and the colour couplers may be considered separately.

(b) *Homocyclic amino primary intermediates* A wide range of benzenoid primary intermediates is described in the literature giving rise on oxidation to a range of brown and related shades. The most commonly used compounds were first used for hair dyeing very many years ago and no new amines appear to have been adopted. Corbett (1971) lists some fifteen compounds, the majority of which were in use in the last century as hair colourants, as the most important compounds of this class.

One limiting factor on any development is of course the carcinogenic activity of aminonaphthylamines particularly α-naphthylamine. The knowledge of a potential danger from aminonaphthalenes would make very extended testing of such compounds essential with no clear indication of a product of any particular merit at the end of the programme. This is the factor which probably lies at the heart of the relatively small investigative effort in this field.

The chemistry of the oxidation of the homocyclic amines in hair dyeing has not been extensively studied. However the behaviour of *p*-phenylenediamine under oxidation conditions in solution has been studied by several workers thus giving some indications of the possible origins of the brown colour produced.

The results of oxidation of *p*-phenylenediamine depend upon whether vigorous or mild oxidation is involved. The former leads to the colourless *p*-benzoquinone but under mild conditions a coloured compound is obtained. This was first studied by Bandrowski (1894) after whom the coloured base product is named. The structure of Bandrowski's base was suggested by Erdmann (1894) was thought to be formed by trimerization of *p*-phenylenediimine the first product of the oxidation of the diamine. However, the imine can be prepared in the pure state and dissolved in an alkaline buffer to give a quite different compound (Wilstatter and Meyer, 1904) suggesting that Erdmann's proposed route was incorrect. In addition the proposed structure of Bandrowski's base (XV) was soon rivalled by an alternative proposed by Green (1913).

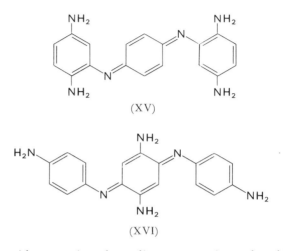

(XV)

(XVI)

The main evidence against the earlier structure is produced by the work of Lauer and Sunde who produced the compound (XV) by an unambiguous route and showed that it was not the same as Bandrowski's base. Further evidence has been produced by Corbett (1969) who starting with Bandrowski's base has shown that it hydrolyses to give 2:5 dihydroxy-benzoquinone, p-phenylenediamine and ammonia. Such products point strongly to structure (XVI). Additionally Corbett demonstrated that the yields of p-phenylenediamine and 2:5 dihydroxybenzoquinone were in the ratio 2:1. Thus structure (XVI) must be accepted. Erdmann's suggested route i.e. trimerization of benzoquinone diimine is supported by kinetic studies (Corbett, 1969) although the important catalytic role of p-phenylene-diamine was unsuspected by Erdmann. The reaction scheme is shown on page 199.

Thus the diamine participates in the reaction both directly and by involvement in the transitional diphenylamine. Not unexpectedly, other reactions occur on a small scale (Dolinsky et al., 1968) giving rise to a number of other products including p-nitroaniline, 4:4'diaminoazobenzene and an amino anilino benzoquinone diimine.

There is, however, very little evidence that the interesting and complex sequence of reactions discussed above actually occurs in the hair itself. Early experiments by Cox (1940) reportedly produced small quantities of Bandrowski's base from wool oxidation dyed with p-phenylenediamine.

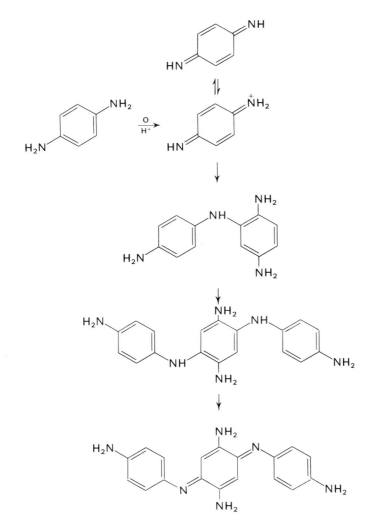

However, later experiments by Altman and Rieger (1959) failed to show the presence of any of the base in dyed hair. Similar results were obtained by Brody and Burns (1968). It is distinctly possible that the presence of amino- and guanidinyl groups in wool and hair could lead to side reactions and a brown colouration due to some other base. The hair itself could act in a sense as a colour coupler leading to coloured products resisting normal extraction procedures. It would be premature to regard the problem as intractable since relatively little work has been done on the in-fibre reaction.

(c) *Heterocyclic primary intermediates*   The potential dermatological hazards of the use of the benzenoid diamines have led to the search not only for conventional primary intermediates with lower sensitizing action leading to numerous substituted N-substituted phenylene diamines (L'Oreal, 1965) but also for quite new compounds. In the sixties dyes based on pyridine were reported to be weaker sensitizers (Lange, 1965, 1966) and a number of interesting products have emerged in the basis of the research thus stimulated. The possible diamino pyridines have been described and also dihydroxy pyridines. Corbett (1971) lists the colours yielded by pyridine and quinoline derivatives. Generally the shades are lighter than those given by the homocyclic diamines and lacking in dark brown shades. Thus, the use of the heterocyclic compounds may be safer but it is also of less value for the majority of cases where hair requires to be dyed.

(d) *Colour couplers and colour coupling reactions*   The use of colour couplers to modify the shades produced by primary intermediates is clearly an attractive method of extending the available colour gamut based on a restricted group of compounds. The colour coupling reactions are related to those of the colour formers used in photography. The reactions are less clear cut however since the primary intermediates themselves produce a colour effect depending upon relative concentrations. Colour couplers may be used to produce a very wide range of shades ranging from yellows (using β-diketones) through blues (using m-diamines) to magenta (with 3-methyl-1-aminophenols). The chemistry of reactions in solution has been extensively studied but as in the case of the work on Bandrowski's base, the relevance of such work to actual results in the hair remains to be established.

The controlling reaction, as in the formation of Bandrowski's base, would appear to be the formation of the protonated benzoquinonediimine. This can react with m-diamines to give a leuco indamine which may be oxidized to give a bluish coloured dye (XVII).

Similarly the reaction with phenols leads to the formation of indoaniline dyes (Heller, 1921) by coupling para to the hydroxyl group (Corbett, 1970). Corbett has also suggested that oxidative coupling by the same diimine is involved in the formation of the magenta and yellow colours produced in the presence of pyrazolones and β-diketones (Corbett, 1968).

6. *Autooxidative Hair Colourants*

(a) *General*   The application of oxidative hair colourants involves the separate application of the primary intermediate with or without added colour couplers followed by the oxidizing agent, normally hydrogen peroxide. This can create problems of control and, in certain cases, difficulty due to oxidation damage to the hair. The two components have to be

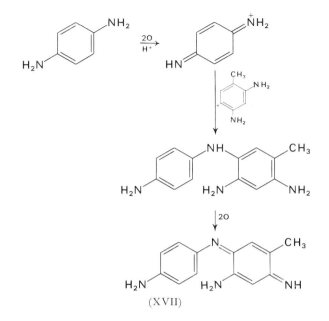

(XVII)

applied uniformly in each case. It is obvious that at some time attempts should be made to use atmospheric oxygen as the oxidizing agent thus reducing the system involving one colouration component. Inevitably the primary intermediates used in this, so called, autooxidation procedure are less stable and more readily oxidized than those employed in regular oxidative hair colouration unless the colouring procedure is to be prolonged to an undesirable degree.

The oxidation in the atmosphere of p-phenylenediamine is slow but 2:4 diaminophenol, which is more readily oxidized, is mentioned in the early patents of Erdmann and Erdmann (1888). However, the use of this compound and other related amines does not offer a sufficiently good basis for autooxidative hair colouration and it was not until some 60 years later when it was observed that 1,2,4-benzenetriol and derivatives provided an excellent basis for such a process that there was significant commercial development of this approach (Winthrop, 1939; Burton and Stores, 1950, 1951). This has been limited however by the stability problems previously mentioned.

(b) *The chemistry of autooxidative systems* As is readily deduced from first principles, the autooxidative colouration systems are based on compounds which are more powerful reducing agents than is, for example, p-phenylene-diamine. This is, of course, not the only property required since the colour forming reactions are essential. Attention has concentrated on compounds related to hydroquinone or alkoxy and hydroxy amines. Typical compounds and the colours produced are shown in Table II.

The chemistry of colour formation is even less well understood than is the case with the oxidative hair colourants previously discussed.

Corbett (1967) has shown that the first step in the oxidation of benztriols in solution involves oxidation to hydroxyquinones and the formation of hydrogen peroxide and that considerable free radical formation occurs. There have been several studies of the colours formed by the autooxidation of various autooxidative colourants in solution (Von Auers and Borsh, 1915, 1921; Kehrmann and Mattison, 1906; Möhlaü, 1892; Horner and Sturm, 1956). Inside the hair, complex side reactions are possible and may

Table II
Typical autooxidative colourants

General type	Substitution position								Colour produced
	1	2	3	4	5	6	7	8	
	OH	OH	H	OH	H	H	—	—	Mid brown (Winthrop, 1939)
	OH	OH	H	OCH$_3$	H	H	—	—	Auburn (L'Oreal, 1956)
Benzenoid	OH	NH$_2$	H	NH$_2$	H	H	—	—	Red brown (L'Oreal, 1956a)
	OH	NH$_2$	OH	H	OH	H	—	—	Golden brown (Gillette, 1962)
	Br	NH$_2$	OH	H	NH$_2$	H	—	—	Purple (Gillette, 1961)
	OH	OH	H	OH	H	H	H	H	Orange red (Winthrop, 1939)
Naphthalene	NH$_2$	OH	H	NH$_2$	H	H	H	H	Blue (Corbett, 1971)
	OH	NH$_2$	H	H	H	OH	H	H	Black (Thera-chemie, 1964)
Quinoline	—	H	H	H	OH	OH	H	OH	Orange brown (Corbett, 1971)
	—	N$_2$H		NH$_2$	H	OH	H	H	Violet (Lange, 1967)
Pyridine	—	NH$_2$	NH$_2$	H	H	NH$_2$	—	—	Green (Lange, 1967)

occur to a degree which casts doubt on conclusions drawn from "in solution" studies. Hampton (1976) has shown that the swelling of wool produced by hydroquinone falls from over 10% to less than 1% with time as colour formation reactions proceed indicating direct reaction with the wool. Reaction in the presence of ammonia has been demonstrated by Lantz and Michel (1961) and reactions with amino groups in fibres is likely.

7. Direct Hair Colourants

(a) *General* The use of oxidative and autooxidative hair colourants involves several complex chemical reactions and is based on compounds which, while they may be very carefully screened, are always open to criticism on the grounds of skin sensitization and even carcinogenicity as will be discussed later. Although the complexity of the human hair precludes the concept of any colouration process being simple, it is clear that the use of a direct dye i.e. a colouring matter giving rise to a coloured effect by virtue of its structure and adsorption rather than by chemical reactions inside the hair, offers the basis for simpler, more controllable, possibly safer hair colouration procedures.

Some of the difficulties of direct hair dyeing have been discussed already in general terms. The problem is to find a satisfactory resolution of the following factors:

(a) difficulties of fibre penetration require that small low affinity dye molecules should be used;

(b) the low degrees of dye uptake achieved require the use of dye molecules of high absorbance i.e. high colour value;

(c) the absorbance of a dye molecule generally is low if the molecular weight is low.

Investigation into the direct dyeing of human hair has consequently taken two directions. Firstly the attempt to accelerate dye diffusion rates so as to maximize dye uptake in useful dyeing times. This has been discussed already (see D.3). The second approach has been to develop low molecular weight dyes with as high an absorbance as possible.

The first direct hair colourants were introduced at the turn of the century and were based on the nitro diphenylamines. They were intended for use in conjunction with oxidation hair dyes. The scale of demand for hair colourants was not high enough to support special developments particularly for that end use and little work was carried out until the 1950 period. In the intervening period there was some exploration of the use of selected acid and basic dyes which found some outlet as temporary colourants. The reasons for the upsurge in interest are not too clear. These were the developments in solvent assisted dyeing processes (Peters and Stevens, 1956) of the mid 1950 period which may have encouraged the view that previously unsolved problems were about to be resolved. On the other hand and probably more influential was the growth in the hair colourant market including that for domestic use, this providing a more secure basis for research investment. The direct hair colourants fall into four main categories from the chemical point of view and these are discussed in turn.

(b) *Nitrodiphenylamine and related dyes*   The early products and the majority of the dyes of this type examined subsequently have been based on nitro-benzene bearing two electron donating substituents. The latter were in the first instance amino groups as in the dyes (XVIII) and (XIX) below.

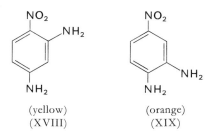

(yellow)   (orange)
(XVIII)   (XIX)

Corbett (1967a) who has studied the relationship between the colour of this group of compounds and their chemical constitutions has shown an additivity rule governs the spectral shifts produced by auxochromic groups. By suitable selection of such groups a full colour gamut can be achieved from the shade of (XV) to those of (XX) and (XXI).

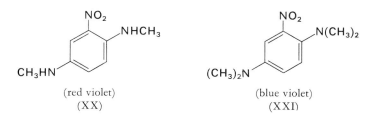

(red violet)   (blue violet)
(XX)   (XXI)

There is a strong correlation between the propensity of molecules to become involved in dispersion force interactions and their absorbance of relatively low energy radiation such as that provided within the visible spectrum (Longuet Higgins, 1965). Thus it is not surprising that dyes of high extinction show low solubility and high affinity unless some counter-vailing influence is built into their structures. Hair dyes based on very polarisable small structures such as those discussed fall into this category. This low solubility results in a low degree of adsorption and their high affinity for the hair (arising from the same cause) results in slow diffusion. The problem facing the chemist is thus one of increasing the solubility by reducing the tendency for intermolecular binding without excessively lowering the affinity and without increasing the molecular size and so putting a further constraint on diffusion in the hair. Some successes have been reported (Unilever, 1952) based on hydroxyalkylamino dyes such as (XXII) and (XXIII) below.

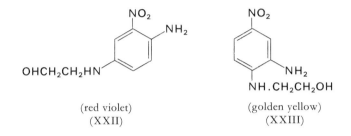

(red violet)	(golden yellow)
(XXII)	(XXIII)

Numerous related dyes have been reported since the early 1950s in which the obvious variations on this theme have been explored. An alternative approach has been to use the ε-aminoalkylamino substituents as in (XXIV) (L'Oreal, 1956a). The effect of such a substituent would not be expected to be very great. On the other hand by quaternizing the amino substituent as in (XXV) an element of charge repulsion is introduced which is helpful and at the same time the dye will show enhanced affinity for the negatively charged hair.

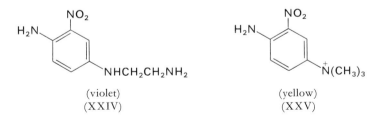

(violet)	(yellow)
(XXIV)	(XXV)

A more useful alternative is to increase the hydrophilic nature of the phenyl residue by substitution with hydroxyl to give nitroaminophenols and derivatives. Such derivatives are used fairly widely, picramic acid derivatives being particularly useful. The most important products are shown below, (XXVI–XIX).

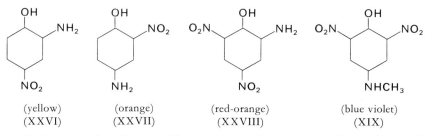

(yellow)	(orange)	(red-orange)	(blue violet)
(XXVI)	(XXVII)	(XXVIII)	(XIX)

(c) *Polynuclearquinonoid dyes*   The essential colouring ingredient of one of the most venerable hair colourants, henna is the naphthoquinone Lawsone. A number of derivatives have been reported designed to give a wider range of shades. Examples are given below,

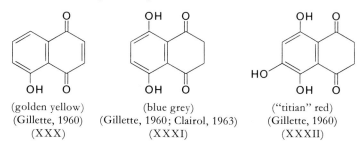

(golden yellow)	(blue grey)	("titian" red)
(Gillette, 1960)	(Gillette, 1960; Clairol, 1963)	(Gillette, 1960)
(XXX)	(XXXI)	(XXXII)

The corresponding naphthoquinoneimine dyes have also been prepared (Clairol, 1965).

The anthraquinone dyes were not seriously considered until nearly twenty years ago when there was a brief interest resulting in several patents. The anthraquinoid chromogen provides an excellent basis for blue shades which are of relatively limited interest in hair colouration. Yellow, orange and red dyes can be prepared but these tend to be of low absorbance. The molecules are in addition large and diffusion rates slow as a consequence. Two approaches have been taken, namely to produce basic dyes such as XXXIII and acid dyes from the reaction of the standard intermediate, bromamine acid, with various amines as in XXXIV.

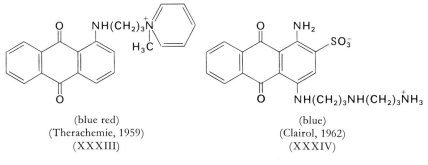

(blue red)	(blue)
(Therachemie, 1959)	(Clairol, 1962)
(XXXIII)	(XXXIV)

(d) *Azo dyes* The azo chromogen provides the basis for a full range of shades from yellow to black. If nitrodiphenylamine is diazotized and coupled with an appropriate compound then the product can be seen as a further example of a nitro dye with an aryl azo substituent (XXXV).

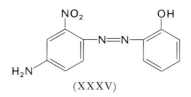

(XXXV)

However, such a large substituent inevitably brings with it problems of solubility, high affinity etc. The solubility problem has been partially solved by quaternization of the free amino group as in (XXXVI) (Therachemie, 1959).

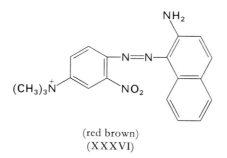

(red brown)
(XXXVI)

However, it is clear that ready diffusion of such large dye molecules in hair under salon dyeing conditions must be slow unless special means such as solvent assistance are used to accelerate the process. Thus dyes of the azo type tend to be limited in use to more temporary surface colourations as is the case with the quinonoid type of molecule previously discussed.

(e) *Reactive dyes* Dyes capable of covalent binding onto hair offer, in principle, one means of obtaining a colouration of high enough fastness to shampooing, water etc. with dye molecules of low enough molecular weight to achieve reasonable penetration of the hair in appropriate dyeing times. Investigations into the utilization of this approach have been limited, in general, to the application of the reactive dyes and the reactive systems developed for textile dyeing. Not surprisingly little success has resulted and the situation has not changed at all since Broadbent (1963) expressed the view that problems of application prevented the effective use of the reactive dye concept.

The development of reactive dyes to date has involved the use of reactive systems which operate by nucleophilic substitution or nucleophilic addition by the appropriate groups in the fibre. Such investigations as have taken place have shown that the best chance of producing rapid and efficient reaction between dyes of these types and human hair is to react with reduced thiol groups. Corbett (1965) showed that with vinyl sulphonyl reactive dyes such as (XXXVII) the ratio of reactivities of thiol, amino and hydroxy groups is $SH:NH_2:OH = 10^4:10^2:1$. The importance of the thiol groups for the production of reasonable results was also shown by Shansky who showed that reduction of the disulphide bonds in the hair and the incorporation of an antibonding solute such as urea were both necessary to produce adequate results with a monochlorotriazinyl amino azo dye (Shansky, 1966).

Generally speaking it seems improbable that dyes which will possess the necessary reactivity for fixation to be achieved in the short times available for a hair colouring operation will have the necessary stability for use as hair colourants. It seems improbable that without some surprising new discovery in fibre reactive dye technology the contribution of reactive dyes to hair colouration will remain marginal.

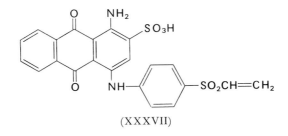

(XXXVII)

8. Superficial Hair Colouration

There is a continuing interest, as yet largely unsatisfied, in temporary or short term hair colouration whereby the applied colour may be brushed or combed out of the hair. This has stimulated cosmetic interest in a branch of colour chemistry which has been developing in recent years, the intrinsically coloured polymers. These may be produced by either of two approaches.

A polymer containing reactive side chains may be reacted with a suitable coloured compound to give a coloured substitution product. This approach is clearly related to fibre reactive dye technology since the end result of a reactive dyeing process is an intrinsically coloured cellulose protein or polyamide molecule albeit with a low degree of substitution. Polymeric bases which have been studied for hair colouration include alginic acid

(Schwarzkopf, 1967), polyacryoylchloride (L'Oreal, 1962) and glycidyl monomers (L'Oreal, 1966). In the case of alginic acid a fibre reactive dye is reacted with the hydroxyl groups of the polymer whereas in the latter two instances a dye containing an amino or a hydroxyl group may be reacted with reactive substituents in the polymer. Extensions of this approach are a matter of general organic chemistry.

A second approach is provided by using a bifunctional coloured monomer to form the polymer. Bifunctional vinylsulphonyl dyes have been used by Batty and Guthrie (Batty and Guthrie, 1975) to produce intensely coloured sulphonated polymers with interesting properties. Polyvinylanthraquinones have also been prepared (Gradwell and Guthrie, 1976). None of these products have been examined specifically for cosmetic purposes although it would not be expected that their use would involve any special considerations.

Alternatively a monofunctional dye of appropriate structure may be used in a copolymerization reaction. The second approach has been more widely explored in the cosmetic field. Typical of the cosmetic intrinsically coloured polymers are those prepared using the Primazine dyes as the coloured component (BASF, 1960) e.g. (XXXVIII).

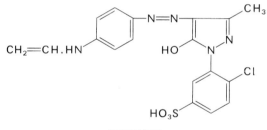

(XXXVIII)

Such dyes are copolymerized either with vinylpyrrolidone or a mixture of vinylpyrrolidine with acrylamide. Dyes containing vinylsulphonyl reactive groups e.g. (XXXVII) may be similarly used.

The incorporation of polymers of this type into hair sprays has met with some consumer resistance due to the difficulties of ensuring that coloured spray does not land on the clothing and elsewhere. For reasons which are not altogether clear this factor has not been of such importance in Australia where coloured hair sprays were at one time accepted (Root, 1960) by the consumer.

9. *Health Factors in Hair Colouration*
It has long been recognized that certain colouring matters and other organic chemicals brought into contact with the skin for significant

periods of time possess the property of sensitization in the case of individuals. The resultant skin irritation may be mild or very severe to the point of strong allergic reaction or even skin cancer. Sensitization caused by some potential hair colourants was observed in the early days and since the 1920s new products have been subjected to rigorous sensitization tests before marketing. Calman (1967) reporting on allergic reactions to cosmetic materials did not include hair colourants among his list of major complaint sources and this may arise from the care taken by hair colourant producers. However dyes remain a hazard albeit avoidable. Weissler (1974) has found in a survey of cosmetic injury complaints that dyes and colour rinses provided the basis of less than 10% of complaints in 1971 and only 3.5% in 1970. This situation is susceptible to improvement but the low level is a product of care, control and vigilance by the market leaders.

Recently great interest has been aroused by a hitherto unsuspected possible source of hazards, the absorption of hair colourants through the skin into the metabolism and possible carcinogenicity as shown by their mutagenic activity. This has led to the industry adopting a voluntary carcinogenicity testing programme in the last year or so in the absence of any official regulation (Heenan, 1974; Nader, 1974).

A study carried out by Kiese and Rauscher (1968) showed that absorption of some hair colourants through the scalp when using a simplified hair dye preparation was significant. Among the compounds studied was 2:5 diaminotoluene and its diacetyl derivative. It was found that the diacetyl derivative, for example, was excreted in the urine for two days after hair dyeing. In another study Kiese et al. (1968) demonstrated that dogs could absorb Bandrowski's base through the skin. Five years later Marshall and Palmer (1973) reported that dark urine occurred regularly following the use of some hair dyes. No evident distress or long term effects were observed. Later Wernwick et al. (1975) reported the receipt of reports of a similar nature relating to hair colourant absorption through the scalp.

The study by Wernwick et al. went on to examine the effects of feeding dyes and base components used in semipermanent hair colourants i.e. nitro dyes to various animals over a two year period. No chronic toxicity was observed in connection with dogs fed with the dyes. No effect on reproductive performance or teratologic effect was observed. However, studies by Ames et al. (1975) have produced important indirect evidence of possible carcinogenicity on the part of many hair colourant products. As with most evidence of its kind the problem remains of deciding the relationship between the undoubted laboratory observations of a particular effect and the actual medical effects involving human subjects. Ames has developed a sensitive and simple test for the detection of chemical mutagens (Ames, 1971; Ames *et al.*, 1973a; Ames *et al.*, 1973b) which has been shown to correlate very well with known carcinogenic activity. The test has been applied to a broad range of 30 commercial oxidative hair dyeing preparations. Most of the compounds used were found to be mutagenic either on their own or after peroxidation.

A number of common hair colourants such as *p*-phenylenediamine, *p*-aminodiphenylamine and *m*-aminophenol were found to be mutagenically inactive on their own against a number of Salmonella typhimurium mutants. However if the agents were pretreated with peroxide they became very active and it was found that Bandrowski's base formed by *p*-phenylenediamine under such conditions was also mutagenically active. The significance of the formation of Bandrowski's base in connection with actual hair dyeing remains unclear as has been stated previously so that the significance of the observation of peroxide activation also becomes somewhat uncertain. However 4-nitro *o*-phenylenediamine and several other compounds were active mutagens. Partial confirmation of these results has been reported by Benedict (1976) using another tester stain and also by Searle *et al.* (1975) using several tester stains. The latter investigators comment on the uncertainties regarding the relevance of mutagenic testing to human reaction but consider that a comprehensive study is needed in view of the observed indications of possible carcinogenicity.

The conclusions to be drawn from this recent work are as yet unclear since experimentation is necessarily indirect and no direct ascription of carcinogenic activity in human beings is likely to be produced. Nevertheless, the existence of a hazard has been recognized and investigation is being actively pursued.

REFERENCES

Albers, J. (1973). "Interactions of Color". Yale University Press.
Alex, W. (1975). *J. Soc. Cosmetic Chem.* **26**, 389.
Altman, M. and Rieger, M. (1968). *J. Soc. Cosmetic Chem.* **19**, 141.
Ames, B. N. (1971). *In* "Chemical Mutagens" (Ed. A. Hollaender) Vol. 1, 267. Plenum Press, New York.
Ames, B. N., Lee, F. D. and Durston, W. E. (1973a). *Proc. Nat. Acad. Sci. USA* **70**, 782.
Ames, B. N., Durston, W. E., Yamasaki, E. and Lee, F. D. (1973b). *Proc. Nat. Acad. Sci. USA* **70**, 2281.
Ames, B. N., Kammen, H. O. and Yamasaki, E. (1975). *Proc. Nat. Acad. Sci. USA* **72**, 2423.
Atkinson, J. C., Filson, A. and Speakman, J. B. (1959). *Nature* **184**, 444.

Austrian, J. A., Van Bommel, C. and Schwarz, N. (1964). *J. Soc. Cosmetic Chem.* **15**, 465.

von Auwers, K. and Borsch, E. (1915). *Ber.* **48**, 1710.

von Auwers, K. and Borsch, E. (1921). *Ber.* **54***B*, 1291.

Bandrowski, E. (1894). *Ber.* **27**, 480.

BASF A. G. (1960). British Patent Specification 877402.

Bassin, A. (1975). Proceedings Symposium "A Sensory Approach to Cosmetic Science". Soc. Cosmetic Chemists, Manchester.

Batty, N. S. and Guthrie, J. T. (1975). *Polymer* **16**, 370.

Beasley, J. K., Atkins, J. T. and Billmeyer, F. W. (1965). Proceedings 2nd Interdisciplinary Conf. "Electromagnetic Scattering". Amherst, Mass.

Benedict, W. F. (1976). *Nature* **260**, 368.

Billmeyer, F. W. and Saltzmann, M. (1968). "Principles of Color Technology". Interscience, NY.

Broadbent, A. D. (1963). *Am. Perfumer Cosmetics* **78**, 21.

Brody, F. and Burns, M. S. (1968). *J. Soc. Cosmetic Chem.* **19**, 361.

Burton, H. and Stoves, J. L. (1950). *J. Soc. Dyers & Colourists* **66**, 474.

Burton, H. and Stoves, J. L. (1951). *J. Soc. Cosmetic Chem.* **2**, 240.

Butcher, B. H. and Cussler, E. (1972). *J. Soc. Dyers & Colourists* **88**, 398.

Calman, C. D. (1967). *J. Soc. Cosmetic Chem.* **25**, 99.

Calman, C. D. (1967a). *J. Soc. Cosmetic Chem.* **18**, 215.

Cassie, A. B. D. (1960). *J. Soc. Dyers & Colourists* **76**, 617.

Clairol (1962). British Patent Specification 969377.

Clairol (1963). British Patent Specification 1003600.

Clairol (1965). British Patent Specification 1097271.

COLOUR 73 (1973). Proceedings 2nd Congress Internat. Colour Ass. York. Adam Hilger, London.

Cooley, A. J. (1868). "The Toilet in Ancient and Modern Times". Hardwicke, London.

Corbett, J. F. (1965). Proceedings 3rd Internat. Wool Res. Conf. Paris, Section 3, 321.

Corbett, J. F. (1967). *J. Chem. Soc. (C)*, 611.

Corbett, J. F. (1967a). *Spectrochem. Acta* **23A**, 2315.

Corbett, J. F. (1968). Chimia (Proceedings 3rd Internat. Symp. on Colour Chemistry) 140.

Corbett, J. F. (1969). *J. Soc. Dyers & Colourists* **85**, 71.

Corbett, J. F. (1969a). *J. Chem. Soc. (B)*, 818.

Corbett, J. F. (1970). *J. Chem. Soc. (B)* 1418.

Corbett, J. F. (1970a). *J. Chem Soc. (C)*, 2101.

Corbett, J. F. (1971). *In* "The Chemistry of Synthetic Dyes", Vol. V, (Ed. K. Venkataraman). Academic Press, New York.

Cox, H. E. (1940). *Analyst* **65**, 393.

Cronin, E. (1967). *J. Soc. Cosmetic Chem.* **18**, 681.

Cussler, E. L. and Breuer, M. M. (1972). *Nature Phys. Sci.* **235**, 74.

Cussler, E. L. and Breuer, M. M. (1972a). *A.I. Chem. E. J.* **18**, 812.

Den Beste, M. and Moyer, A. (1968). *J. Soc. Cosmetic Chem.* **19**, 595.

Dolinsky, M., Wilson, C. H., Wisneski, H. H. and Dauers, F. (1968). *J. Soc. Cosmetic Chem.* **19**, 41.

Duliere, W. L. and Raper, H. S. (1930). *Biochem. J.* **24**, 239.

Erdmann, E. (1894). *Ber.* **37**, 2906.

Erdmann, H. and Erdmann, E. (1888). German Patent Specifications 47349: 51073: 80814: 92006; 98431.

Fattorusso, E., Miniale, L. and Sodano, G. (1970). *Gazz. Chim. Ital.* **100**, 452.

Fujiwara, M., Kato, S., Yuasa, S., Morita, K. and Fujita, A. (1973). *Cosm. and Perfumer* **88**, 49.

Garn, G. M. (1948). Harvard University, Ph.D Thesis.

Gillette (1962). British Patent Specification 99210.

Gillette (1961). British Patent Specification 1012793.

Gillette (1960). British Patent Specification 889813.

Gillette (1964). British Patent Specification 959132.

Gloag, J. and Walker, C. T. (1927). "Home Life in History". Benn Bros., London.

Gradwell, A. J. and Guthrie, J. T. (1976). *Polymer* **17**, 643.

Green, A. G. (1913). *J. Chem. Soc.* **103**, 933.

Greenstein, L. M. and Bolomey, R. S. (1971). *J. Soc. Cosmetic Chem.* **22**, 161.

Hampton, G. M. (1976). University of Leeds, Ph.D. Thesis

Hardy, J. (1973). *J. Soc. Cosmetic Chem.* **24**, 423.

Head, R. D. H. and Raper, H. S. (1933). *Biochem. J.* **27**, 36.

Heenen. J. (1974). *F.D.A. Consum.* November, p. 22.

Heller, G. (1921). *Annalen* **392**, 25, 43.

Hofmann, A. W. (1863). *Jahrchem* 42.

Holmes, A. W. (1964). *J. Soc. Cosmetic Chem.* **15**, 595.

Horner, L. and Sturm, K. (1956). *Annalen* **608**, 128.

Hunter, L. D. and Wall, R. A. (1974). *Perfumer and Cosmetics* **87**, 31.

Judd, D. B., MacAdam, D. L. and Wyszecki, G. (1964). *J. Opt. Soc. Amer.* **54**, 1031, 1382.

Judd, D. B. and Wyszecki, G. (1963). "Color in Business, Science and Industry". 2nd ed. Wiley, New York.

Karrholm, M. (1956). *Text. Res. J.* **26**, 528.

Karrholm, M. (1960). *J. Text. Inst.* **51**, T1323.

Kehrmann, F. and Mattison, M. (1906). *Ber.* **39**, 135.

Kieser, M. and Rauscher, E. (1968). *Toxicol. Appl. Pharmacol.* **13**, 325.

Kieser, M., Rauscher, E. and Rachor, M. (1968). *Toxical. Appl. Pharmacol.* **12**, 495.

Kubelka, P. and Munk, F. (1931). *Z. Tech. Physik,* **12**, 593.

Kubelka, P. (1948). *J. Opt. Soc. Amer.* **38**, 1067.

Kubelka, P. (1954). *J. Opt. Soc. Amer.* **44**, 330.

Lange, F. W. (1965). *Am. Perfumer Cosmetics* **80**, 33.

Lange, F. W. (1966). *Arch. Biochim. Cosmetol* **9**, 185.

Lange, F. W. (1967). *Perfumer Ess. Oil Record* 447.

Lautz and Michel, E. (1961). *Bull. Soc. Chim. France* 2402.

Longuet-Higgins, H. C. (1965). Faraday Soc. Discussions No. 40 "Intermolecular Forces".

L'Oreal (1956). British Patent Specification 802554.

L'Oreal (1956a). British Patent Specification 812211.

L'Oreal (1957). British Patent Specification 840904.

L'Oreal (1959). British Patent Specification 857070.

L'Oreal (1962). British Patent Specification 993181.

L'Oreal (1965). Belgian Patent Specification 650836.

L'Oreal (1966). Neth. Patent Application 6605588.

Marshall, S. and Palmer, W. S. (1973). *J. Amer. Med. Ass.* **226**, 1010.

Medley, J. A. and Ramsden (1960). *J. Text. Inst.* **51**, T1311.

Möhläu, R. (1892). *Ber.* **25**, 1055.

Monnet, P. (1883). French Patent Specification 158558.

Monsegur, P. A. (1915). "Hair Dyes and their Application". Obsorne, Garrett, London.

Nader, R. (1974). *In* "Consumer Health and Product Hazards: Cosmetics and Drugs, Pesticides and Food Additives" (Eds S. S. Epstein and R. D. Grundy). MIT, Cambridge, Mass.

Newton, I. (1730). "Opticks". 4th Edn. London.

Nicolaus, R. A., Prota, G. Santacroce, C., Scherillo, G. and Sica, D. (1969). *Gazz, Chim. Ital.* **99**, 323.

Patterson, D. and Blacker, J. G. (1969). *J. Soc. Dyers & Colourists* **85**, 598.

Peters, L. and Stevens, C. B. (1957). British Patent Specification 826479.

Peters, L. and Stevens, C. B. (1956). *Dyer*, **115**, 327.

Peters, L. and Stevens, C. B. (1956a). *J. Soc. Dyers & Colourists* **72**, 100.

Peters, L. and Stevens, C. B. (1957). *J. Soc. Dyers & Colourists* **73**, 23.

Peters, L. and Stevens, C. B. (1958). *J. Soc. Dyers & Colourists* **74**, 183.

Peters, R. H. (1976). "Textile Chemistry" Vol. 3. Elsevier, Amsterdam.

Porter, J. and Fouweather, C. (1975). *J. Soc. Cosmetic Chem.* **26**, 299.

Prota, G. (1972). *In* "Pigmentation: Genesis and Biological Control" (Ed. V. Riley). Appleton-Century-Crofts, New York.

Prota, G. and Nicolaus, R. A. (1967). *Adv. Biol. Skin* **8**, 823.

Raper, H. S. (1927). *Biochem. J.* **21**, 89.

Rapidol (1959). British Patent Specification 918597.

Rattee, I. D. and Breuer, M. M. (1975). "The Physical Chemistry of Dye Adsorption". Academic Press, London.

Root, M. J. (1975). *Amer. Perf. Aromat.* **75**, 43.

Schlossmann, M. L. and Feldman, A. J. (1971). *J. Soc. Cosmetic Chem.* **22**, 599.

Schrier, E. E., Sheraga, H. A. and Ingwall, R. T. (1965). *J. Phys. Chem.* **69**, 298.

Schwarzkopf, A. G. (1967). German Patent Specification 1247552.

Searle, C. E., Hamden, D. G., Venitt, S. and Gyde, O. H. B. (1975). *Nature* **255**, 506.

Shansky, A. (1966). *Amer. Perfumer Cosmetics*, **81**, 23.

Sidi, E. and Zviek, C. (1966). "Problems of Capillaries". Gauthier Villars, Paris.

Speakman, J. B. and Smith, S. C. (1936). *J. Soc. Dyers & Colourists* **52**, 121.
Therachemie, A. G. (1959). British Patent Specification 909700.
Therachemie, A. G. (1964). British Patent Specification 1023327.
Thomson, R. H. (1974). Angewandte Chemie Internat. Edn. 13, 308.
Unilever (1952). British Patent Specification 707618.
Unilever (1965). British Patent Specification 1096943.
Wall, F. E. (1974). *In* "Cosmetics—Science and Technology" (Eds M. S. Balsan and E. Sagarin) 2nd Edn. Vol. 3. Wiley, New York.
Weissler, A. (1974). *J. Soc. Cosmetic Chem.* **25**, 99.
Wernwick, T., Lauman, B. M. and Fraux, J. L. (1975). *Toxicol. App. Pharmacol.* **32**, 450.
Wheeler, D. A., Moyler, D. A. and Thirkettle, J. T. (1975). Proceedings Symp. "A Sensory Approach to Cosmetic Science" Soc. Cosmetic Chem. Manchester.
Wilmsmann, H. (1961). *J. Soc. Cosmetic Chem.* **12**, 490.
Wilstatter, R. and Meyer, E. (1904). *Ber.* **37**, 1494.
Winthrop Chemical Co. (1939). US Patent Specification 2162458.
Wolfram, L. J. (1968). *Text Res. J.* **38**, 1144.
Wolfram, L. J., Hall, K. and Hui, I. (1970). *J. Soc. Cosmetic Chem.* **21**, 875.
Wolfram, L. J. and Lindemann, M. K. O. (1971). *J. Soc. Cosmetic Chem.* **22**, 839.
Zahn, H. and Blankenburg, G. (1964). *Text. Res. J.* **34**, 176.

DETERMINATION AND ANALYSIS OF SEBUM ON SKIN AND HAIRS

Max Gloor
Department of Dermatology,
Universitäts-Hautklinik,
Heidelberg, West Germany

I. BIOCHEMISTRY AND PHYSIOLOGY OF THE SKIN SURFACE LIPIDS AND HAIR LIPIDS

A. The Amount of the Skin Surface Lipids and Hair Lipids

The amount of skin surface lipids varies from individual to individual and from location to location. People producing large amounts of skin surface lipids are called seborrhoics, those with only slight amounts of skin surface lipids are sebostatics. The skin surface lipids are a mixture of sebaceous gland and epidermal lipids. The sebaceous gland lipids are present to a much greater quantity than the epidermal lipids. Therefore, it depends almost entirely on the amount of sebum secretion whether somebody is a seborrhoic or sebostatic. The amount of epidermal lipids is of no special importance.

The terms seborrhoea and sebostasis describe conditions which cannot be called diseases. There is no clear distinction between the so-called normal persons and either seborrhoics or sebostatics. A definition of the boundaries, of necessity, is only arbitrary. Besides, it must be emphasized that seborrhoea and sebostasis are not conditions which last an entire lifetime. Moreover, reference must already be made at this point to the fact that numerous physiological parameters and environmental factors have a decisive influence on the amount of lipid secreted during different stages of a life span. Studies by Gloor and Schnyder (1977) have shown that the amount of skin surface lipids secreted is controlled, to a great extent, by the genetic make-up of the individual.

When determining the amount of the skin surface lipids, we must take the body area into account. Most investigators are in agreement that the highest skin surface lipid concentrations are on the scalp skin and on the forehead. Apart from that, many skin lipids are also demonstrable on the face, the back and the chest. Slight amounts can be found on the extremities and on the abdomen. It is, therefore, understandable that seborrhoea manifests itself only on the scalp skin, the face, back and chest, whereas sebostasis is to be found above all on the extremities and on the abdomen (Herrmann and Prose, 1951; Jadassohn, 1963).

When determining the lipid amounts, it is important to gauge the rate of the re-fatting after de-fatting has occurred. Herrmann and Prose (1951) determined the amounts of lipid half an hour after a de-fatting of the skin has occurred, and repeated the measurement afterwards four consecutive times. By adding these values, they estimated the total lipid secretion in two hours. Secondly, they also determined the amount of lipid collected in one extraction two hours after a previous de-fatting of the skin. It could be shown that the amounts that were determined by the first method were considerably larger than those obtained by the second method. This result suggested that lipids which are present on the skin surface, inhibit the re-secretion (Gloor, Weidemann and Friederich, 1974). The replacement of the lipids after de-fatting is rapid at first and then slows down until a constant level is finally established after about 4–5 hours (Kuhn-Bussius, 1974) (Fig. 1). Similar conditions apply to the scalp skin and proximal hair parts. Figure 2 shows that replacement of oils after de-fatting by hair-washing is rapid at first, but becomes gradually slower until the pre-wash level is again reached

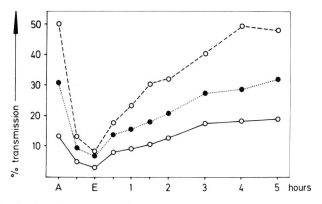

Fig. 1.   Re-fatting situation on the hairless skin of the seborrhoic type, the so-called normal type and the sebostatic type after de-fatting with plastic foil. Transmission corresponds to the lipid amounts using the frosted glass method (Kuhn-Bussius, 1974).

                    – – – – High sebaceous secretion;
                    · · · · · · Normal sebaceous secretion;
                    ——— Low sebaceous secretion.

in about 3–5 days. The re-fatting situation in the distal hair parts, also shown in the figure, indicates that the re-fatting situation is, in principle, the same, except that a time delay exists between the scalp skin and the distal hair parts (Gloor, Rietkötter and Friederich, 1973).

Interesting viewpoints have arisen when comparing the re-fatting situation in the seborrhoic and the sebostatic type: Fig. 1, taken from a publication by Kuhn-Bussius (1974), demonstrates that the pre-wash lipid levels are reached more quickly on the hairless skin by sebostatics than by seborrhoics. Gloor and Kohler (1977a) made similar findings in their investigations of the scalp.

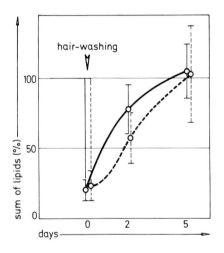

Fig. 2. Re-fatting situation of the hair-bearing scalp after hair washing. The upper line (———) demonstrates the re-fatting situation on the scalp and proximal hair portions, the lower line (– – – –) on the distal hair portions (Gloor, Rietkötter and Friederich, 1973).

The sebum excretion is greater in the seborrhoic cases than in the case of sebostatics (Fig. 3). In Fig. 4 one can see that initial lipid level in a sebostatic is reached on the fifth day after hair-washing on an average. On the other hand, the lipid values found in seborrhoic cases on the fifth day are very much lower than the initial lipid levels were before washing. We may conclude, therefore, that the re-fatting rate of the seborrhoics is more intensive, and a longer period of time passes before the initial lipid levels are again reached.

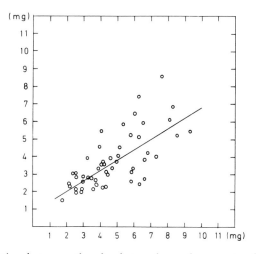

Fig. 3. Correlation between the absolute values of amounts of scalp and hair lipids and the lipids replaced within 5 days after hair washing. One may observe that there is a greater sebum secretion in the seborrhoic than in the sebostatic type (Gloor and Kohler, 1977a).

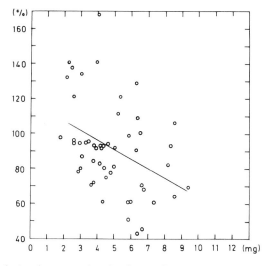

Fig. 4. Correlation between the absolute values of the amount of scalp and hair lipids and the percentage lipids replaced within five days after hair washing, expressed in percentage of the amount of removed lipids. The initial lipid level is reached on the fifth day in the sebostatic but not in the seborrhoic type (Gloor and Kohler, 1977a).

B. Composition of the Skin Surface and Hair Lipids

Skin surface lipids contain a heterogenic mixture of diverse lipids. Among these, squalene and cholesterol can be defined chemically (Fig. 5). Squalene is a precursor in the cholesterol synthesis. It has in its molecule different positions for the unsaturated groups, and no hydrophilic group at all. In contrast, cholesterol has a hydrophilic OH-group.

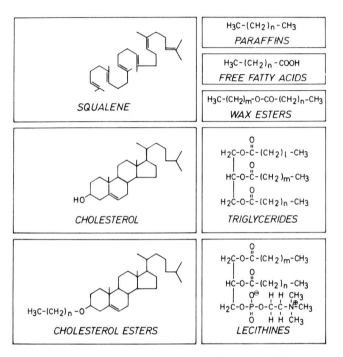

Fig. 5.   Formulae of the main compounds consisting of skin surface lipids.

Unlike squalene and cholesterol, other skin lipids are all very heterogeneous. This applies especially to the triglycerides and free fatty acids (Fig. 5). In Fig. 6, a gas chromatogram of the fatty acids is shown in skin lipids (Gloor, Kionke and Friederich, 1973). The variety of fatty acids is, in fact, even greater than depicted in the figure; it is possible to demonstrate even shorter and longer chain fatty acids, shown in Fig. 6, by means of special gas chromatographical methods. Thus, the chain length of fatty acids can vary from C8 to C22. The results, taken from the above figure, agree essentially with investigation results of numerous other authors which will, however, not be discussed in detail in this study.

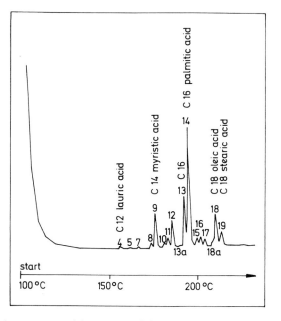

Fig. 6.   Gas chromatographic pattern of the free fatty acids of skin surface lipids (Gloor, Kionke and Friederich, 1973).

The wax and cholesterol esters are also a very heterogeneous group (Fig. 5). The chain lengths of wax esters seem to vary from C26 and C42. The gas chromatogram of wax esters (Fig. 7), taken from one of our publications (Gloor and Kionke, 1972), shows that chain lengths between C34 and C36 are regular. Grimmer, Jacob and Kimmig (1971) state that the chain lengths C16 and C18 are to be found both in acids as well as in alcohols, and that saturated as well as unsaturated alcohols and fatty acids are present. Another very exact analysis of wax esters was made by Haahti (1961), who found that the composition of the fatty acid components of the cholesterol esters were just as heterogenous as those of the wax esters.

The paraffins are another heterogenic group (Figs 5 and 8). Haahti (1961) as well as Gloor, Kionke, Strack and Friederich (1972) demonstrated by means of gas chromatography that paraffins contained chain lengths of C16 to C32 and that the distribution was almost symmetrical. (For a typical gas chromatographic pattern see Fig. 8.)

Triglycerides and cholesterol esters represent a group of substances which is mainly lipophilic and only slightly hydrophilic. Squalene and paraffins are lipophilic. Free cholesterol and the free fatty acids, on the other hand, contain a hydrophilic group as well. Therefore, they have

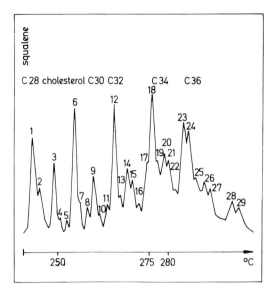

Fig. 7.   Gas chromatographic pattern of the wax esters of skin surface lipids (Gloor and Kionke, 1972).

tenside-like properties. This is of great importance for the physiology of the skin surface lipids.

The phospholipids are another fraction of skin lipids. They cannot be detected by simple thin layer chromatographic methods. Therefore, relatively little is known about this group. Important compounds in this group are the lecithines and kephalines (Fig. 5). These are glycerides in which one or two OH-groups of glycerine are linked to fatty acids. The third OH-group is linked via phosphoric acid to an alcohol—either choline (Lecithine) or cholamine (kephaline). Similarly, there is a great variety of fatty acids here. Chain lengths from C16 to C18 are mainly found. Phospholipids are relatively hydrophilic. It seems that they are only to be found in small quantities in the skin surface lipids.

The quantitative determination of the composition of skin surface lipids is mainly based on investigations by thin layer chromatography. For technical reasons, the presence of the phospholipids, as a rule, cannot usually be demonstrated by thin layer chromatography. A summary of the composition of the skin surface lipids, based on many investigations of two different age groups, can be found in Table I (Gloor, Kionke and Friederich, 1975). Considerably more free fatty acids are found in the scalp lipids than in the skin sebum. It must be re-emphasized, however, that the percentage

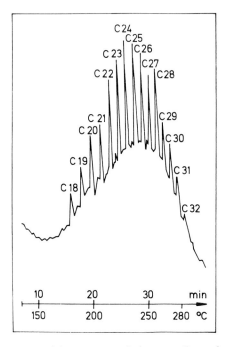

Fig. 8. Gas chromatographic pattern of the paraffins of skin surface lipids (Gloor, Kionke, Strack and Friederich, 1972).

amount can only be evaluated in relation to the test method used since differences in methods can lead to considerable differences in the results.

A detailed description of the lipogenesis would be too involved within the framework of this study. One must, however, stress that as a rule it is not possible for lipids to reach the sebaceous gland via the blood. On the contrary, nearly every single lipid molecule is re-synthesized in the sebaceous gland or in the epidermis. The lipogenesis itself seems to resemble that of other organs. Details of this cannot, however, be discussed here and can be found in the review by Downing and Strauss (1974). A dietary origin of trans-unsaturated fatty acids is discussed by Morello and Downing (1976).

Whereas all the other lipid fractions are obviously subjected to biosynthesis in the sebaceous gland and the epidermis, respectively, it is doubtful whether this also applies to paraffins. At any rate, the greatest part of paraffins contained in the skin surface lipids reach the skin through the fumes in the air. This problem has been thoroughly investigated by Gloor, Josephs and Friederich (1974). These authors found evidence for the fact that the fraction of paraffins in the skin surface lipids is greater in fume-filled areas than in fumeless areas and, moreover, that there is a great

Table I
Amount and composition of skin surface lipids in two age groups

	Male (years)		Females (years)		Total group A (n = 103)
	8–12 (n = 9)	18–80 (n = 42)	8–12 (n = 9)	18–80 (n = 38)	
Lipid level (mg/16 cm²)	0·40 (0·21)	1·50 (0·84)	0·96 (0·46)	1·57 (0·82)	1·37 (0·85)
Free cholesterol (%)	10·50 (5·75)	8·81 (2·42)	7·81 (2·93)	8·49 (3·87)	8·72 (3·43)
Free fatty acids (%)	5·71 (3·16)	24·82 (6·93)	13·49 (5·73)	21·96 (6·15)	20·89 (8·81)
Triglycerides (%)	47·60 (5·99)	30·74 (5·96)	40·28 (6·61)	34·68 (5·30)	34·65 (8·04)
Wax and cholesterol esters (%)	15·26 (33·3)	20·45 (2·34)	17·61 (3·16)	18·60 (2·95)	19·02 (3·15)
Squalene (%)	13·87 (2·11)	9·30 (3·40)	13·51 (1·15)	11·31 (5·16)	10·92 (4·23)
Paraffins (%)	6·94 (3·96)	5·84 (2·50)	7·24 (6·00)	4·99 (2·67)	5·75 (3·14)

According to Gloor, Kionke and Friederich, 1975.

dependence on the weather. Mention must also be made to the fact that the paraffins demonstrated are undoubtedly caused partly by contamination of the solutions (Josephs, Gloor and Friederich, 1974).

Free cholesterol needs special attention. Cholesterol is above all a component of the epidermal lipids; it is contained only in smaller quantities in the sebum lipids (Greene, Downing, Pochi and Strauss, 1970; Gloor, Kionke, Strack and Friederich, 1972). An increase in the percentage of free cholesterol indicates, therefore, an increase in the amount of epidermal lipids in the total lipid mixture. It is thus probable than an increase in free cholesterol can be correlated to an acceleration of the cell turnover in the epidermis and to a thickening of the stratum corneum. This is of special interest from a pharmacological point of view. A change in cell turnover in the epidermis can, thus, be estimated by the amount of cholesterol in the skin surface lipids. In certain cases this method can also be used to measure the "keratolytic" effect of drugs. This would express itself in an increase in cholesterol.

The relationship between fatty acids and triglycerides is of further importance. There are very few free fatty acids in pure sebum. Evidence for this can be found in investigations by Kellum (1967), Peter *et al.* (1970) as well as Peter *et al.* (1971). Using a special method (Kellum, 1966), these authors isolated pure sebum from skin of corpses and examined it by thin layer and gas chromatography, respectively. It seems that the free fatty acids are released from triglycerides in the sebaceous gland secretory ducts. A splitting of wax esters and cholesterol esters hardly seems to occur. This result has been documented especially in investigations by Gloor, Schultz, Wieland and Wiegand (1972) who demonstrated an indirect correlation between the amounts of free fatty acids and triglycerides but not between those of the free fatty acids and wax esters. Moreover, Haahti and Horning (1961) and Nicolaides (1961) could not demonstrate wax alcohols to any great extent on the skin surface.

By histochemical methods, Steigleder (1960) and Nicolaides and Wells (1957) found the presence of lipases in the sebaceous gland secretory ducts and on the skin surface. Essentially, these lipases are ectoferments of the saprophytic skin flora; the skin flora consists mainly of corynebacterium acnes, propionibacterium granulosum and different staphylococcus types. Extensive studies on this theme have been carried out by Pablo *et al.* (1974) and Roberts (1975). Amongst the lipases there are also lipases which are not of microbial origin and lipolytic enzymes which are released by other

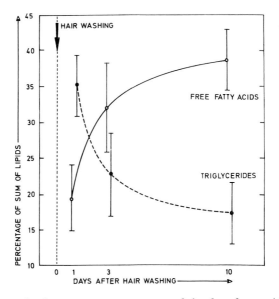

Fig. 9.   Changes in the percentage amounts of the free fatty acids and triglycerides in the scalp and hair lipids after hair washing. (Gloor and Kohler, 1977a.)

microorganisms (Brabant and Delmotte, 1959; Holt, 1971; Horáček and Pospišil, 1965; Downing, 1970). It must be stated, however, that the ectoferments of the above bacteria play a most important part.

Only relatively slight lipolysis takes place on the skin surface after the sebum have passed through the secretory ducts. It is quite different on the scalp. Numerous lipase-releasing bacteria and fungi are to be found there. For a review, see Noble and Somerville (1974). On the scalp, these bacteria cause the triglycerides to split to a much greater extent (Nicolaides and Rothman, 1953). Figure 9 shows the physiological conditions after hair washing (Gloor and Kohler, 1977a). A similar, almost complete splitting of triglycerides can also be observed in the comedone (Nicolaides *et al.*, 1970; Peter and Eichenseher, 1973; Gloor and Friederich, 1974a). Correspondingly, bacteria which release lipases can also be demonstrated in the comedone (Marples *et al.*, 1973; Whiteside and Voss, 1973).

It seems that similarly to the splitting of triglycerides, the esterification of free cholesterol in the epidermis is mainly caused by bacteria (Puhvel, 1975; Freinkel and Fiedler-Weiss, 1974). Many bacteria and fungi which release lipases can also be found on the scalp and therefore the triglycerides are split up to a considerable extent, on the scalp. In contrast, an esterification of free cholesterol by the scalp bacteria and fungi cannot be found on the scalp (Gloor and Kohler, 1977b).

C. Physiological Importance of the Skin Surface Lipids

Kligman (1963) expressed the opinion that no special role should be attributed to the skin surface lipids. To a certain extent this is correct. In particular, the protective function of the skin surface lipids against chemicals and bacteria seems to be rather weak. Although investigations by Schmidt, *et al.* (1964) support a protective function of the lipids against chemical substances, according to Gloor, Strack, Oschmann and Friederich (1972) the alkali resistance of the skin does not seem to be particularly influenced by the presence of skin lipids. The antimicrobial effect of skin lipids seems also to be small. A slight antimicrobial effect of free fatty acids has been indicated by Miescher (1960) and by other authors' work. However, this effect seems to be relatively slight under physiological conditions. It is probable that other factors play a more important part in the antibacterial and antimycotic effect on the skin surface.

Contradicting Kligman (1963), however, we are of the opinion that the skin surface lipids are not without significance as far as the water content of the stratum corneum is concerned. This is also assumed by Sulzberger and Herrmann (1960) as well as Schneider (1970). By means of resonance frequency measurement Schneider could demonstrate that skin abundant in sebum is also abundant in water, and that skin lacking in sebum is at the same time lacking in water.

It is difficult to interpret Schneider's findings. Using a variety of ointment bases, Tronnier (1962) was able to show that waterless ointments increase the water content of the stratum corneum more than do emulsions containing water. This is due probably to a semi-occlusive effect of the oil. However, it is hard to imagine that this semi-occlusive effect is also brought about by skin surface lipids. Findings by Kligman and Shelley (1958), Dvorken *et al.* (1966) and Gloor, Franz and Friederich (1973) suggest that the ability of the skin surface lipids to spread is exceptionally slight and therefore it is difficult to imagine that a continuous film similar to the one which covers the skin when lipophilic ointments are used, is formed by the skin surface lipids.

Investigations by Schneider and Schuleit (1951) have revealed another phenomena of importance. These authors found that the more skin surface lipids are present, the better the skin is moistened with water. Kleine-Natrop (1960) confirmed this in later studies. Hopf and Winkler (1959) have assumed, on the basis of *in vitro* tests, that the free fatty acids in the skin surface lipids are responsible for this effect. Using *in vivo* tests Gloor, Franz and Friederich (1973) confirmed these findings. One may, therefore, suppose that the influence on the water content of the stratum corneum by the skin lipids can be accounted for by the influence on the moistening of the horny layer keratins. It is a known fact that other factors are also responsible for the water content of the skin. In particular, hygroscopic substances must be taken into consideration.

II. ANALYSIS OF THE AMOUNTS AND COMPOSITIONS OF THE SKIN AND HAIR LIPIDS

In describing the methods of analysis, a discussion of those methods which are no longer employed will be deliberately omitted.

A. Determination of the Amount of Skin Surface Lipids and Hair Lipids

Before the different methods of quantitative lipid determination are discussed separately, the general nomenclature will be explained. Essentially, this is based on the publication by Herrmann and Prose (1951).

When using analytical methods, one must first decide whether it is necessary to consider the lipids resting on the skin, or the amounts of skin surface lipids, which are replaced as a function of time after the initial de-fatting, are to be determined.

If the amount of the skin surface lipids is measured, then one can distinguish between casual levels, total levels and retained levels of lipids. If the skin is protected from any kind of contact before lipid determination, then the total level is evaluated. If this protection is abandoned, then the casual level is measured. If the skin is wiped before determination, then the retained value is estimated. The true physiological parameter is the casual level. The casual level is, of course, always considerably lower than the total level, since even from a bare skin surface a continual abrasion of the skin surface lipids takes place. As a rule, the retained level is smaller than the casual level.

If the replacement of skin surface lipids after defatting is to be determined as a function of time, according to Herrmann and Prose (1951), we quantify the "replacement amount." However, different authors define replacement lipids in various ways. Most differences result from the fact that the period of time chosen is different. Herrmann and Prose use four time intervals of half an hour each, whereas other authors, e.g., Strauss and Pochi (1961) and Cunliffe and Shuster (1969), use three hour intervals in their determinations. As a rule, we chose two hours in our own investigations as a time limit. It is important that the interval should be taken into consideration when calculating the replacement rate since the effect of sebum secretion is greatly decreased when the amount of lipids on the skin surface is increased. Thus, the maximal secretion cannot be determined by any of these methods; perhaps Hermann and Prose's values come the nearest to the maximal secretion.

When using different determination methods for skin surface and hair lipids, distinction should be made between the physical and the extraction methods.

1. *Physical Determination Methods*

(a) *Osmium acid method*   The method was first described by Brun *et al.* (1953). It is based on the principle that a suitable absorbent paper is pressed on to the skin and then subsequently exposed to osmium acid vapours. The osmium acid stains the skin surface lipids. This staining can then be evaluated by quantitative photometric methods. Many modifications of this method can be found in the literature.

(b) *Frosted glass method*   Schäfer and Kuhn-Bussius (1970) have described a method which is based on frosted glass being pressed on to the skin and then the light permeability of the frosted glass measured. The more lipids adhere to the frosted glass, the greater the light permeability of this frosted glass will be. An exact description of this method can be found in a paper by Schäfer (1973). In the meantime, this method has become very popular. Its greatest advantage is that it is extremely simple to perform. Another advantage is that only the lipids on the skin surface are collected; there is no absorbent effect which could reach the lipids in the sebaceous gland secretory ducts.

Two important modifications of the frosted glass method must be mentioned. Eberhardt and Kuhn-Bussius (1975) have used thinner frosted glass in order to measure the lipids on hair. They pressed the frosted glass on to the hair and then, according to the original method measured the light permeability of the frosted glass. Tronnier and Kuhn-Bussius (1974) have made yet another important modification, the foil method, in which plastic foil is pressed on to the skin and the skin surface lipids adhering to the foil are measured photometrically. This technique is particularly simple and also serves as a basis for equipment on the market.

It is equally applicable to all the above physical methods for determining skin lipids that the results, obtained by various authors can only be compared with one another when exactly the same test conditions have been employed. This applies especially to the quality of paper used in the osmium acid test and to the quality of frosted glass used in the frosted glass method.

2. Extraction Methods

In contemplating the extraction methods, one must distinguish between the direct and the indirect extraction methods. In the direct extraction methods the solvent is brought into direct contact with the skin. In the indirect extraction methods the lipids are removed from the skin by other means and then collected by extraction from the corresponding material.

The direct extraction method was originally described by Carrié (1936) and also Emanuel (1936). Various modifications—which will not be described here—have been made, mainly with regards to the kind of solvent used. Honsig (1967) has published a critical discussion on this theme. He advocates the use of petrol ether. We used Honsig's technique in all our investigations.

Gloor, Rietkötter and Friederich (1973) have described a modification of the direct extraction method. They removed hair of up to 4·5 cm in length from the head and then extracted the lipids from the scalp and from the remaining 4·5 cm of hair. It is therefore possible with this method to estimate those lipids which adhere to the scalp and to the proximal 4·5 cm of hair. The method has proved to be easily reproducible in many other own experiments.

The same authors have also determined the amounts of lipid adhering to the distal hair parts by direct extraction of the hair. The hair was cut to a length of 8·5 cm and then discarded. The hair was then cut to a length of 4·5 cm and collected. The lipids adhering to these distal 4 cm of hair were estimated by extraction with petrol ether.

The paper absorption method according to Strauss and Pochi (1961) is a widely used indirect extraction method. This method has also been subjected to modification. Good variations have been described by Cunliffe and Shuster (1969). The test procedure is based on the principle that a filter paper is pressed on to the skin twice and then thrown away. Then the lipid absorbed on to a filter paper which has been in contact with the skin for 3 hours is determined. The lipids are removed from the filter paper by extraction with a solvent. It must be emphasized that the choice of paper used in this test is of extreme importance since the absorbency of different types of paper varies considerably (Cunliffe et al., 1975). Essentially, the direct extraction methods obtain higher results than the paper absorption method.

For quantitative measurement of the extracted lipids, almost all the authors employ gravimetrical measuring techniques. Other methods are no longer utilized.

3. *Morphometrical Estimation of the Size of the Sebaceous Gland*
Only brief mention will be made of these methods as they are practically only of importance in animal experiments. The amount of lipid secretion from a sebaceous gland correlates well (as a rule) with its size. In particular, the sebum secretion after test by drugs generally depends on the size of the sebaceous glands. For this reason numerous authors have studied the size change of glands.

B. Estimation of the Composition of the Skin Surface Lipids and Hair Lipids

1. *Collection of the Investigation Material*
The direct extraction method and the indirect extraction method according to Strauss and Pochi (1961) may be equally employed in obtaining the material to be examined. However, other methods may also be considered. As early as 1927 Schnur and Goldfarb obtained lipids by wiping the skin with a fat-free sponge soaked in a suitable solvent. This method has been utilized by other authors. Horáček (1953) objected to the fact that uncontrolled extractions occur with this technique, especially from the lower parts of the epidermis. Despite this objection, Cunliffe has used this method recently (1976) on a large scale in order to analyse the composition

of skin surface lipids. According to Cunliffe (1976), this procedure provides reproducible results.

Recently Gloor and Kohler (1977c) have utilized the frosted glass method with the aim of gaining material for the analysis of the composition of the skin surface lipids. As opposed to other methods, this procedure has the advantage that it only includes the surface lipids on the skin. All the other methods include the epidermal lipids and the lipids in the sebaceous gland secretory ducts to a more or less greater extent. Mention should also be made to the fact that the direct extraction method can also be used in a modified form in order to obtain lipids from animals: the greatest part of the skin surface of the animal is extracted (Archibald and Shuster, 1970).

It is of extreme importance to consider the manner in which the lipids are recovered if the lipid composition is to be evaluated. Cunliffe *et al.* (1971) and Josephs *et al.* (1974) compared the direct extraction method with the paper absorption method. They agreed that the epidermal lipids, and especially free cholesterol, are recovered to a lesser extent by paper absorption than by direct extraction methods. This also applies to the paraffins which are concentrated in the stratum corneum although they are of exogenous origin (Gloor, Josephs and Friederich, 1974). On the other hand, the sebum lipids, and of these especially squalene and wax esters, are obtained to a greater extent by the paper absorption method.

The sponge method fundamentally provides results similar to those obtained by the direct extraction method. The frosted glass method has not yet been investigated in this respect. From latest investigations by Gloor and Kohler (1977c), it may be assumed that epidermal and sebaceous duct lipids are gained to an even lesser extent by the frosted glass method than by the paper method and that more sebaceous duct than epidermal lipids can be extracted by the paper absorption method.

2. *Thin Layer Chromatography*

In the analysis of skin surface lipids the method of thin layer chromatography has proved itself to be of great significance. Since this method has been available a vast amount of investigations dealing with the composition of the skin surface lipids has been published. On the one hand, this is due to the fact that thin layer chromatography makes an accurate quantitative analysis of the total lipid mixture possible and, on the other hand, to the fact that the investigation procedure is relatively simple. The procedures used by the various authors do not basically differ very much. The variations refer mainly to the different preparation of the plates and to the choice of solutions. An example of such investigations may be found in the publications of Greene *et al.* (1970), Cotterill *et al.* (1971b) as well as Gloor, Schulz, Wieland and Wiegand (1972). The procedure which we employ is fundamentally based on the micro-slide method according to Van Gent (1968).

The following fractions can be clearly differentiated by thin layer chromatographical analyses: free cholesterol, free fatty acids, triglycerides, wax and cholesterol esters, squalene and paraffins. One disadvantage of this procedure is that the fraction of wax esters cannot be clearly distinguished from the fraction of cholesterol esters. Moreover, it is common to all thin layer chromatographical methods that a further separation of the fatty acids, triglycerides, wax esters and cholesterol esters is not possible. It must be noted furthermore, that other lipids, although in small amounts, can be contained in the above fractions.

Haahti et al. (1963) have described a modification to this procedure which is worthy of mention because it allows a separation of the phospholipids. They employed silicic gel plates impregnated with silver nitrate. Mention must also be made of a modification which is widely used at present in East European countries, i.e., chromatography is carried out on silicic gel bound to glass fibres (Černiková, 1960).

3. Gas–Liquid Chromatography

The main advantage of gas–liquid chromatography, as opposed to thin layer chromatography, is above all in the fact that it allows a much more differentiated separation of the skin surface lipids than does thin layer chromatography. On the other hand, it is much more difficult to obtain a quantitative evaluation and determination of percentages of the lipid fractions of the total lipid mixture, since it is generally necessary to isolate the lipid class to be examined prior to gas chromatography. Finally, the investigation procedure requires more time and outlay than the technique of thin layer chromatography.

4. Other Chromatographical Methods

Nowadays, paper chromatographical methods are basically of historical importance only. This also applies to column chromatographic investigations. These are, however, used for the pre-fractioning of the lipids for gas–liquid chromatography.

5. Infra-red Spectroscopy

With regards to the technique of infra-red spectroscopy reference is made to the publication of Anderson and Fulton (1973). Infra-red spectroscopy enables a particularly good determination of the percentage amounts of free fatty acids and triglycerides. Thus, one can estimate the relationship between these two fractions relatively well. Shalita et al. (1975) have reported on comparative investigations between thin layer chromatography and infra-red spectroscopy. These authors are of the opinion that thin layer chromatography is more accurate. It must, however, be noted that infra-red spectroscopy is important in particular for extensive investigations, as it is simple and can be performed without much time and outlay.

III. INFLUENCE OF HEREDITARY AND ENVIRON-MENTAL FACTORS ON THE SKIN SURFACE LIPIDS

A. Amount of the Skin Surface and Hair Lipids

It is necessary to assume right from the beginning that genetic factors influence the amount of skin surface lipids. However, it is not definitely clear whether these genetic influences are of any great importance or not. This problem can only be resolved by means of investigating twins. Recently, Gloor and Schnyder (1977) reported such an investigation and found that the differences between identical twins are significantly less than in the case of binovular twins, suggesting that a genetic influence on the amount of skin surface lipid excretion does exist. Moreover, the data indicate that these influences are of considerable magnitudes.

On the other hand there is no doubt that environmental factors are of great importance on skin surface lipids. This becomes evident on contemplating investigation results by Gloor, Handke, Baumann and Friederich (1975). These authors were able to demonstrate that the amount of skin surface lipid is subjected to considerable changes depending on the time of year. The values can be seen in detail in Fig. 10. In particular, the amount of skin surface lipid is much less in winter than in summer. Kuhn-Bussius (1974) also found similar results.

The dependence of sebum excretion on temperature can be taken as an explanation for this finding. This dependence has been confirmed by numerous authors. Amongst the many publications, mention must be made of Miescher and Schönberg (1944), Dünner (1946) as well as Cunliffe et al. (1970). It may thus be supposed that this influence on sebum excretion is brought about in the first place by changes in the consistency of the lipids dependent on the skin temperature. The opinion that perspiration essentially influences sebum excretion can no longer be accepted (Kligman and Shelley, 1958; Ikai and Nitta, 1962).

Climatic factors can, however, influence sebum secretion in different ways. This has been impressively demonstrated by Williams et al. (1974). They revealed that the diameter of the sebum secretory ducts is also de-

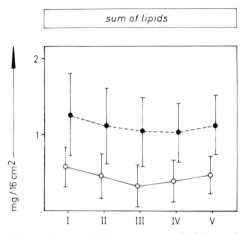

Fig. 10.   Seasonal dependence of the amount of skin surface lipids (Gloor, Handke, Baumann and Friederich 1975) – – – Casual level ———Replacement sum. I: 16.8.1973; II: 20.10.1973; III: 18.1.1974; IV: 22.3.1974; V: 24.6.1974.

pendent on the humidity of the air. This dependence can be explained by the influence on hydration of keratin.

Another important factor influencing sebum secretion is light. Korenev (1965) was able to show in animal experiments that radiation therapy with ultraviolet light can have an inhibiting as well as a stimulating effect on sebum secretion. Corner (1966) was of the opinion that a high dose of light radiation in the Antarctic can produce an inhibition of the sebum secretion. According to Okido *et al.* (1974) a single dose of ultraviolet-light in humans can increase the sum of epidermal lipids with unchanged sebum secretion. By means of light application, closely corresponding to that used in acne therapy, Gloor and Karenfeld (1977) could demonstrate that sebum lipids and epidermal lipids increase after such a treatment.

Besides the environmental factors other factors assuredly play a part in sebum secretion. This is especially indicated by the fact that sebum secretion is strongly dependent on age. Gloor, Kionke and Friederich (1975) and Gloor, Oschmann and Friederich (1973) have presented findings referring to wide-spread investigation material. They were able to show that sebum secretion is slight in a child, increases in puberty and then decreases with age. This finding is in agreement with clinical experiences and results of numerous other authors who will, however, not be discussed in detail here. The influence of the sex is the most interesting finding in the above paper. Whereas, no significant differences could be demonstrated in adults between men and women, there were fewer skin surface lipids in the males than in the females of the 8–12 year old group. One can only interpret these results by the fact that puberty sets in later in the male sex than in the female. These results can be found in detail in Table I. As opposed to our findings, Cotterill *et al.* (1972b) found in adults lower lipid amounts in women than in men. This was probably caused by the fact that we evaluated the steady state, whereas these authors determined the secretion rate. In addition results of Agache *et al.* (1977) must be pointed out which are showing that in the first week of life sebum secretion is relatively high.

All these results indicate an influence of endocrine factors on sebum secretion. Extensive literature exists on this problem. Recent good reviews can be found by Ebling (1974) and Pochi and Strauss (1974). All these findings have shown that, in principle, androgens effect a stimulation of sebum secretion. However, this influence of androgen application remains ineffective in a healthy young man since his sebum secretion has obviously had maximum stimulation (Winkler, 1972). In contrast, sebum secretion can be stimulated by the application of androgens to senior males and to castrates (Smith and Brunot, 1961; Pochi and Strauss, 1974). This also applies to women. This is indicated by the clinical observation that application of anabolics to women frequently causes an increase in sebum secretion (Winkler, 1972). With regards to this, it must also be stressed that androgens in the skin are subjected to physiological changes and that this metabolism is definitely of special importance for the physiology of sebum secretion (Ebling *et al.*, 1973; Hay and Hodgins, 1974).

On the other hand oestrogens seem to inhibit sebum secretion. It is not so much that the oestrogens reduce the mitotic rate in the sebaceous gland but that they intervene with the lipogenesis. Amongst the female sex hormones it is the gestagens which also influence sebum secretion. This influence of gestagens cannot be evaluated as a whole. It does seem at least that many gestagens stimulate sebum secretion. It is probable that this is the cause of stimulation of sebum secretion during pregnancy (Burton *et al.*, 1975b).

Recently, anti-androgens have been the subject of especial interest. Anti-androgens do not occur under physiological conditions. They can, however, be used for experimental and also therapeutic purposes. They have an inhibiting effect on sebum secretion. The mechanism of anti-androgens differs from that of oestrogens in that the mitotic rate in the sebaceous gland is reduced more and the lipogenesis influenced less (Ebling, 1970). Extensive literature exists on anti-androgens but only the publications by Lutsky *et al.* (1975) and Burton *et al.* (1973) will be mentioned here.

Moreover, other hormones exert influence on sebum secretion. The mechanism has been described in many different ways and will not be discussed any further here. Striking clinical observations on acromegaly and hypopituitarism have documented this (Burton *et al.*, 1972; Goolamali *et al.*, 1973; Goolamali *et al.*, 1974). There are also numerous publications dealing with the influence of the hormones of the thyroid and adrenal gland. There is, however, no uniform opinion on this problem. Finally, reference is made to the publication of Goolamali and Shuster (1974) who were able to demonstrate that tumours of the breast effect an increase in sebum secretion. The above paper reveals that other hormone-like substances exist which also influence sebum secretion.

The influence of nutrition on sebum secretion has not yet been clarified. According to Pochi *et al.* (1970) extensive fasting may lead to a decrease in sebum secretion. In contrast, a diet rich in fats and carbohydrates causes an increase in sebum secretion (Förster *et al.*, 1973). It is, however, questionable whether nutritional habits which are described as "normal" are of influence on sebum secretion. From our own results one may assume the opposite (Gloor, Oschmann and Friederich, 1973).

Finally, the influence of the central nervous system claims our interest. Sebum secretion is, in fact, independent of the nervous system. This has been especially emphasized by investigations of Gloor and Friederich (1970) on the human skin grafts. On the other hand, increased sebum secretion can be found in Parkinson's disease and in epilepsy (Grasset and Brun, 1959; Burton *et al.*, 1973a). Publications by Burton *et al.* (1971) and Summerly *et al.* (1971) indicate a possible influence of pareses.

In this respect, factors influencing the hair lipids are of particular importance. Gloor, Weidemann and Friederich (1974) were able to show that sebum secretion is greater on the head of males when the hair is longer. Gloor, Schemel and Friederich (1975) have shown that re-fatting of the hair occurs to a much greater extent when the hair has been blown dry than when it has been left to dry in the air. These results can be explained by the re-fatting control situation on the head. One part of the lipids, however, seems to cling to the hair pilum. This "wick" effect seems to be effective long enough for the hair to be completely re-fatted. As long as this "wick" effect exists the lipids present on the scalp cannot lead to a complete subsidence of sebum depletion.

This interpretation would explain our findings: The longer the hair, the longer time is needed until the hair is completely re-fatted and correspondingly the "wick" effect of the hair remains longer. Moreover, blowing the hair dry with a hair dryer seems to slow the replacement of the lipids on the hair. Accordingly, the "wick" effect of the hair remains longer after blow drying the hair and thus sebum secretion is stimulated more than when the hair is left to dry in the air.

B. Composition of the Skin Surface Lipids

As yet no information has been given in the literature as to the influence of genetic factors on the composition of the skin surface lipids. The only method, suitable for clarifying such questions, is an investigation carried out on twins. As there are definite correlations between the amount of skin surface lipids and the composition of the lipids (Gloor, Schulz, Wieland and Wiegand, 1972b; Gloor, Kionke, Strack, and Friederich, 1972) and as, on the other hand, the lipid amount is subjected to genetic influences (Gloor and Schnyder, 1977) it is not possible to approach this problem with the above method because a dependence of sebum composition on genetic factors results from these facts alone.

On the other hand, the importance of environmental factors is demonstrated in investigations by Gloor, Handke, Baumann and Friedrich (1975). As can be seen in Fig. 11, seasonal factors produce great changes in all the fractions of the skin surface lipids. It is difficult to interprete these changes separately. This also applies to the concentration of the free fatty acids which is dependent on the time of day, as has been pointed out by Cotterill et al. (1973).

Amongst the environmental factors an essential influence on the lipid composition has been mainly attributed to light reactions. Investigators are in agreement that ultraviolet radiation of the skin obviously produces an increase in the free and also total cholesterol (Ohkido et al., 1974; Gloor and Karenfeld, 1977). It is probable that this finding is correlated with the thickening of the stratum corneum under the influence of light which Miescher already indicated in 1931. Furthermore, it is not a reduction in the free fatty acids that is achieved by ultraviolet-radiation—as would theoretically be expected on account of the bactericide effect of light and on account of the significance of bacterial lipases for the release of free fatty acids from triglycerides—but an increase in free fatty acids is produced instead (Gloor and Karenfeld, 1976).

It is a well-known fact that light influences the vitamin D_3 synthesis in the epidermis. This has been documented for example in investigations by Rauschkolb et al. (1969) and Wheatley and Reinertson (1958). In this respect it is worth noting that lipoperoxydes are released under the influence of ultraviolet-light (Meffert and Reich, 1969). Other results referring to the influence of light on lipid composition have not produced uniform opinions and will not be discussed further in this study.

Age and sex are also of influence on lipid composition. This is evident in investigation findings by Gloor, Kionke and Friederich (1975), as described in Table I. One may observe that there are considerable differences

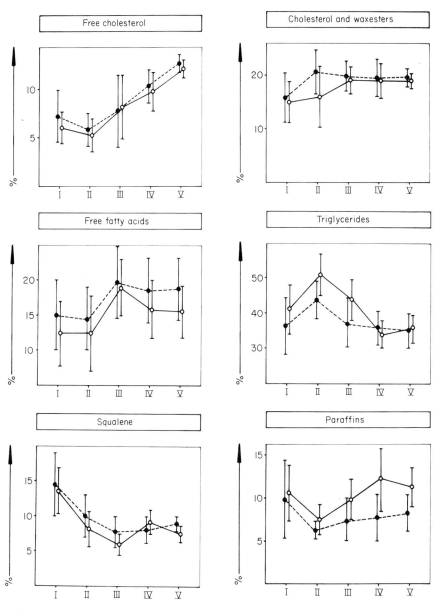

Fig. 11.　Seasonal dependence of the composition of skin surface lipids (Gloor, Handke, Baumann and Friederich, 1975)

I: 16.8.1973;
II: 20.10.1973;
III: 18.1.1974;
IV: 22.3.1974;
V: 24.6.1974.

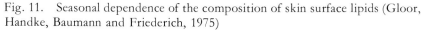

– – – Causal level　――― Replacement sum.

between children and adults and that moreover differences in the children can also be demonstrated between the sexes. The high reduction of free fatty acids in childhood before puberty is particularly impressive. This can be correlated to the occurrence of corynebacterium acnes which undergoes a great elevation during puberty. Next to the koagulase-negative staphylo-cocci and propionibacterium granulosum, corynebacterium acnes is known to be the bacteria which mainly releases lipases into the sebaceous gland secretory ducts. Attention must be given to the publication by Peter *et al.* (1971) who revealed a vast amount of alterations in the composition of the pure content of the sebaceous glands during the course of a lifetime. For details one must refer to the original publication.

Hormones have also been described as having an influence on the lipid composition. The findings are, however, still debatable but it does seem that essential importance is attributed to insulin. This is particularly evident in studies by Gloor, Marckardt and Friederich (1975) which reveal that the free fatty acids are increased in a badly adapted diabetic but that this increase can be almost normalized by a better adaptation of the metabolic disturb-ance.

As yet the literature has not presented a uniform description of the influence of nutrition on the lipid composition. Attention must be given in this respect firstly to the publication by McDonald (1973) who demon-strated that a diet mainly containing unsaturated carbohydrates, produces a reduction in glycerides and cholesterol in males and secondly to Pochi *et al.* (1970) who showed that fasting not only produces a reduction in sebum secretion but also a reduction in the relative amounts of all the lipid fractions to the advantage of squalene. There are also psychosomatic influences on the release of free fatty acids (Kraus, 1970).

It must also be noted in this context that exact data and systematic investigations *in vivo* on the influence of various environmental factors on the bacterial lipolysis still need to be carried out. There are no accurate results in the literature which could estimate the influence of environ-mental factors on the saprophytic skin flora in the sebaceous gland secretory ducts which in their turn are essential for bacterial lipolysis. It is still an unsolved problem as to how far genetic factors influence the saprophytic skin flora. From investigations by Roberts (1975) dependence on environ-ment seems very likely.

IV. SKIN SURFACE LIPIDS UNDER PATHOLOGICAL CONDITIONS

A. Changes in the Skin Surface Lipids in Seborrhoea Oleosa and Seborrhoea Sicca

Restrictively speaking, it must be re-emphasized—as stressed in a previous chapter—that the classification of seborrhoea oleosa and seborrhoea sicca as pathological conditions is not justified, but that they are rather extreme variants. Nevertheless, these changes will be discussed in this chapter.

In the past importance of seborrhoea oleosa and seborrhoea sicca has been greatly overrated. One spoke of a so-called seborrhoic syndrome into which those diseases, attributed to be correlated with seborrhoea, were classified. Nowadays, it can be accepted as certain that there is only a correlation between acne vulgaris and seborrhoea. However, the significance of seborrhoea oleosa and seborrhoea sicca, respectively, is far greater for cosmetic chemistry than for the pathogenesis of dermatological diseases. Persons with seborrhoea oleosa complain of enlarged pores and a greasy shine to the facial skin. Whereas seborrhoea oleosa thus induces the persons in question to consult a doctor or beautician, seborrhoea sicca has no such relevant importance for the appearance of the skin. In contrast to seborrhoea oleosa the facial skin has no greasy shine.

Statements in the literature on the amount and composition of the skin surface lipids are contradictory. This partly results from the fact that corresponding investigations were performed at a time when there were no adequate and accurate methods for the analysis of lipid composition, and because it requires a great deal of experience to classify test persons accurately as persons suffering from seborrhoea oleosa and seborrhoea sicca. The most exact statements on this problem may be found in the publication by Gloor, Breitinger and Friederich (1973). These authors cooperated with an experienced beautician and used the opinion of this beautician in the clinical classification of the definite skin types of the test persons.

Figure 12 shows the results of these authors from which one may see that the lipid amounts are practically identical in seborrhoea oleosa and seborrhoea sicca. In both cases they are considerably greater than the average amount expected in control persons of corresponding age and sex. In each case one must therefore determine that seborrhoea sicca is not identical with sebostasis.

When considering the composition of the skin surface lipids, it is striking that free cholesterol as well as free fatty acids increase in persons with

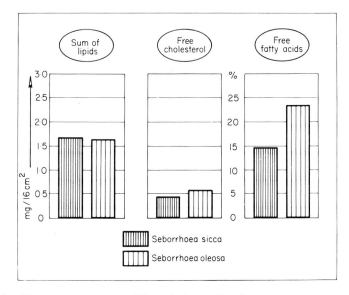

Fig. 12. Percentage amount of free cholesterol and percentage amount of free fatty acids on the non hair-bearing skin of persons with seborrhoea oleosa and seborrhoea sicca (according to Gloor, Breitinger and Friederich, 1973).

seborrhoea oleosa compared with persons with seborrhoea sicca. There is also a considerable difference in the quantity of free fatty acids. The other lipid fractions are increased more in seborrhoea sicca than in seborrhoea oleosa. Free cholesterol and free fatty acids are the only fractions in the skin surface lipids which demonstrate hydrophilic components and thus possess tenside-like qualities. Accordingly, one may assume that this can produce the differing clinical symptoms for seborrhoea oleosa and seborrhoea sicca. This is probable, especially since we know from studies by Gloor, Franz and Friederich (1973a) that the moistening of the skin with water depends on the percentage amounts of these tenside-like components.

Korolev (1958) arrived at similar results based on paper chromatographical investigations. This author also found an increased amount of free fatty acids in seborrhoea oleosa and a reduced amount in seborrhoea sicca. The opinion of this author that more cholesterol can be found in seborrhoea sicca than in seborrhoea oleosa is not consistent with our findings. Horáček (1965) states that the lipids are significantly reduced in seborrhoea sicca compared with a control group. One must therefore suspect that in these studies, test persons with sebostasis were included in the group of seborrhoea sicca. Therefore, the analysis of lipid composition by this author will not be discussed further.

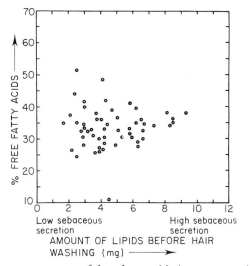

Fig. 13.   Percentage amounts of free fatty acids in persons with high and low sebaceous secretion in the scalp and hair lipids (Gloor and Kohler, 1977a).

It is also worth noting the analyses dealing with the composition of fatty acids in seborrhoea oleosa and seborrhoea sicca. From gas chromatographical investigations by our group of workers, it may be assumed that there are no significant differences between seborrhoea oleosa and seborrhoea sicca (Gloor, Kionke and Friederich, 1973). Thus, they were not able to confirm the results of Korolev (1958) who had found a varying fatty acid composition in test persons with seborrhoea oleosa as compared with test persons with seborrhoea sicca.

The situation on the scalp skin is different. Figure 13 taken from a publication by Gloor and Kohler (1977a) documents that the free fatty acids always demonstrate relatively high values in a seborrhoic type. The clinical picture of seborrhoea sicca with fatty acid values around 15% only occur rarely under physiological conditions but relatively often under the influence of drugs.

B. Acne Vulgaris

Correlations between the amounts and composition of skin surface lipids and acne vulgaris have long been subject of discussions. It is generally known that acne vulgaris manifests itself mainly in regions containing numerous sebaceous glands and that it especially afflicts those age groups where sebum secretion is particularly high.

According to the literature, it is debatable whether seborrhoea is present in acne vulgaris. Recent studies have clarified this question definitely. It may now be accepted that the amounts of lipid are significantly greater in persons with acne vulgaris than in healthy people of the same age and sex. The articles by Burton and Shuster (1971), Tronnier and Brunn (1972), Gloor, Graumann, Kionke, Wiegand and Friederich (1972), Azar et al. (1975) and Cooper et al. (1976) are but a few of the numerous publications on this theme. All the investigators are of the opinion that it is the rule for correlations to exist between the degree of severity of the acne and the extent of the seborrhoea. There are by all means cases of acne where a seborrhoea is not present. Seborrhoea must, therefore, be a partial factor in the pathogenesis of acne vulgaris. It is possible that the increased fraction of squalene in the skin surface lipids of the seborrhoic type plays a part (Summerly et al., 1976). From animal studies it may be assumed that squalene has a comedonogenic effect (Kligman et al., 1970).

Great interest has been given to the free fatty acids in the skin surface lipids, especially since studies have shown that free fatty acids, and among these, mainly the saturated medium-chained ones, have a comedonogenic effect (Lorincz et al., 1968; Kligman et al., 1970). Moreover, another series of studies document that free fatty acids with chain lengths less than C12 can cause inflammatory stimulation (Strauss and Pochi, 1965 and 1968; Kellum, 1968). As a result of these experiments, it was deduced in the past that essential pathogenetic importance for acne vulgaris could be attributed to the free fatty acids.

Doubts about this hypothesis have arisen since investigations on the amount of free fatty acids in the skin surface lipids of patients with acne. All the investigators agree that the free fatty acids are not increased in acne vulgaris; they are reduced instead (Vecova and Picin, 1971; Tronnier and Brunn, 1972; Gloor, Graumann, Kionke, Wiegand and Friederich, 1972; Cotterill et al., 1972a). The complete lipolysis in the comedo, which has been demonstrated by numerous authors (Nicolaides et al., 1970; Felger, 1969; Gershbein et al., 1970; Peter and Eichenseher, 1973; Gloor and Friederich, 1974b), cannot be taken as an explanation for the formulation of inflammatory acne efflorescences, since any blockage in the sebaceous gland secretory duct can lead to a similar result without any inflammatory changes near the comedo and sebaceous gland, respectively. This has been indicated by studies of Gloor and Friederich (1974a and b) on Morbus Favre Racouchot and on the Nevus sebaceous where inflammatory changes are never seen. The same applies to the content of large sebaceous glands on the nose (Nicolaides, 1965). In this context it must be briefly mentioned that numerous authors have demonstrated Corynebacterium acnes and Propionibacterium granulosum in the comedo content of acne vulgaris as well as of

Morbus Favre Racouchot (Marples *et al.*, 1973; Whiteside and Voss, 1973; Izumi *et al.*, 1973).

There has also been discussion as to whether changes in the composition of fatty acids play an important part in acne vulgaris (Gloor and Kionke, 1972; Tronnier and Brunn, 1972). This must, however, be rejected as a result of more recent studies by various authors (Runken *et al.* (1969), Kellum and Strangfeld, 1972; Lantz *et al.*, 1972; Gloor, Kionke and Friederich, 1973). Thus, in agreement with the early publication by Boughton *et al.* (1959) one may assume nowadays that the composition of the fatty acids is not altered in acne vulgaris.

New studies on free fatty acids have appeared recently. Gloor and Haberdank (1976) have applied *C. acnes* and *P. granulosum* orally. As a result they found a great reduction in the inflammatory and an increase in the non-inflammatory acne efflorescences. A considerable increase in the free fatty acids at the cost of the triglycerides corresponded to this. Based on these investigations, it may be assumed that the comedonogenic effect of the free fatty acids, which was demonstrated in model studies, also applies *in vivo*. On the other hand, it does not seem probably that the free fatty acids produce a stimulatory effect on inflammation. The latter mentioned is also consistent with findings by Fulton *et al.* (1975) which revealed that local application of a lipase inhibitor does reduce the free fatty acids considerably but does not effect a clinical improvement in the acne vulgaris *per se*, and with findings by Puhvel and Sakamoto (1977) which showed that intra-cutaneous injection of free, fatty acids in concentrations corresponding to the physiological concentrations in sebaceous gland ducts does not produce more than a very mild inflammatory reaction.

On the other hand, it appears that *C. acnes* and *P. granulosum* are of importance for the pathogenesis of acne vulgaris in a different, still unknown way. This is emphasized by the fact that numerous therapeutic measures leading to a reduction in the number of germs of these bacteria also produce a clinical improvement in the inflammatory acne efflorescences. It is possible that immunological mechanisms are involved here. It has also been discussed that other ectoferments than the lipases or a chemotactic factor can play a part (Haegele *et al.*, 1973; Gloor and Haberdank, 1976; Edwards *et al.*, 1975b; Gould *et al.*, 1977). Since the lipases responsible for splitting the free fatty acids are in the first place ectoferments of the above bacteria, a reduction in free fatty acids by a therapeutic measure can indicate the therapeutic efficacy of this drug on inflammation although no fundamental significance can be attributed to free fatty acids for the pathogenesis of inflammatory acne efflorescences. It may, however, suggest that the number of germs in *C. acnes* and *P. granulosum* is reduced.

Moreover, numerous publications have appeared dealing with other fractions of the skin surface lipids in acne vulgaris. The results of these publications are difficult to interpret and are at times conflicting and will therefore not be discussed any further.

C. Dysseborrhoic Dermatitis and Rosacea

Numerous authors have studied the skin surface lipids in dysseborrhoic dermatitis. Mention must be made in this context to the investigations by Hodgson-Jones *et al.* (1952 and 1953); Horacek (1965); Gloor, Wiegand and Friederich (1972); Marchionini *et al.* (1938); Konrád and Černiková (1963); Pye *et al.* (1977). These investigators are in agreement in that a seborrhoea does not have to be present in dysseborrhoic dermatitis and, except for Pye *et al.* (1977), that the epidermal lipids—and these of especially free cholesterol and paraffins—are increased on the healthy skin of patients with dysseborrhoic dermatitis whereas the relative fraction of the sebum lipids—and here especially squalene, and wax esters—is reduced in the skin surface lipids (Fig. 14). Moreover, a reduction in the fraction of free fatty acids to the advantage of the triglycerides could be determined (Fig. 15). This result could probably account for the fact that the skin of patients with dysseborrhoic dermatitis seems to be dry. Besides, this result could also indicate a disturbance in the microflora of the skin which at the present moment is being considered as a pathogenetic factor in dysseborrhoic dermatitis. Emphasis must again be placed on the fact that in analyses of the composition of fatty acids (Boughton *et al.*, 1959; Hodgson-Jones *et al.*, 1953) a decrease in the saturation degree of fatty acids has been demonstrated. It does, however, seem difficult to find an interpretation for this result which would be of any significance for the pathogenesis of dyssseborrhoic dermatitis.

Studies on the skin surface lipids in rosacea, as reported by Gloor, Wiegand, Baumann and Friederich (1974), Burton *et al.* (1975a) and Pye *et al.* (1976) are of interest. As a result of our investigations, it must be assumed that the amount of lipids and the ratio of epidermal lipids to sebaceous gland lipids are almost identical to that of dysseborrhoic dermatitis (Fig. 14). On the other hand the relation free fatty acids/triglycerides seems to be different in these diseases (Fig. 15). These findings seem to be of particular interest since Unna (1921) was able to demonstrate as early as 1921 that a distinct correlation exists between rosacea and dysseborrhoic dermatitis. Our results were, however, only confirmed by results of Burton *et al.* (1975) and Pye *et al.* (1976) as far as the amounts of lipids were concerned.

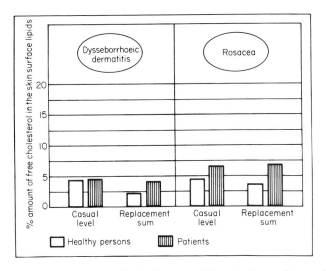

Fig. 14. Percentage amounts of the fraction of free cholesterol in patients with dysseborrhoic dermatitis and patients with rosacea, compared with healthy persons of the same age and sex (according to Gloor, Wiegand and Friederich, 1972 and Gloor, Wiegand, Baumann and Friederich, 1974).

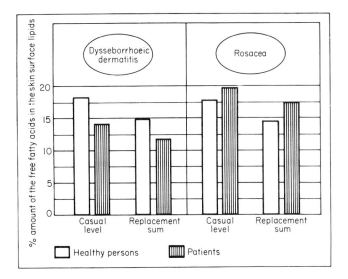

Fig. 15. Percentage amounts of the fraction of free fatty acids in patients with dysseborrhoic dermatitis and patients with rosacea, compared with healthy persons of the same age and sex (according to Gloor, Wiegand and Friederich, 1972 and Gloor, Wiegand, Baumann and Friederich, 1974).

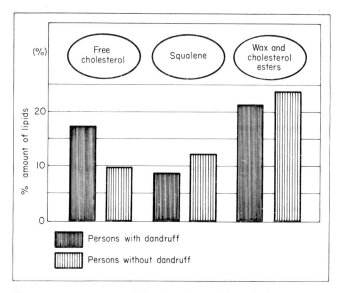

Fig. 16. Percentage amounts of the fractions of free cholesterol, squalene and wax and cholesterol esters in the scalp and hair lipids in persons with and without dandruff (Gloor and Kohler, 1977b).

D. Alopecias

According to Schweikert (1967/68) a reduction in sebum secretion takes place after a long duration of the alopecia areata. The opposite is said to be the case in androgenetic alopecias.

E. Dandruff

Gloor and Kohler (1977b) demonstrated that more epidermal and less sebaceous gland lipids can be found in the scalp and hair lipids of persons with dandruff (Fig. 16).

F. Atopic Eczema

Articles on atopic eczema are to be found mainly by Rajka (1974) and Mustakallio *et al.* (1967). These authors documented a pronounced sebostasis in endogenous eczema. Moreover, they demonstrated that the sebum lipids are greatly reduced and lastly, they all found an increase in the free fatty acids at the cost of triglycerides.

G. Allergic Contact Eczema

As a result of investigations by Gloor, Strack, Geissler and Friederich (1972) the predisposition of a seborrhoic type towards allergic contact eczema, as assumed earlier by numerous authors, must be rejected.

H. Tumours of the Skin

Gloor, Klaubert and Friederich (1974) and Gloor and Kriett (1976) were able to show that the epidermal lipids are reduced in the healthy skin not only of persons with squamous cell carcinoma but also of persons with basal cell carcinoma. Analogous to this is a reduction in the light protective function of the stratum corneum. It is probable that this finding is caused by a thinning of the stratum corneum and by a reduction in the cell turnover in the epidermis which must inevitably lead to a decrease in the light protective effect of the stratum corneum.

I. Infectious Skin Diseases

It is interesting to note that even after extensive investigations by our team, neither seborrhoea nor sebostasis represent predisposing factors for a microbial skin infection. On the other hand, we demonstrated that an increase in free cholesterol is characteristic for impetigo contagiosa. This is clearly understandable since it indicates a thickening of the stratum corneum, and a thickened, slack stratum corneum could by all means improve survival conditions for microorganisms on the skin (Gloor, Weigel and Friederich, 1975). A finding more difficult to interprete, is the increase in squalene which we determined not only in cutaneous candidiasis but also in pityriasis versicolor (Gloor, Kümpel, Friederich, 1975; Gloor, Geilhof, Ronnenberger and Friederich, 1976). It is worth noting that there was no alteration in the amount of free fatty acids in any of the examined skin diseases.

J. Psoriasis Vulgaris

According to investigations by various authors (Rothman, 1950; Meffert et al., 1969; Wilkinson and Farber, 1967a) the esterification of cholesterol seems to be altered in the healthy skin of the psoriatic. Since for this esterification bacteria are responsible (according to Puhvel, 1975; Freinkel and Fiedler-Weiss, 1974) it must be assumed that in psoriasis vulgaris it is a case of a disturbance in the skin flora. This has been indicated also by results which show that less free fatty acids are demonstrable on the healthy skin of the psoriatic than of a healthy person (Rothman, 1950; Wilkinson and

Farber, 1967b; Coon *et al.*, 1961). It is, however, not probable that correlations exist between these findings and the pathogenesis of psoriasis. Moreover, the literature describes a changed composition of the fatty acids in the psoriatic, changes in the melting point of the lipids, changes in cholesterol and others. These findings will not be discussed in detail because a correlation between the pathogenesis of psoriases is not recognizable and besides, the findings are still subject of controversy.

V. PHARMACOLOGICAL INFLUENCE ON THE SKIN SURFACE AND HAIR LIPIDS

A. Influence on the Lipid Secretion

A drug can influence the production of lipids in the sebaceous gland. Similarly the depletion of the sebum lipids can also be influenced. If the production of the lipids is increased, then a reduction in the skin surface lipids always occurs after a period of more than one week (Weinstein, 1974). If the depletion is influenced, then the effect can be observed immediately after application of the drug.

1. Influence on the Production of Sebum Secrete
The production of sebum secretion can be fundamentally altered by influencing the mitosis in the sebaceous gland or by influencing the lipogenesis. Up till now, it has not been possible in most cases to determine whether a drug influences the mitosis rate or the lipogenesis. It is only known that oestrogens mainly react on the lipogenesis whereas anti-androgens mainly reduce the mitoses in the sebaceous glands (Ebling, 1974). It is probable that in most cases the influence on the mitosis rate correlates with an influence on the lipogenesis.
(a) *Drugs applied therapeutically to reduce sebum secretion*   Oestrogens have a sebosuppressive effect but because of their effect on the whole organism they are only applied systemically in the form of oral contraceptives. The application of oral contraceptives does not bring about a reduction in sebum secretion until they have been applied over a period of several menstrual cycles and then only after application of products containing many oestrogens and few gestagens. This reduction is quantitatively not of great importance (Aron-Brunetière and Robin, 1969; Ludwig, 1972; Tronnier, 1972 and others). Oestrogens can also be used for local therapy. Using a suitable form of application, however, only a relatively slight reduction in sebum secretion can be achieved (Gloor Hübscher, Friederich, 1974).

Up till now anti-androgens have not been applied as a routine method. An excellent sebosuppressive effect has been attributed to those oral

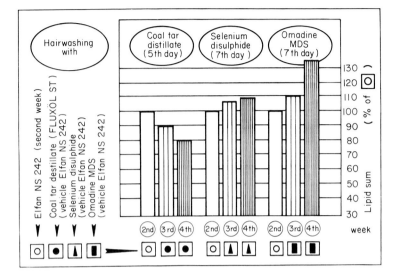

Fig. 17. Change in the amount of scalp and hair lipids in three differently treated test groups (according to Gloor, Mattern and Friederich, 1976; Gloor, Baldes, Lipphardt and Jäger, 1977; Gloor, Mildenberger and Miltenberger, 1977).

contraceptives which contain anti-androgens instead of gestagens. These oral contraceptives do not seem to cause any serious side-effects. The effect is quantitatively much greater than in the traditional oral contraceptives (Winkler and Schäfer, 1973). Anti-androgens have not, as yet, proved effective in local application.

Sodium bituminosulfonates have, on systemic application, a sebo-suppressive effect although it is also only a relatively slight one (Gloor, Steingräber and Friederich, 1973). It must be pointed out that simultaneous application of tetracyclines causes not only the tetracyclines but also the bituminosulfonates to be non-effective (Gloor, Josephs and Friederich, 1975).

The local treatment of a coal tar distillate (FLUX ‡L ST) in shampoos also has a sebosuppressive effect (Gloor, Mattern and Friederich, 1976) (Fig. 17). This sebosuppressive effect could also be impressively demonstrated by means of investigations on the hamster ear (Gloor and Kellermann, 1977). In the local application of bituminosulfonates the resorption of the reagent is not great enough to result in a sebosuppressive effect (Gloor, Wollner and Friederich, 1976).

Benzylthio-2-ethylamine and 6-hydroxy-1,3-benzoxathiol-2-on are used for therapeutic measures but the present findings do not allow a definite judgment of their sebosuppressive effect (Aubin *et al.*, 1974; Tronnier, 1958).

(b) *Drugs, not used for therapeutic measures, but which demonstrate a sebo-suppressive effect* As these drugs are of no particular importance for a cosmetic effect, preference is ony made to the list in Table II. In all cases possible alien effects on the whole organism prevent therapeutic administration. Moreover, the sebosuppressive effect of propanolol and L-Dopa therapy is controversial.

Table II
Drugs not used for therapeutic purposes but which effect a reduction in sebum secretion

Drugs and references
1. Phenothiazine derivates (Stüttgen, 1967)
2. 5:8:11:14 tetraynoic acid (Summerly *et al.*, 1972; Burton and Shuster, 1972)
3. Anticholinergics (Cartlidge *et al.*, 1972)
4. Propanolol (Cunliffe and Cotterill, 1970)
5. Leva-Dopa therapy in Parkinson's disease (Cotterill *et al.*, 1971a; Kohn *et al.*, 1973)

(c) *Drugs which increase sebum secretion* Hereby selenium disulphide plays the most important part for cosmetic results. Selenium disulphide is widely used in shampoos on account of its reducing effect on dandruff production. The increase in sebum secretion is an undesired side-effect. Skog (1958) demonstrated a stimulating effect of selenium disulphide in animal experiments. Goldschmidt and Kligman (1968) showed in humans that a shampoo containing selenium disulphide produces an increase in sebum secretion in a third of their test persons. This increase in secretion sets in after several applications and disappears within 12 weeks even if the treatment is continued. Bereston (1954) made similar findings. On the other hand, Gloor, Baldes, Lipphardt and Jäger (1977) found an increase in secretion in almost all their test persons. Moreover, they were able to demonstrate this effect after the first application. It did, however, become more intensive after several applications (Fig. 17).

We also found that Omadine MDS had a stimulating effect to sebum secretion. This effect could be demonstrated in animal experiments on the hamster ear and in experiments on humans (Gloor, Mildenberger and Miltenberger, 1977) (Fig. 17). Omadine MDS is employed in shampoos on account of its excellent effect on dandruff. Thus, the stimulating effect on sebum secretion is—as in selenium disulphide—an important undesired side-effect.

The other substances, attributed to increase secretion, are of less interest as far as the cosmetic effect is concerned. Mention must be made to andro-gens and barbiturates. Androgens affect an increase of secretion of sebum in women and men in senium but not in healthy younger men (Winkler, 1972). The stimulation on secretion by barbiturates may be of importance as a side-effect (Stüttgen, 1967). Recently, Ueda *et al.* (1976) described a stimu-latory effect on secretion by γ-oryzanole.

2. Influence on the Depletion of the Sebaceous Gland

By means of comparative investigations with the frosted glass test and the direct extraction method Gloor, Derichs and Friederich (1976) demon-strated that pyrollidon carbon acid hexadecyl ester produces an inhibition of sebum depletion as a result of its unspecific qualities as a lipophilic substance. Inhibition of sebum depletion can be determined by the frosted glass test since pyrollidon carbon acid hexadecyl ester does not influence this method (Eberhardt, 1974) (Fig. 18). A physical influence on depletion seems to have taken place since the effect sets in rapidly.

These results are not so much of interest on account of practical thera-peutic importance but more on account of the mechanism. If one were

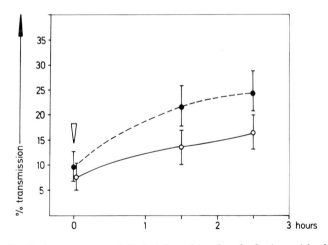

Fig. 18.   Re-fatting situation of the hairless skin after de-fatting with plastic foil, after application of pyrollidone carbon acid hexadecyl ester (———) and the situation after nonapplication of the same (– – – –). The transmission corres-ponds to the amounts of lipids by the frosted glass method (Gloor, Derichs and Friederich, 1976).

successful in finding lipophilic substances tolerated better by the patient than his own skin surface lipids, then an inhibition of sebum depletion could thus be achieved. Pyrollidon carbon acid hexadecyl ester does not fulfill these expectations.

In contrast, there is another mechanism which is of practical importance, although the effect is not known by most consumers. Gloor, Fichtler and Friederich (1973) could demonstrate that the application of 70% isopropyl alcohol as a hair tonic leads to a displacement of the scalp lipids from the scalp on to the hair. This effect produces a distinct inhibition of sebum depletion.

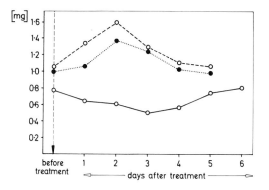

Fig. 19.   Influence of hyperemisating drugs (Nicotinan percutan[R] ······, Propyl nicotinicum 10% – – – –) and Aerosil 1% (————) on the sum of skin surface lipids (Rätz and Mattheus, 1975).

There is another mechanism also of importance. Hyperemisating substances are widely used in cosmetic chemistry. Rätz and Mattheus (1975) showed that the increase in temperature caused by these substances lead to an increase in sebum depletion (Fig. 19). Here again it is a physical mechanism because the effect sets in immediately after the first application. The reaction represents a frequent side-effect of cosmetic therapy.

B. Influence on the Composition of the Skin Surface and Hair Lipids

1. *Influence on the Relationship Between Epidermal Lipids and Sebum Lipids*
Ackermann and Kligman (1969) have shown that the production of dandruff is caused by an acceleration of the cell turnover in the epidermis. A reduction in the cell turnover must lead to a thinning of the stratum corneum in persons without dandruff. This, in its turn, causes a reduction

in the amount of epidermal lipids in the scalp and hair lipid mixture. If a drug thus produces a reduction in free cholesterol and an increase in squalene and wax esters in a healthy person, it may be accepted that the drug will reduce dandruff production in the patient with dandruff. Because—as stated above—the amount of epidermal lipids in the total lipid mixture is increased in the patient with dandruff, this is the case not only in healthy persons but also in patients with dandruff. Since a bacterial cholesterol esterification does not occur on the scalp—as mentioned above—one may assume the same with regards to the testing of antimicrobial substances.

An increase in epidermal lipids on the hair-bearing head must also be of interest. Since no acceleration of the cell turnover in the human epidermis is known by any drug under the conditions of therapy, one may normally accept that a "keratolytic" effect increases epidermal lipids.

On testing external substances, aimed at influencing dandruff production, one must distinguish between the effect of the reagent and the effect of the basic components. It is possible that tensides which are contained in shampoos demonstrate a "keratolytic" effect (Fig. 20). For example, the tenside polyethylene glycol lauryl ether sulphate, sodium salt (Elfan NS 242) possibly causes an increase in the epidermal lipids. In order to demonstrate the dandruff-inhibiting effect of a drug we have almost always used this

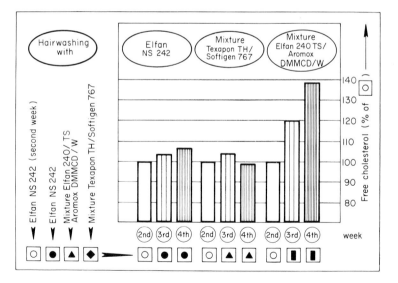

Fig. 20.   Changes in the amount of free cholesterol in the scalp and hair lipids in three differently treated test groups. One can see that tensides can have a "keratolytic" effect (Gloor, Jäger and Baldes, 1977).

tenside as a vehicle in our own experiments. A reduction in the epidermal lipids, demonstrated here, can by no means be simulated by the basic component. Conversely, the increase in epidermal lipids, determined by such an investigation, must be evaluated carefully (Gloor, Jäger and Baldes, 1977).

Figures 21 and 22 show our results with various substances which cause a reduction in the epidermal lipids. Hereby the concentrations were closely based on those concentrations in commercial products. This effect seems to be present in a coal tar distillate (FLUXÖL ST), in cadmium sulphide, ichthyol-sodium and in selenium disulphide (Gloor, Mattern and Friederich, 1976a; Gloor, Woläner and Friederich, 1976b; Gloor Baldes, Lipphardt and Jäger, 1977). We could not achieve a similar result with Omadine MDS as the strong "keratolytic" effect obviously conceals the dandruff-inhibiting effect after the first few applications (Gloor, Mildenberger and Miltenberger, 1977).

This corresponds to animal experiments in which a reduction of the mitosis in the epidermis could be found after treatment with a coal tar distillate (FLUXÖL ST), ichthyol-sodium, cadmium sulphide, Omadine MDS (Gloor, Dressel and Schnyder, 1977) and selenium disulphide (Plewig and Kligman, 1970).

For the sake of entirety, it must also be mentioned that all the drugs which influence sebum secretion also indirectly influence the relationship between epidermal lipids and sebum lipids. This effect is, however, usually so slight, quantitatively speaking, that it is of no significance from a pharmacological point of view.

2. Influence on the Relationship between Free Fatty Acids and Triglycerides

Gloor (1977b) demonstrated that one may expect a reduction in free fatty acids, caused by a drug, to have a clinically favourable influence on the inflammatory and non-inflammatory efflorescences of the acne patient even if no other effect is attributed to the drug employed. Bearing in mind the previous remarks on the pathophysiology of acne vulgaris it becomes evident that such an assumption correlates with the present pathophysiological opinions on acne vulgaris.

On the other hand, different effects, which could be of importance in the treatment of acne, are attributed to numerous antimicrobial substances, and mainly to antibiotics. In this context, the antiphlogistic effect of tetracyclines and erythromycine must be mentioned (Plewig and Schöpf, 1976). It thus seems evident that there are no exact correlations between reduction in free fatty acids and clinical influence of acne for example by tetracyclines (Anderson *et al.*, 1976).

The importance of bacterial lipolysis for seborrhoea oleosa capitis has

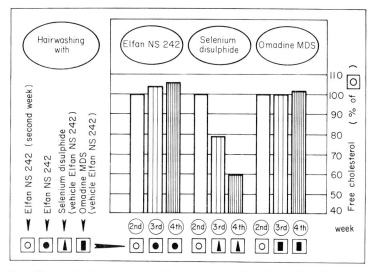

Fig. 21.   Change in the amount of free cholesterol in the scalp and hair lipids in three differently treated test groups. Selenium disulphide but not Omadine MDS reduce the amount of free cholesterol (according to Gloor, Baldes, Lipphardt and Jäger, 1977 and Gloor, Mildenberger and Miltenberger, 1977).

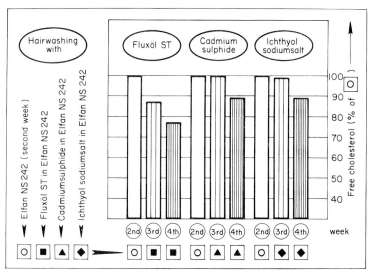

Fig. 22.   Change in the amount of free cholesterol in the scalp and hair lipids in three differently treated test groups. The three drugs tested reduce the amount of free cholesterol (according to Gloor, Mattern and Friederich, 1976 and Gloor, Wollner and Friederich, 1976).

already been emphasized. A reduction in the free fatty acids by means of a drug leads to a conversion of the seborrhoea oleosa—which is almost always present on the hair-bearing head of the seborrhoic type—into a seborrhoea sicca. The reduction in free fatty acids is therefore a desirable aim in the treatment of seborrhoea oleosa capitis. Since the lipolysis on the hair-covered scalp takes place to a great extent outside the sebaceous gland secretory ducts on the scalp, externally applied substances are assuredly of greater importance than systemically administered pharmaca.

The concentration of the antimicrobial drug at the site of its influence on the lipase-releasing bacteria is of essential importance. Locally applied anti-microbial substances on the hair-bearing scalp always come in direct contact with the lipase-releasing microbes. This is by no means the case on the hairless skin since the antimicrobial agent must invade the sebaceous gland secretory duct. It depends on the basic components of the pharmacon as to whether this occurs or not.

This becomes evident in the example of antibiotics. Gloor, Hübscher and Friederich (1974) and Fulton and Pablo (1974) discovered a much greater reduction in the free fatty acids by tetracycline hydrochloride than Anderson et al. (1976). Whereas Fulton and Pablo (1974) demonstrated a great reduction by erythromycine, Cotterill and Cunliffe (1973) did not make any similar findings. Since the agents were identical in both cases, but the basic components different, it must be assumed that the latter are responsible for the differing results.

It is probable that the concentration of the agent is also an essential criterion in systemic antibiotic therapy. The antibiotics tetracycline, erythromycine and clindamycine, which are regularly employed in clinical practice, are excreted in relatively large amounts in the sebum (Cunliffe and Cotterill, 1975). For literature on the reducing effect on free fatty acids by different antibiotics refer to the Ad hoc Committee Report (1975) and to the book by Cunliffe and Cotterill (1975) as well as the review article by Gloor (1977a).

The mechanism must also be mentioned. In most antimicrobial stimulants, with the exception of antibiotics, it is only a case of an antimicrobial effect on the lipase-releasing microorganisms. However, a lipase inactivation is also possible with the antibiotics tetracycline, erythromycine and clindamycine (Hassing, 1971; Edwards et al., 1975a) and with ethyl lactate (Swanbeck, 1972). Moreover, an inhibition of the lipase synthesis is debatable (Edwards et al., 1975a). Usually, one can not decide in one particular case whether it is the antimicrobial effect which is responsible in the first place for the reduction in free fatty acids or whether it is the lipase-inactivating effect or the effect inhibiting the release of lipases.

It is difficult to give a quantitative impression of the conditions after varying treatments. Figure 23 has attempted to do so. It is based exclusively on our own results. Nevertheless, the values stated only represent a rough picture of the situation on the hairless skin since the test models were different. As a result of our findings, however, we assume that the local therapy with antimicrobial pharmaca in the treatment of acne has most probably been generally underrated.

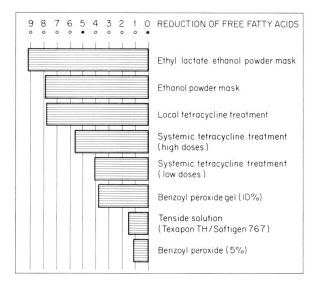

Fig. 23. Reduction of the amount of free fatty acids by varying treatments (according to Gloor, Mendel, Baumann and Friederich, 1975; Gloor, Hübscher and Friederich, 1974; Gloor, Graumann, Wiegand and Friederich, 1972; Gloor, Hummel and Friederich, 1975; Gloor, Döring and Kümpel, 1976).

More accurate quantitative conclusions may be drawn from our investigations on the hair-bearing scalp since the studies were carried out under comparable test conditions. Figure 24 shows that there are tensides without a fatty acid reducing effect but that tenside mixtures can also be produced which cause not only a slight but also an extremely great reduction in free fatty acids. The fatty acid reducing effect of drugs also varies. Figure 25 shows that colloidal sulphur, selenium disulphide and Omadine MDS have a more or less pronounced reducing effect on the free fatty acids (Gloor and Mattern, 1976; Gloor, Jäger and Baldes, 1977; Gloor, Mildenberger and Miltenberger, 1977).

However, it is also possible that pharmaca accelerate the release of free fatty acids from triglycerides. Gloor and Mildenberger (1977) proved this

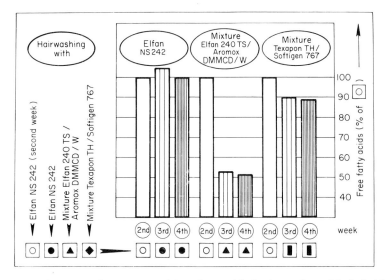

Fig. 24. Change in the amount of free fatty acids in the scalp and hair lipids in three differently treated test groups. Tensides can partly reduce the free fatty acids (Gloor, Jäger and Baldes, 1977).

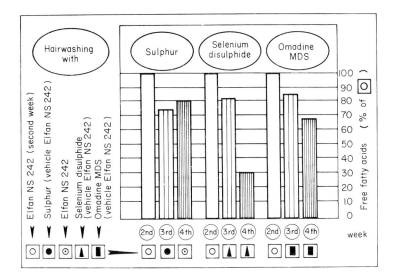

Fig. 25. Change in the amount of free fatty acids in the scalp and hair lipids in three differently treated test groups. The three drugs tested reduce the amount of free fatty acids (Gloor and Mattern, 1976; Gloor, Baldes, Lipphardt and Jäger, 1977; Gloor, Mildenberger and Miltenberger, 1977).

with the example of a local application of a corticosteroid. These findings could explain the development of the steroid acne. The differences documented by these authors are relatively slight in quantity. It is, however, probable that the differences could be more intensive on application of other vehicles or by systemic application. Moreover, the lack in insulin seems to affect the bacterial lipolysis. Gloor, Marckardt and Friederich (1975) determined that the bacterial lipolysis is increased in a diabetic; after sufficient treatment of the diabetes this increase in bacterial lipolysis proved itself to be partly reversible.

REFERENCES

Ackermann, A. B. and Kligman, A. M. (1969). Some observations on dandruff. *J. Soc. Cosmetic Chem.* **20**, 81–101.

Ad hoc Committee Report (1975). Systemic antibiotica for treatment of acne vulgaris. *Arch. Derm.* **111**, 1630–1636.

Agache, P., Barrand, C., Colette, C., Ratti, A. and Laurent, R. (1977). Sebum levels in the first year of life. Annual Meeting of the European Society for Dermatological Research, Amsterdam.

Anderson, R. L., Cook, C. H. and Smith, S. E. (1976). The effect of oral and topical tetracycline on acne severity and on skin surface lipid composition. *J. invest. Derm.* **66**, 172–177.

Anderson, A. S. and Fulton, J. E. (1973). Sebum: Analysis by infrared spectroscopy. *J. invest. Derm.* **60**, 115–118.

Archibald, A. and Shuster, S. (1970). The measurement of sebum secretion in the rat. *Br. J. Derm.* **82**, 146–151.

Aron-Brunetière, R. and Robin, J. (1969). Donées nouvelles sur le traitement de la séborrhée et de l'acne vulgaire feminine par les inhibiteurs d'ovulation. *Rev. méd. franç.* **20**, 85–106.

Aubin, G., Brod, J. and Manoussos, G. (1971). Inhibition of seborrhea by means of specific metabolic blocking. *Amer. Parf. Cosm.* **86**, 29–34.

Azar, G., Barrand, C., Laurent, R. and Agache, P. (1975). Le dosage des lipides cutanées superficiels (LCS) dans l'acne. *Ann. Derm. (Paris)* **102**, 532–534.

Bereston, E. S. (1954). Use of selenium sulfide shampoo in seborrhoic dermatitis. *J. Amer. med. Ass.* **156**, 1246–1247.

Boughton, B., McKenna, R. M. B., Wheatley, V. R. and Wormall, A. (1959). The fatty acid composition of the surface skin fats ("sebum") in acne vulgaris and seborrhoeic dermatitis. *J. invest. Derm.* **33**, 57–64.

Brabant, H. and Delmotte, A. (1959). Inoculation expérimentale et activité lipolytique de candida albicans. Activité fungicide du borate de phenyl-mercure. *Arch. belges Derm.* **15**, 138–139.

Brun, R., Enderlin, K. and Kull, E. (1953). A propos de sebum tests. *Dermatologica (Basel)* **106**, 165–170.

Burton, J. L., Cartlidge, M., Cartlidge, N. E. F. and Shuster, S. (1973a). Sebum excretion in Parkinsonism. *Br. J. Derm.* **89**, 263–266.

Burton, J. L., Cunliffe, W. J., Saunders, J. G. G. and Shuster, S. (1971). The effect of facial nerve paresis on sebum excretion. *Br. J. Derm.* **84**, 135–138.

Burton, J. L., Laschet, U. and Shuster, S. (1973b). Reduction of sebum excretion in man by the antiandrogen, cyproterone acetate. *Br. J. Derm.* **89**, 487–490.

Burton, J. L., Libman, L. J., Cunliffe, W. J., Wilkinson, R., Hall, R. and Shuster, S. (1972). Sebum excretion in acromegaly. *Br. med. J.* **1**, 406–408.

Burton, J. L., Pye, R. J., Meyrick, G. and Shuster, S. (1975a). The sebum excretion rate in rosacea. *Br. J. Derm.* **92**, 541–543.

Burton, J. L. and Shuster, S. (1971). The relationship between seborrhoea and acne vulgaris. *Br. J. Derm.* **84**, 600–602.

Burton, J. L. and Shuster, S. (1972). The effect of topical tetraynoic acid on the seborrhoea of acne. *Br. J. Derm.* **86**, 66–67.

Burton, J. L., Shuster, S. and Cartlidge, M. (1975b). The sebotrophic effect of pregnancy. *Acta derm. venerol. (Stockh.)* **55**, 11–13.

Carrié, C. (1936). Untersuchungen über die chemischen Substanzen auf der Haut. I. Mitteilung: Methode zur Bestimmung chemischer Substanzen auf der Haut. *Arch. Derm. Syph. (Berl.)* **173**, 604–606.

Cartlidge, M., Burton, J. L. and Shuster, S. (1972). The effect of prolonged topical application of an anticholinergic agent on the sebaceous glands. *Br. J. Derm.* **86**, 61–63.

Černiková, M. (1960). Chromatographische Lipid-Trennung auf Glasfaserpapier. *Fette, Seifen* **62**, 587–589.

Coon, W. M., Herrmann, F. M. and Mandol, L. (1961). Acid number of skin surface lipids in psoriatics. *Arch. Derm.* **83**, 619–626.

Cooper, M. F., McGrath, H. and Shuster, S. (1976). Sebaceous lipogenesis in human skin. *Br. J. Derm.* **94**, 165–172.

Corner, R. W. (1966). Sebaceous gland activity of young men in the antarctic. *Br. J. Derm.* **78**, 444–450,

Cotterill, J. A. and Cunliffe, W. J., 1973, quoted by Cunliffe, W. J. and Cotterill, J. A. (1975). "The Acnes-Clinical Features, Pathogenesis and Treatment". W. B. Saunders Comp. Ltd., London–Philadelphia–Toronto.

Cotterill, J. A., Cunliffe, W. J. and Williamson, B. (1973). Variation in skin surface lipid composition and sebum excretion rate with time. *Acta derm.-venerol. (Stockh.)* **53**, 271–274.

Cotterill, J. A., Cunliffe, W. J., Williamson, B., Arrowsmith, W. A., Cook, J. B. and Sumner, D. (1971a). Sebum excretion rate and skin surface lipid composition in Parkinson's disease before and during therapy with levadopa. *Lancet* **1**, 1271–1272.

Cotterill, J. A., Cunliffe, W. J., Williamson, B. and Bulusu, L. (1972a). Further observations on the pathogenesis of acne. *Br. med. J.* **3**, 444–446.

Cotterill, J. A., Cunliffe, W. J., Williamson, B. and Bulusu, L. (1972b). Age and sex variation in skin surface lipid composition and sebum excretion rate. *Br. J. Derm.* **87**, 333–340.

Cotterill, J. A., Cunliffe, W. J., Williamson, B. and Forster, R. A. (1971b).

A semiquantitative method for the biochemical analysis of sebum. *Brit. J. Derm.* **85**, 35–39.

Cunliffe, W. J. (1976). Personal communication.

Cunliffe, W. J., Burton, J. L. and Shuster, S. (1970). The effect of local temperature variations on the sebum excretion rate. *Br. J. Derm.* **83**, 650–654.

Cunliffe, W. J. and Cotterill, J. A. (1970). The effect of propanolol on acne vulgaris and the rate of sebum excretion. *Br. J. Derm.* **83**, 550–551.

Cunliffe, W. J. and Cotterill, J. A. (1975). *In* "The acnes-clinical features, pathogenesis and treatment". W. B. Saunders Comp. Ltd., London–Philadelphia–Toronto.

Cunliffe, W. J., Cotterill, J. A. and Williamson, B. (1971). Variations in skin surface lipid composition with different sampling techniques. *Br. J. Derm.* **85**, 40–45.

Cunliffe, W. J. and Shuster, S. (1969). The rate of sebum excretion in man. *Br. J. Derm.* **81**, 697–704.

Cunliffe, W. J., Williams, S. M. and Tan, S. G. (1975). Sebum excretion rate investigations. *Br. J. Derm.* **93**, 347–350.

Downing, D. T. (1970). Lipolysis by human skin surface debris in organic solvents. *J. invest. Derm.* **54**, 395–398.

Downing, D. T. and Strauss, J. S. (1974). Synthesis and composition of surface lipids of human skin. *J. invest. Derm.* **62**, 228–244.

Dünner, M. (1946). Der Einfluß physikalischer Faktoren (Druck, Temperatur) auf die Talgabsonderung des Menschen. *Dermatologica (Basel)* **93**, 249–271.

Dvorken, L., Maggiora, A. and Jadassohn, W. (1966). The problem of sebum spread on the surface of the skin. *Dermatologica (Basel)* **132**, 59–63.

Eberhardt, H. (1974). Zur Regulation der Hautfettung. *Kosmetologie* **3**, 93–95.

Eberhardt, H. and Kuhn-Bussius, H. (1975). Bestimmung der Ruckfettungskinetik der Haare. *Arch. Derm. Res.* **252**, 139–145.

Ebling, F. J. (1970). Steroid hormones and sebaceous secretion. *In* "Advances in Steroid Chemistry and Pharmacology" (Ed. Briggs), Vol. 2. Academic Press, London.

Ebling, F. J. (1974). Hormonal control and methods of measuring sebaceous gland activity. *J. invest. Derm.* **62**, 161–171.

Ebling, F. J., Ebling, E., McCaffery, V. and Skinner, J. (1973). The responses of the sebaceous glands of the hypophysectomized castrated male rat to 5 Androstane-3-β-17 Diol. *J. invest. Derm.* **60**, 183–187.

Edwards, J. C., Williams, S. M., Tan, G. and Cunliffe, W. J. (1975a). Quoted by W. J. Cunliffe, J. A. Cotterill. *In* "The Acnes-Clinical Features, Pathogenesis and Treatment". W. B. Saunders Comp. Ltd., London–Philadelphia–Toronto.

Edwards, J. C., Williams, S., Tan, G., Holland, K. T., Roberts, C. D. and Cunliffe, W. J. (1975b). Physiology of *C. acnes* exoenzymes: lipase, protease, hyaluronidase—a comparison. *J. invest. Derm.* **64**, 290.

Emanuel, Sv. (1936). Quantitative determinations of the sebaceous glands function with particular mention of the method employed. *Acta derm.-venerol. (Stockh.)* **17**, 444–456.

Felger, C. B. (1969). The etiology of acne. I. Composition of sebum before and after puberty. *J. Soc. Cosm. Chem.* **20**, 565–575.

Förster, F. J., Henckel, S., Balikoioglu, S. Harth, P., Heller, G. and Förster, H. (1973). Einfluß einer bilanzierten fettfreien synthetischen Diät auf die Hautoberflächenlipide. *Arch. Derm. Res.* **248**, 191–200.

Freinkel, R. K. and Fiedler-Weiss, U. (1974). Esterification of sterols during differentiation and cornification of developing rat epidermis. *J. invest. Derm.* **62**, 458–462.

Fulton, J. E. and Pablo, G. (1974). Topical antibacterial therapy for acne-study of the family of erythromycine. *Arch. Derm.* **110**, 83–86.

Fulton, J. E., Weeks, J. G. and McCarty, L. (1975). The inability of a bacterial lipase inhibitor to control acne vulgaris. *J. invest. Derm.* **64**, 281–282.

van Gent, C. M. (1968). Separation and microdetermination of lipids by thin layer chromatography followed by densiometry. *Z. anal. Chem.* **236**, 344–350.

Gershbein, L. L. Haeberlin, J. B. and Singh, E. J. (1970). Composition of human comedone lipids. *Dermatologica (Basel)* **140**, 264–274.

Gloor, M. (1977a). Antimikrobielle Pharmaka in der Therapie der Acne vulgaris. *Zbl. Haut-Geschl. Kr.* **138**, 1–12.

Gloor, M. (1977b). Über die Reduktion der freien Fettsäuren in den Hautoberflächenlipiden als Kriterium für die therapeutische Wirksamkeit antimikrobieller Acnetherapeutica–Untersuchungen mit äthyllactat- und äthanolhaltigen Filmmasken. *Drug Res.* (in the press).

Gloor, M., Baldes, G., Lipphardt, B. A. and Jäger, B. (1977). Über den Effekt von Selendisulfid auf Menge und Zusammensetzung der Kopfhautlund Haarlipide. *Therapiewache* (in press).

Gloor, M., Breitinger, J. and Friedrich, H. C. (1973). Über die Zusammensetzung der Hautoberflächenlipide bei Seborrhoea oleosa und Seborrhoea sicca. *Arch. Derm. Res.* **247**, 59–64.

Gloor, M., Derichs, R. D. and Friedrich, H. C. (1976). Über die Beeinflussung der Talgdrüsensekretion durch Pyrollidoncarbonsäurehexadecylester. *Ärztl. Kosm.* **6**, 4–8.

Gloor, M., Döring, W. J. and Kümpel, D. (1976). Über den Einfluß synthetischer Tenside auf die Zusammensetzung der Hautoberflächenlipide. *Fette–Seifen–Anstrichmittel,* **78**, 40–43.

Gloor, M., Dressel, M. and Schnyder, U. W. (1977). The effect of coal tar distillate, cadmium sulfide, ichthyol sodium and Omadine MDS on the epidermis of the guinea pig. *Dermatologica* (Basel) (in the press).

Gloor, M., Fichtler, C. and Friederich, H. C. (1973). Über den Einfluß alkoholischer Haarwässer auf das Nachfetten der Haare nach der Kopfwäsche. *Kosmetologie* **3**, 193–194.

Gloor, M., Franz, P. and Friederich, H. C. (1973). Untersuchungen über die Physiologie der Talgdrüsen und über den Einfluß der Hautoberflächenlipide auf die Benetzbarkeit der Haut. *Arch. Derm. Res.* **248**, 79–88.

Gloor, M. and Friederich, H. C. (1970). Experimentelle Untersuchungen über die Talgsekretion auf freien autologen Epidermis-Cutistransplantaten beim Menschen. *Hautarzt* **21**, 219–221.

Gloor, M. and Friederich, H. C. (1974a). Über die Zusammensetzung der Talgdrüsenlipide bei Naevus sebaceus Jadassohn. *Z. Hautkr.* **49**, 45–49.

Gloor, M. and Friederich, H. C. (1974b). Über die Zusammensetzung der Comedonenlipide bei Morbus Favre-Racouchot. *Hautarzt* **25**, 439–441.

Gloor, M., Geilhof, A., Ronneberger, G. and Friederich, H. C. (1976). Biochemical and physiological parameters on the healthy skin surface of persons with candidal intertrigo and of persons with tinea cruris. *Arch. Derm. Res.* **257**, 203–211.

Gloor, M., Graumann, U., Kionke, M., Wiegand, I. and Friederich, H. C. (1972). Menge und Zusammensetzung der Hautoberflächenlipide bei Patienten mit Acne vulgaris und gesunden Vergleichspersonen. I. Mitteilung. *Arch. Derm. Res.* **242**, 316–322.

Gloor, M., Graumann, U., Wiegand, I. and Friederich, H. C. (1972). Über den Einfluß der Tetracyclintherapie bei Acne vulgaris auf Menge und Zusammensetzung der Hautoberflächenlipide bei verschiedener Dosierung. I. Mitteilung. *Arch. Derm. Res.* **242**, 309–315.

Gloor, M. and Habedank, W. D. (1976). Zur Pathogenese der Acne vulgaris. *Münch. med. Wschr.* **118**, 649–652.

Gloor, M., Handke, J., Baumann, C. and Friederich, H. C. (1975). Über den Einfluß jahreszeitlicher und klimatischer Faktoren auf die Hautoberflächenlipide. *Derm. Mschr.* **161**, 996–1002.

Gloor, M., Hübscher, M. and Friederich, H. C. (1974). Untersuchungen zur externen Behandlung der Acne vulgaris mit Tetracyclinen und Östrogenen. *Hautarzt* **25**, 439–441.

Gloor, M., Hummel, A. and Friederich, H. C. (1975). Experimentelle Untersuchungen zur Benzoylperoxydtherapie der Acne vulgaris. *Z. Hautkr.* **50**, 657–663.

Gloor, M., Jäger, B. and Baldes, G. (1977). Zum Wirkungseffekt von Tensiden Waschaktiver Substanzen in Kopfwaschmitteln. *Hautarzt* (in press).

Gloor, M., Josephs, H. and Friederich, H. C. (1974). Über den Einfluß der Luftverschmutzung auf den Paraffingehalt der Hautoberflächenlipide. *Arch. Derm. Res.* **250**, 277–284.

Gloor, M., Josephs, H. and Friederich, H. C. (1975). Über den Einfluß einer speziellen Zubereitung von Oxytetracyclin und Natriumbituminosulfonaten auf Menge und Zusammensetzung der Hautoberflächenlipide bei Acne vulgaris. *Drug. Res.* **25**, 1944–1947.

Gloor, M. and Karenfeld, A. (1977). Effect of ultraviolet light therapy, given over a period of several weeks, on the amount and composition of the skin surface lipids. *Dermatologica (Basel)* **154**, 5–13.

Gloor, M. and Kellermann, H. (1977). Tierexperimentelle Untersuchungen zur sebosuppressiven Wirkung von Steinkohlenteer. *Derm. Mschr.* **163**, 557–554.

Gloor, M. and Kionke, M. (1972). Gaschromatographische Analysen der Wachsesterfraktion der Hautoberflächenlipide bei Acne vulgaris. *Arch. Derm. Res.* **244**, 165–168.

Gloor, M., Kionke, M. and Friederich, H. C. (1973). Über Menge und Zusammensetzung der Hautoberflächenlipide bei Patienten mit Acne vulgaris und gesunden Vergleichspersonen. Gaschromatographische Analysen der Zusammensetzung der freien Fettsäuren. *Z. Hautkr.* **48**, 987–994.

Gloor, M., Kionke, M. and Friederich, H. C. (1975). Biochemical and physiological parameters on the skin surface of healthy test persons. A contribution towards the interpretation of the results obtained by a screening program. *Arch. Derm. Res.* **252**, 317–330.

Gloor, M., Kionke, M., Strack, R. and Friederich, H. C. (1972). Untersuchungen über einen Zusammenhang zwischen Menge und Zusammensetzung der Hautoberflächenlipide. II. Mitteilung. *Fortschr. Med.* **90**, 1271–1274 and 1278.

Gloor, M., Klaubert, W. and Friederich, H. C. (1974). Funktionelle Minderwertigkeit der Haut als praedisponierender Faktor für das Spinaliom. *Arch. Derm. Res.* **249**, 373–379.

Gloor, M. and Kohler, H. (1977a). On the physiology and biochemistry of scalp and hair lipids. *Arch. Derm. Res.* **257**, 273–279.

Gloor, M. and Kohler, H. (1977b). A contribution to a new test method for dandruff inhibiting and "keratolytic" action of drugs. *Europ. J. clin. Pharm.* **11**, 377–380.

Gloor, M. and Kohler, H. (1977c). Über den Einfluß der Materialgewinnung auf die Analyse der Zusammensetzung der Hautoberflächenlipide. Vergleichende Untersuchungen mit der Mattglasmethode und der Papierabsorptionsmethode. *J. Soc. Cosmet. Chem.* **28**, 211–217.

Gloor, M. and Kriett, P. (1976). Experimentelle Untersuchungen zur Physiologie und Biochemie der Haut bei Basaliomträgern. *Hautarzt, Suppl.* **1**, 126–128.

Gloor, M., Kümpel, D. and Friederich, H. C. (1975). Predisposing factors on the surface of the skin in persons with pityriasis versicolor. *Arch. Derm. Res.* **254**, 281–286.

Gloor, M., Marckardt, V. and Friederich, H. C. (1975). Biochemical and physiological particularities on the skin surface of diabetics. *Arch. Derm. Res.* **253**, 185–194.

Gloor, M. and Mattern, E. (1976). Über die Wirkung eines Zusatzes von kolloidalem Schwefel zu Haarwaschmitteln auf die behaarte Kopfhaut. *Drug. Res.* **26**, 1724–1726.

Gloor, M., Mattern, E. and Friederich, H. C. (1976). Über den therapeutischen Effekt eines Steinkohlenteerzusatzes zu Kopfwaschmitteln. *Derm. Mschr.* **162**, 678–683.

Gloor, M., Mendel, R. Baumann, Ch. and Friederich, H. C. (1975). Untersuchungen zur Äthyllactattherapie der Acne vulgaris. Einfluß von Wirkstoff und alkoholischer Grundlage auf die Hautoberflächenlipide. *Hautarzt* **26**, 149–152.

Gloor, M. and Mildenberger, H. (1977). Unpublished results.

Gloor, M., Mildenberger, H. and Miltenberger, G. (1977). Unpublished results.

Gloor, M., Oschmann, H. and Friederich, H. C. (1973). Über den Einfluß endogener und exogener Faktoren auf die Hautoberflächenlipidmenge. *Z. Haut-Geschl. Kr.* **48**, 413–418.

Gloor, M., Rietkötter, J. and Friederich, H. C. (1973). Entfettung und Nachfettung der Kopfhaut und der Haare nach Kopfwäsche mit verschiedenen Tensiden. *Fette–Seifen–Anstrichmittel* **75**, 200–202.

Gloor, M., Schemel, A. and Friederich, H. C. (1975). Über den Einfluß des Fönens der Haare und der Anwendung von Haarsprays auf das Nachfetten der Haare und der Kopfhaut nach der Kopfwäsche. *Kosmetologie* **4**, 10–12.

Gloor, M. and Schnyder, U. W. (1977). Verebung funktioneller Eigenschaften der Haut. *Hautarzt* **28**, 231–234.

Gloor, M., Schulz, U., Wieland, G. and Wiegand, I. (1972). Untersuchungen über einen Zusammenhang zwischen Menge und Zusammensetzung der Hautoberflächenlipide. I. Mitteilung. *Fortschr. Med.* **90**, 325–327.

Gloor, M., Steingräber, V. and Friederich, H. C. (1973). Über den antiseborrhoischen Effekt von Bituminosulfonaten bei Acne vulgaris. *Hautarzt* **24**, 288–290.

Gloor, M., Strack, R., Geißler, H. and Friederich, H. C. (1972). Quantity and composition of skin surface lipids and alkaline resistance in subjects with contact allergy and in healthy controls. *Arch. Derm. Res.* **245**, 184–190.

Gloor, M., Strack, R., Oschmann, H. and Friederich, H. C. (1972). Über den Einfluß der Hautoberflächenlipide auf das Ergebnis der Alkaliresistenzbestimmung nach Burckhardt. *Berufsdermatosen* **20**, 105–110.

Gloor, M., Weidemann, J. and Friederich, H. C. (1974). Über den Einfluß der Haarlänge auf die Talgdrüsensekretion am behaarten Kopf. *Derm. Mschr.* **160**, 730–734.

Gloor, M., Weigel, H. J. and Friederich, H. C. (1975). Predisposing factors of the skin surface in persons with impetigo contagiosa. *Arch. Derm. Res.* **254**, 95–101.

Gloor, M., Wiegand, I., Baumann, C. and Friederich, H. C. (1974). Über Menge und Zusammensetzung der Hautoberflächenlipide bei Rosacea. *Derm. Mschr.* **160**, 468–473.

Gloor, M., Wiegand, I. and Friederich, H. C. (1972). Über Menge und Zusammensetzung der Hautoberflächenlipide beim sogenannten seborrhoischen Ekzem. *Derm. Mschr.* **158**, 759–764.

Gloor, M., Wollner, B. and Friederich, H. C. (1976). Beitrag zur Wirkung eines Cadmiumsulfid- und eines Ichthyol-Natriumzusatzes zu Kopfwaschmitteln auf die behaarte Kopfhaut. *Therapiewoche* **26**, 7503–7510.

Goldschmidt, H. and Kligman, A. M. (1968). Increased sebum secretion following selenium sulfide shampoos. *Acta derm.-venerol. (Stockh.)* **48**, 489–491.

Goolamali, S. K., Burton, J. L. and Shuster, S. (1973). Sebum excretion in hypopituitarism. *Br. J. Derm.* **89**, 21–24.

Goolamali, S. K., Plummer, N., Burton, J. L., Shuster, S. and Thody, A. J. (1974). Sebum excretion and melanocyte-stimulating hormone in hypoadrenalism. *J. invest. Derm.* **63**, 253–255.

Goolamali, S. K. and Shuster, S. (1974). A sebotrophic stimulus in benign and malignant breast tumours. *Br. J. Derm.* **91** (Suppl. 10), 21–22.

Gould, D. J., Cunliffe, W. J. and Holland, K. T. (1977). Chemotaxis and acne. Annual Meeting of the Society for Dermatological Research. Amsterdam.

Grasset, N. and Brun, R. (1959). Etude du film sébacé de sujets sains et de patients atteints d'épilespsie ou de maladie de Parksinson. *Dermatologica (Basel)* **119**, 232–237.

Greene, R. S., Downing, D. T., Pochi, P. E. and Strauss, J. S. (1970). Anatomical variation in the amount and composition of human skin surface lipid. *J. invest. Derm.* **54**, 240–247.

Grimmer, G., Jacob, J. and Kimmig, J. (1971). Difference between the composition of positional isomeric fatty acids from psoriatic scales and normal human skin. *Z. klin. Chem. klin. Biochem.* **9**, 111–116.

Haahti, E. (1961). Major lipid constituents of human skin surface with special reference to gas-chromatographic methods. *Scand. J. clin. Lab. Invest.* **13** (Suppl. 59), 1–108.

Haahti, E. and Horning, E. C. (1961). Separation of human skin waxes by gas chromatography. *Acta chem. scand.* **15**, 930–931.

Haahti, E., Nikkari, T. and Juva, K. (1963). Fractionation of serum and skin sterol esters and skin waxes with chromatography on silica gel impregnated with silver nitrate. *Acta. chem. scand.* **17**, 538–540.

Hägele, W., Schäfer, H. and Stüttgen, G. (1973). Über die Bedeutung der Triglyceridspaltung durch Corynebacterium acnes für die Acne vulgaris. *Arch. Derm. Res.* **246**, 328–334.

Hassing, G. S. (1971). Inhibition of corynebacterium acnes lipase by tetracycline. *J. invest. Derm.* **56**, 189–192.

Hay, J. B. and Hodgins, M. B. (1974). Metabolism of androgens by human skin in acne. *Br. J. Derm.* **91**, 123–133.

Herrmann, F. and Prose, P. H. (1951). Studies on the ether-soluble substances on the human skin. I. Quantity and "replacement sum". *J. invest. Derm.* **16**, 217–230.

Hodgson-Jones, I. S., MacKenna, R. M. B. and Wheatley, V. R. (1952). The study of human sebaceous activity. *Acta derm.-venerol. (Stockh.)* **32** (Suppl. 29), 155–161.

Hodgson-Jones, I. S., MacKenna, R. M. B. and Wheatley, V. R. (1953). The surface skin fat in seborrhoeic dermatitis. *Br. J. Derm.* **65**, 246–251.

Holt, R. J. (1971). The esterase and lipase activity of aerobic skin bacteria. *Br. J. Derm.* **85**, 18–23.

Honsig, Chr. (1967). Vergleichende Untersuchungen über Lipidgehalt und Regenerationszeit an der Innenseite von Hand und Vorderarm unter Berücksichtigung des Spreiteffektes. MD-Thesis Munich.

Hopf, G. and Winkler, A. (1959). Untersuchungen über die Spreitwirkung des Hauttalges. *Fette–Seifen–Anstrichmittel* **61**, 974–978.

Horáček, J. (1953). Mikroby kuže ve vztahu k lipoidnimu profilu povnchu kožniho. (The microbes of the skin in relation to the skin surface lipids.) *Bratisl. lék. Listy* **33**, 687–695.

Horáček, J. (1965). "Ochranné mechanismy epidermálni". (Protective mechanisms of epidermis.) Dissert. Karl's Universität, Praha.

Horáček, J. and Pospišil, L. (1965). Lipázy stafylokoků kožniho povrchu. (The lipases of the skin surface staphylococci.) *Bratisl. lék. Listy* **45**, 193–197.

Ikai, K. and Nitta, H. (1962). Thermogenic, hormonal and neural control in the sebaceous excretion. Proc. 12th int. Congr. Derm. Washington, Exc. Med. Found. Amsterdam–New York–London–Milan–Tokyo, 2, 1215–1216.

Izumi, A. K., Marples, R. R., Path, M. R. C. and Kligman, A. M. (1973). Senile (solar) comedones. J. invest. Derm. 61, 46–50.

Jadassohn, W. (1963). Hautanhangsgebilde. Arch. klin. exp. Derm. 219, 63–82.

Josephs, H., Gloor, M. and Friederich, H. C. (1974). Über den Einfluß der Lipidsammelsammelmethode auf den Nachweis von Paraffinen in den Hautoberflächenlipiden. Derm. Mschr. 161, 97–103.

Kellum, R. E. (1966). Isolation of human sebaceous gland. Arch. Derm. 93, 610–612.

Kellum, R. E. (1967). Human sebaceous gland lipids. Analysis by thin layer chromatography. Arch. Derm. 95, 218–220.

Kellum, R. E. (1968). Acne vulgaris, Studies in pathogenesis. Relative irritancy of free fatty acids from C2 to C16. Arch. Derm. 97, 722–726.

Kellum, R. E. and Strangfeld, K. (1972). Acne vulgaris. Studies in pathogenesis: Fatty acids of human surface triglycerides from patients with and without acne. J. invest. Derm. 58, 315–322.

Kleine-Natrop, H. E. (1960). Talgspiegel und Benetzbarkeit der Haut. Proc. 11th Int. Congr. Derm. Stockholm 1957. Acta derm.-venerol. (Stockh.) 3, 248–253.

Kligman, A. M. (1963). The uses of sebum? In "Advances in biology of skin" (Eds W. Montagna, R. A. Ellis and A. F. Silver), Vol. 4, 110–124. Pergamon Press, Oxford–London–New York–Paris.

Kligman, A. M. and Shelley, W. B. (1958). An investigation of the biology of the human sebaceous gland. J. invest. Derm. 30, 99–126.

Kligman, A. M., Wheatley, V. R. and Mills, O. H. (1970). Comedogenicity of human sebum. Arch. Derm. 102, 267–278.

Kohn, St. R., Pochi, P. E., Strauss, J. S., Sax, D. S., Feldman, R. G. and Timberlake, W. T. (1973). Sebaceous gland secretion in Parkinson's disease during L-Dopa treatment. J. invest. Derm. 60, 134–136.

Konrád, B. and Černiková, M. (1963). Biochemische Untersuchungen bei Dermatitis seborrhoica. Derm. Wschr. 147, 383–385.

Korenev, I. P. (1965). Izmenenije salnych željez koži krolikov pod vlijanijem ultravioletovych lučej. Vestn. Derm. Vener. 38, 42–45.

Korolev, J. F. (1958). Izmenenije sostava koznovo sala pri seboreje. Vestn. Derm. Vener. 32, 9–14.

Kraus, J. S. (1970). Stress, acne and skin surface free fatty acids. Psychosom. Med. 32, 503–508.

Kuhn-Bussius, H. (1974). Messungen von Regeneration und jahreszeitlichen Schwankungen des Hautfettes beim Menschen. Kosmetologie 3, 96–98.

Lantz, J. P., Sutter, M. T. and Tardieu, J. C. (1972). Composition du sébum humain. Édude préliminaire des acides gras totaux par chromatographie en phase gazeuse chez des sujets du sexe féminin acnéiques et normaux avant et après prise d'oestro-progestatifs de synthèse. Ann. Derm. Syph. (Paris) 99, 277–280.

Lorincz, A. L., Krizek, H. and Brown, S. (1968). Follicular hyperkeratinization induced in the rabbit ear by human skin surface lipids. XIII. Int. Congr. Derm., Munich 1967, Vol. II, pp. 1016–1017, Springer-Verlag, Berlin Heidelberg, New York.

Ludwig, E. (1972). Behandlung der Seborrhoea oleosa und Acne mit kontrazeptiven Hormonen. In "Ovulationshemmer in der Dermatologie. Therapeutische Anwendung und Nebenwirkungen an der Haut" (Ed. H. Zaun), 27–35. Georg Thieme, Verlag, Stuttgart.

Lutsky, B., Budak, M., Koziol, P., Monahan, M. and Neri, R. O. (1975). The effects of a nonsteroid antiandrogenflutamide on sebaceous gland activity. *J. invest. Derm.* **64**, 412–417.

MacDonald, I. (1973). Some effects of fats with dietary carbohydrates on the lipids on the surface of the skin. *Brit. J. Derm.* **88**, 267–271.

Marchionini, A., Manz, E. and Huss, F. (1938). Der Cholesteringehalt der Hautoberschicht bei der Seborrhoea und bei der Psoriasis: Beitrag zur Kenntnis der pathochemischen Hautkonstitution der Status seborrhoicus. *Arch. Derm. Syph. (Berl.)* **176**, 613–645.

Marples, R. R., McGinley, K. J. and Mills, O. H. (1973). Microbiology of comedones in acne vulgaris. *J. invest. Derm.* **60**, 80–83.

Meffert, H., Geschwendt, G. and Reich, P. (1969). Über Cholesterin und Cholesterinester im Oberflächenfett von Psoriasis-vulgaris-Kranken. *Derm. Mschr.* **155**, 161–168.

Meffert, H. and Reich, P. (1969). Lipoperoxide und Dithranol-(Cignolin)-Effekt bei Psoriasis vulgaris. *Derm. Mschr.* **155**, 157–161.

Miescher, G. (1931). Die Schutzfunktion der Haut gegenüber Lichtstrahlen. *Strahlentherapie* **39**, 601–618.

Miescher, G. (1960). Antibacterial effects of sebum and the inhibition of these effects by free amino acids. Proc. 11th int. Congr. Derm. Stockholm 1957. *Acta derm.-venerol. (Stockh.)* **2**, 9–13.

Miescher, G. and Schönberg, A. (1944). Untersuchungen über die Funktion der Talgdrüsen. *Bull. schweiz. Acad. med. Wissenschaft* **1**, 101–108.

Morello, A. M. and Downing, D. T. (1976). Trans-unsaturated fatty acids in human skin surface lipids. *J. invest. Derm.* **67**, 279–272.

Mustakallio, K. K., Kiistala, U., Piha, H. J. and Nieminen, E. (1967). Epidermal lipids in Besnier's prurigo. *Ann. Med. Exper. Fenn.* **45**, 323–325.

Nicolaides, N. (1961). Gas chromatographic analysis of the waxes of human scalp skin surface fat. *J. invest. Derm.* **37**, 507–510.

Nicolaides, N. (1965). Skin lipids. IV. Biochemistry and function. *J. Amer. Oil Chem. Soc.* **42**, 708–712.

Nicolaides, N., Ansari, M. N. A., Fu, H. C. and Lindsay, D. G. (1970). Lipid composition of comedones compared with that of human skin surface in acne patients. *J. invest. Derm.* **54**, 487–495.

Nicolaides, N. and Rothman, S. (1953). Studies on the chemical composition of human hair fat. *J. invest. Derm.* **21**, 9–14.

Nicolaides, N. and Wells, G. C. (1957). On the biogenesis of the free fatty acids in human skin surface fat. *J. invest. Derm.* **29**, 423–433.

Noble, W. C. and Somerville, D. A. (1974). "Microbiology of the human skin". W. B. Saunders Comp. Ltd., London–Philadelphia–Toronto.

Ohkido, M., Suzuki, K., Sugihara, I. and Minzono, N. (1974). Effects of ultraviolet irradiation of human skin lipids—in vivo and in vitro studies. *Acta derm.-venerol. (Stockh.)* **54**, 223–226.

Pablo, G., Hammons, A., Bradley, S. and Fulton, J. E. (1974). Characteristics of the extracellular lipases from corynebacterium acnes and staphylococcus epidermidis. *J. invest. Derm.* **63**, 231–238.

Peter, G. and Eichenseher, K. (1973). Relation in der Lipidzusammensetzung von Comedonen, palmarer Hautoberfläche und Talgdrüsen. *Arch. Derm. Res.* **247**, 329–336.

Peter, G., Ritter, W., Schröpl, F. and Peter, R. (1971). Gaschromatographische Untersuchungen der Talgdrüsenlipide. II. Zusammensetzung der Talgdrüsenlipide im Altersablauf. *Arch. Derm. Res.* **241**, 22–32.

Peter, G., Schröpl, F., Lippross, R. and Weiss, G. (1970). Gaschromatographische Untersuchungen der Talgdrüsenlipide. I. Bestimmung der Gesamtlipide. *Arch. klin. exp. Derm.* **239**, 12–21.

Plewig, G. and Schöpf, E. (1976). Antiinflammatory effects of antimicrobial agents—an *in vivo* study. *J. invest. Derm.* **65**, 532–536.

Plewig, G. and Kligman, A. M. (1970). Zellkinetische Untersuchungen bei Kopfschuppenerkrankungen (Pityriasis simplex capillitii). *Arch. klin. exp. Derm.* **236**, 406–421.

Pochi, P. E., Downing, D. T. and Strauss, J. S. (1970). Sebaceous gland response in man to prolonged caloric deprivation. *J. invest. Derm.* **53**, 303–309.

Pochi, P. E. and Strauss, J. S. (1974). Endocrinologic control of the development and activity of the human sebaceous gland. *J. invest. Derm.* **62**, 191–201.

Puhvel, S. M. (1975). Esterification of ($L^{14}C$) cholesterol by cutaneous bacteria (staphylococcus epidermidis, propionibacterium acnes and propionibacterium granulosum). *J. invest. Derm.* **64**, 397–400.

Puhvel, M. S. and Sakamoto, M. (1977). A re-evaluation of free fatty acids as inflammatory agents in acne. *J. invest. Derm.* **68**, 93–97.

Pye, J. R., Meyrick, G. and Burton, J. L. (1976). Skin surface lipid composition in rosacea. *Br. J. Derm.* **94**, 161–164.

Pye, R. J., Meyrick, G. and Burton, J. L. (1977). Skin surface lipids in seborrhoeic dermatitis. *Br. J. Derm.* **97** (Suppl. 15), 12–13.

Rajka, G. (1974). Surface lipid estimation on the back of the hands in atopic dermatitis. *Arch. Derm. Res.* **251**, 43–48.

Rätz, K. H. and Mattheus, A. (1975). Beeinflussung der Hautoberflächenlipide durch einige Lokaltherapeutika. *Derm. Mschr.* **161**, 948–951.

Rauschkolb, E. W., Davis, H. W., Fenimore, D. C., Black, H. S. and Fabre, L. F. (1969). Identification of vitamin D_3 in human skin. *J. invest. Derm.* **53**, 289–294.

Roberts, D. (1975). The role of bacteria in acne vulgaris. Ph.D. Thesis, Leeds.

Rothman, S. (1950). Abnormalities in the chemical composition of the skin surface film in psoriasis. *Arch. Derm.* **62**, 814–819.

Runkel, R. A., Wurster, D. E. and Cooper, G. A. (1969). Investigation of normal and acne skin surface lipids. *J. pharm. Sci.* **58**, 582–585.

Sauter, L. S. and Loud, A. V. (1975). Morphometric evaluation of sebaceous gland volume in intact, castrated and testosterone treated rats. *J. invest. Derm.* **64**, 9–13.

Schäfer, H. (1973). The quantitative differentiation of sebum excretion using physical methods. *J. Soc. Cosmet. Chem.* **24**, 331–353.

Schäfer, H. and Kuhn-Bussius, H. (1970). Methodik zur quantitativen Bestimmung der menschlichen Talgsekretion. *Arch. klin. exp. Derm.* **238**, 429–435.

Schmidt, U., Hunziger, N., Brun, R. and Jadassohn, W. (1964). The protective effect of the sebaceous layer. *Br. J. Derm.* **76**, 395–398.

Schneider, W. (1970). Hautkonstitution und Kosmetik. *Cosmetologica* **19**, 231–236.

Schneider, W. and Schuleit, H. (1951). Der Fettmantel der Haut und seine Bedeutung für die Benetzung. *Arch. Derm. Syph. (Berl.)* **193**, 434–459.

Schnur, H. and Goldfarb, L. (1927). Zur Physiologie und Pathologie der Talgsekretion 1. Untersuchungsmethodik und allgemeiner Sekretionsmechanismus (Regulation). *Wien. klin. Wschr.* **40**, 1255–1259.

Schweikert, H. U. (1967). Quantitative Untersuchungen über die Talgdrüsenfunktion bei Alopecia areata. *Arch. klin. exp. Derm.* **230**, 96–110.

Schweikert, H. U. (1968). Quantitative Untersuchungen über die Talgdrüsenfunktion bei androgenetischer Alopecie. *Arch. klin. exp. Derm.* **231**, 200–206.

Shalita, A., Lewis, S. and Lee, W. (1975). Methods for analysis of sebum composition. *J. invest. Derm.* **64**, 293–294.

Skog, E. (1958). The influence of selenium disulfide on sebaceous gland volume in guinea pigs. *Acta derm.-venerol. (Stockh.)* **38**, 15–19.

Smith, J. G. and Brunot, F. R. (1961). Hormonal effects on aged human sebaceous glands. *Acta derm.-venerol. (Stockh.)* **41**, 61–65.

Steigleder, G. K. (1960). Bemerkungen über das Vorkommen von Enzymen auf, unter und in normaler und pathologisch veränderter Hornschicht. *Arch. klin. exp. Derm.* **211**, 203–207.

Strauss, J. S. and Pochi, P. E. (1961). The quantitative gravimetric determination of sebum production. *J. invest. Derm.* **36**, 293–298.

Strauss, J. S. and Pochi, P. E. (1965). Intracutaneous injection of sebum and comedones. *Arch. Derm.* **92**, 443–456.

Strauss, J. S. and Pochi, P. E. (1968). The pathogenesis of acne vulgaris. *J. Soc. Cosmet. Chem.* **19**, 644–648.

Stüttgen, G. (1967). Zum Einfluß pharmakologischer Reize auf die Hautfettregeneration. *Arch. klin. exp. Derm.* **219**, 795–799.

Sulzberger, M. and Herrmann, F. (1960). Some new observations on the biology of the skin surface. *Arch. Derm.* **81**, 235–244.

Summerly, R., Woodbury, S. and Boddie, H. G. (1971). The effect of facial nerve paresis on sebum excretion. *Br. J. Derm.* **84**, 602–604.

Summerly, R., Woodbury, S. and Yardley, H. J. (1972). The effect of eicosa 5:8:11:14 tetraynoic acid on skin lipid synthesis (^{14}C incorporation) *in vitro*. *Br. J. Derm.* **87**, 608–613.

Summerly, R., Yardley, H. J., Raymond, M., Tabiowo, A. and Ilderton, E. (1976). The lipid composition of sebaceous glands as a reflection of gland size. *Br. J. Derm.* **94**, 45–53.

Swanbeck, G. (1972). A new principle for the treatment of acne. *Acta derm.-venerol. (Stockh.)* **52**, 406–410.

Tronnier, H. (1958). Die experimentelle-dermatologische Prüfung des neuen Wirkstoffes 4-Hydroxy-2-oxybenzoxathiol. *Drug Res.* **8**, 647–651.

Tronnier, H. (1962). Über die Quellung und Austrocknung der menschlichen Haut und ihre Bedeutung. *Parf. Kosm.* **43**, 336–342.

Tronnier, H. (1972). Zur Wirkung hormoneller Ovulationshemmer auf die Erythem- und Pigmentempfindlichkeit, die Talg- und Schweißsekretion sowie die Gefäße der Haut. *In* "Ovulationshemmer in der Dermatologie. Therapeutische Anwendung und Nebenwirkungen an der Haut" (Ed. H. Zaun), 1–12. Georg Thieme, Verlag, Stuttgart.

Tronnier, H. and Brunn, G. (1972). Vergleichsuntersuchungen des Haut-oberflächenfettes Hautgesunder und Acnekranker. *Berufsdermatosen* **20**, 79–88.

Tronnier, H. and Kuhn-Bussius, H. (1974). Zur Brauchbarkeit optischer Methoden für die Bestimmung des Hautoberflächenfettes. *Kosmetologie* **3**, 230–234.

Ueda, H., Hayakawa, S., Hoshino, S. and Kobayashi, M. (1976). The effect of topically applied γ-oryzanol on sebaceous glands. *J. Derm.* **3**, 19–24.

Unna, P. G. (1921). Rosacea seborrhoica. *Münch. med. Wschr.* **68**, 701–702.

Vecova, N. and Picin, D. (1971). Quantitative and qualitative investigations of sebaceous secretion of the skin of normal individuals and patients with acne vulgaris. *Derm.-Venerol. (Sofia)* **10**, 14–19.

Weinstein, G. D. (1974). Cell kinetics of human sebaceous glands. *J. invest. Derm.* **62**, 144–146.

Weirich, E. G. and Longauer, J. (1974). Inhibition of sebaceous glands by topical application of oestrogen und antiandrogen on the auricular skin of rabbits. Histometric studies of the activity of the sebaceous glands. *Arch. Derm. Res.* **250**, 81–93.

Wheatley, V. R. and Reinertson, R. P. (1958). The presence of vitamin D precursors in human epidermis. *J. invest. Derm.* **31**, 51–54.

Whiteside, J. A. and Voss, J. G. (1973). Incidence and lipolytic activity of propionbacterium acnes (corynebacterium acnes group I) and *P. granulosum* (c. acnes group II) in acne and normal skin. *J. invest. Derm.* **60**, 94–97.

Wilkinson, D. I. and Farber, E. M. (1967a). Free and esterified sterols in surface lipids from uninvolved skin in psoriasis. *J. invest. Derm.* **48**, 249–251.

Wilkinson, D. I. and Farber, E. M. (1967b). Fatty acids of surface lipids from lipids from uninvolved skin in psoriasis. *J. invest. Derm.* **48**, 249–251.

Williams, M., Cunliffe, W. J. and Gould, D. (1974). Pilosebaceous duct physiology I. Effect of hydration on pilosebaceous duct orifice. *Br. J. Derm.* **90**, 631–635.

Winkler, K. (1972). Talgdrüsenaktivität im Spiegel endokriner Vorgänge. *Z. Haut-Geschl. Kr.* **47**, 925–930.

Winkler, K. and Schäfer, H. (1973). Das Verhalten der Talgsekretion während der Behandlung der Acne mit Cyproteronacetat und Äthinylöstradiol. *Arch. Derm. Res.* **247**, 249–265.

THE MOLECULAR BASIS OF SKIN IRRITATION

C. Prottey
Unilever Research Laboratory,
Port Sunlight, Wirral,
Merseyside L62 4XN, England

I. INTRODUCTION

A. Definitions

The molecular basis of skin irritation is defined as the adverse reactions of the cells and tissues of the skin, in terms of their constituent molecules, to the types of chemicals that may come in contact with the skin as a result of using cosmetics or skin products.

In a volume entitled "Cosmetic Science" in which skin irritation is discussed,[a] it should not be inferred that cosmetics and skin products in general cause skin irritation in man. Due to the stringency of national and international legislation and the social obligation of manufacturers not to market products that are hazardous to man, cosmetics may be considered to be non-irritant to the skin. Here, the phenomenon of skin irritation has been considered from the standpoint of the cosmetic chemist, whose aims include ensuring that products are non-irritant. This may be achieved by means of adequate premarketing safety tests to screen out potential irritants.

These tests usually involve laboratory animals and human panels, often with exaggerated conditions of application, and the total irritation potential is assessed by examination of the resultant skin reactions. Thus, an understanding of the chemical changes taking place in irritated skin may aid the interpretations of such tests.

1. *Primary Irritation*

Primary (non-allergic) irritation reactions are local skin responses that result in inflammation or injury at the site of application. They are elicited

[a] It is assumed that the reader is familiar with the structure and function of skin, which have been described elsewhere to varying degrees of detail (for example, Zelickson, 1967; Breathnach, 1971; Harry, 1973; Jarrett, 1973; Menton and Eisen, 1971; Montagna and Parakkal, 1974; MacKenzie, 1975).

by the direct toxic or cytolytic action of the applied stimuli (physical traumata or irritant chemicals) on the cells and tissues of the skin and do not involve the immunological system. Shelanski and Shelanski (1953) defined *primary* irritants as being toxic at first contact with the skin, and *secondary* irritants as those producing reactions only after repeated cutaneous contact. Whereas primary irritants would overcome the "protective mechanisms" of the skin on first contact and thereby elicit the irritation response of the tissue, other materials might never completely exhaust this protective capacity on single contact, and only repeated application of the latter would gradually and progressively damage the skin. Kligman and Wooding (1967) preferred the expression "strong" and "weak" irritants. As the skin reacts to varying degrees with different irritants (some eliciting no more than weak erythema or mild injury only after prolonged application, others producing erosions or irreversibly damaging the skin after short contact), it is probably more accurate to describe "weak" or "strong" irritation responses.

Primary irritation responses may be *acute*, when the response rapidly develops and rapidly diminishes, as after single or few applications of the irritant, or *chronic*, when tissue reactions persist for many days due to repeated irritant stimuli. Examples are given below of the effects of chemicals such as organic and inorganic electrolytes, solvents, acids, bases, emollients and surfactants, that are common ingredients of cosmetics. Also, certain types of physical traumata (heat, abrasion, ultraviolet ir-radiation, tape stripping) are included when relevant to the action of chemicals upon the skin. Much of current knowledge has been obtained from animal experiments, but the general mechanisms described largely pertain to man. Björnberg (1968) has described instances of primary skin irritation in man due to various chemicals.

2. *Allergic Inflammation*
Although allergic skin reactions (contact dermatitis) to cosmetics can occur, in the context of the vast numbers of cosmetic products sold each year, such reactions are uncommon. Cosmetics are not sources of potent allergens of the type of laboratory standards such as dinitrochlorobenzene, but they may contain weak sensitizers. Cronin (1967) stated that instances of allergic skin irritation mainly concerned certain lipstick dyes, nail varnish resins, lanolin and hair dyes. A more comprehensive list of such compounds has been compiled by Hardy (1973).

Allergic skin inflammations are not discussed in this review, except when relevant to primary irritation reactions. Definitions of various types of allergic reactions and details of mechanisms are covered in reviews by

Turk (1967), Weiss (1972), Hardy (1973), Fregert (1974) and Zweifach *et al.* (1974).

B. The Nature of the Cutaneous Responses to Primary Irritants

Primary irritants may interact with the skin in three broad ways. These are, firstly, superficially upon the dead cells of the stratum corneum, such as by removing lipids, soluble substances, water or cells, or by denaturing proteins, and these interactions lead to flakiness, dryness, loss of plasticity, impaired barrier function etc. Secondly, an irritant may penetrate the stratum corneum to the living cells of the epidermis, with effects ranging from merely stimulating epidermis metabolism that can result in hyperplasia, to frank cytotoxicity. Thirdly, and most easily recognized visually, an irritant may reach the dermis and elicit an inflammatory response. This classification is emphasized as it may be that some irritants act only upon one or two of these compartments, whereas others may act upon all three, and to varying degrees, depending upon concentration and frequency or duration of application. Furthermore, many of the responses of these three components are interdependent.

The total scope of the skin's reaction to primary irritants is illustrated in Fig. 1. The boldly outlined boxes show the three compartments of the skin, and the bold arrows portray their normal interactions.

The stratum corneum is in contact with the external environment. Indeed, it is the interface between man and the environment, and, as such, may be influenced by the environment (A). For example, water content and flexibility of the stratum corneum are known to be dependent upon ambient temperature and relative humidity; its structure is modified by daily wear and tear due to friction or contact with surfaces. But the stratum corneum is also intimately dependent upon the functioning of the epidermis (B), its thickness (number of cell layers) being governed by rates of cell division and differentiation. These latter mechanisms are under a precise homeostatic control, which, when interfered with by chemical irritants, lead to abnormal stratum corneum. In turn, the normal functions of the epidermis depend upon the influence of the dermis (C) for the supply of nutrients, hormones, and for structural specialization. All three cutaneous compartments are ultimately dependent upon the general state of health of the body (D), and may in themselves reflect impaired health or nutrition of the body by the way that they respond to the action of irritants.

Representative effects of irritants upon the three compartments of the skin are indicated in Fig. 1 by numbered arrows (1–19), and some of these interactions can be considered both as discrete and interrelated phenomena:

(1) The initial effects of an irritant chemical coming in contact with the stratum corneum may include its deposition upon the surface, adsorption onto the cell surfaces or penetration into the interior of the squames, and there may be an accumulation or reservoir of the irritant such that deleterious actions proceed long after the irritant stimulus has passed.

(2) In contracting the stratum corneum there may be unfolding of fibrous protines, denaturation of soluble proteins, extraction and loss of intracellular cementing substances, lipids, water binding components etc., with resultant modified structure and function of the stratum corneum, such as decreased flexibility and barrier properties.

(3) With irritants such as keratolytic agents (e.g. salicylic acid) there may be complete loss of portions of the stratum corneum.

(4) A stratum corneum modified by irritants may be further affected by adverse environmental conditions, such as low temperature and humidity (e.g. cold—chapping).

(5) Irritants may penetrate through or around the horny cells of the stratum corneum to the underlying living cells of the epidermis. Also, entry may be gained via the various appendages (hair follicles, apocrine and eccrine sweat glands, sebaceous glands). Penetration can proceed to the dermis (see xiii).

(6) Various responses of the living epidermal cells to penetrated irritants may result, ranging from metabolic stimulation and hypertrophy, to rapid cell death.

(7) A stratum corneum structurally impaired as a result of contact with irritant chemicals may have reduced barrier properties, allowing subsequent increased penetration and greater irritation of the underlying living tissues.

(8) The result of cellular stimulation in the epidermis may be a greatly accelerated cell turnover, that eventually results in a thickened, hyperkeratotic stratum corneum that has impaired flexibility or barrier properties.

(9) When the effect of an irritant stimulus is severe, epidermal necrosis may result, with the failure of the ability to divide and differentiate.

(10) With the failure of mitosis and differentiation there will be no production of new stratum corneum. (Such situations pertain to certain very corrosive or toxic chemicals, and so this interaction is not relevant to the effects of cosmetic ingredients.)

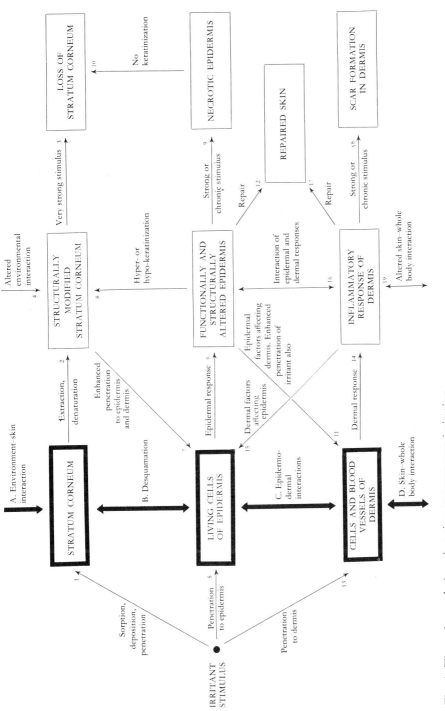

Fig. 1. Tissue interrelations in primary cutaneous irritation.

(11) Irritation of epidermal cells may result in the release of specific factors that subsequently diffuse to the dermis and elicit the inflammatory reaction.

(12) Tissue regeneration and repair generally follow rapidly after irritation of epidermal cells.

(13) Irritants applied to the stratum corneum may also rapidly or ultimately penetrate directly to the dermis, and exert direct effects upon the constituent cells and vessels.

(14) As a result of either epidermal factors (see 11) or penetrated irritants (see 13) the classical dermal inflammatory response may develop.

(15) Dermal inflammatory reactions may, conversely, release mediators or factors that stimulate responses of the overlying epidermal cells.

(16) In severe dermal inflammation, components of dermal oedema, degenerated leucocytes and various products of leucocytic activity may accumulate in the dermis, subsequently exude into the epidermis and be ultimately lost by the process of scab formation and sloughing.

(17) The consequence of acute dermal inflammation is tissue recovery and repair, as occurs in the epidermis (see 12).

(18) In severe or chronic inflammatory reactions, dermal connective tissues are so damaged or destroyed that the ultimate repair processes result in scar formation, with impaired elasticity (such instances are generally not pertinent to the effect of cosmetic ingredients, however).

(19) Products of the inflammation (e.g. inactivated mediators, interstitial fluid) are generally removed from the site of reaction via the lymphatic system and are ultimately excreted.

A point to be emphasized regarding the various reactions depicted in Fig. 1 is that, generally, few or none occur in isolation from others (except, perhaps, for certain chemicals that exert weak effects on the stratum corneum and never extensively penetrate, or when contact times with the stratum corneum are short). Skin irritation by chemicals is a complex and closely interrelated phenomenon. The structure and chemistry of the irritants themselves will determine the nature of the reactions that are possible, but frequency or duration of their contact with the skin will determine the extents of these reactions.

II. THE ACTIONS OF CHEMICALS ON THE STRATUM CORNEUM

The function of the stratum corneum is to act as a flexible and renewable barrier between the external environment and the living cells and tissues of the body. This barrier is bidirectional, preventing both the undue loss of body fluids, that would otherwise cause death of the underlying cells by dehydration, and regulating the percutaneous absorption of toxic materials and pathogenic organisms from the environment. Also the excessive uptake of water is prevented, that would otherwise cause osmotic lysis of the cells of the body. Flexibility of the stratum corneum is necessary in order to accommodate forces of flexion, compression, shear and friction due to movement and contact. Renewal of the stratum corneum by means of regulated epidermal proliferation (see below) is necessary to compensate for daily wear and tear. Thus, irritant chemicals may interact with and unfavourably influence this complex function, such that, at the very least, appearance or "feel" of the stratum corneum may be affected (dryness, roughness, glazing) and at worst, scaliness, fissuring, loss of flexibility and barrier function may result. This range of responses can be described in terms of the structure and chemical composition of the stratum corneum.

A. Structure of the Stratum Corneum

Mammalian stratum corneum is comprised of several flattened sheets of dehydrated, anucleated horny cells. In man these cells, usually hexagonal or pentagonal in shape, range in diameter from 25 μ to 45 μ, and 1000 μ^2 in area (Plewig and Marples, 1970), and are generally up to 1 μ thick. In man these cells are in close lateral contact, separated by intercellular spaces generally ranging from only 150 nm to 400 nm, and the relative surface area of the total intercellular spaces has been calculated to constitute only 0·1% to about 1% of the total surface area of the stratum corneum (Mercer, et al., 1968; Plewig and Marples, 1970). Furthermore, orifices of the pilosebaceous ducts, the eccrine and the apocrine sweat glands open onto the surface of the stratum corneum, and the numbers of these depend upon the body region and animal species. In man, Scheuplein (1967) calculated their contribution to the total surface area of the stratum corneum to be of the order of 0·1%. Clearly, chemicals that come in contact with the skin will, on a statistical basis, react far more so with horny cell surfaces per se than enter appendigeal orifices or intercellular spaces. In the context of skin barrier function and penetration of irritants, however, these minor structural components of the stratum corneum should not be overlooked.

In many regions of mammalian skin the individual horny cells are arranged in ordered, stacked columns, resembling piles of poker chips, with individual cells of the columns and neighbouring columns in close apposition (Mackenzie, 1969). In man, horny cells are about 0·8 μ thick and generally there are 10 to 25 cells stacked one above the other, so that the average thickness of the stratum corneum is about 10 μ, but callus areas of friction surfaces (e.g. plantar and palmar skin) may be much thicker (up to 200 μ). Using a technique of acid or alkali swelling of frozen sections of stratum corneum devised by Christophers and Kligman (1964), Mackenzie (1969) showed that ordered columns were laterally closely interdigitated with their neighbours, with no discrete channels between them. Edges of the hexagonal squames were seen to be stepped, rather like ship-lap timber, thus imparting lateral strength. When viewed from above, the horizontal sheets are seen as regular hexagons, resembling a honey-comb, as would result if horizontally arranged circular plates were packed to give maximal contact of their edges (Menton and Eisen, 1971). This propensity to form ordered columns was shown by MacKenzie (1971) to depend upon low rates of cellular proliferation in the epidermal basal layer. In body regions where epidermal turnover, differentiation and desquamation are relatively higher (e.g. friction surfaces) there is no ordered packing of squames in columns, individual squames are not hexagonal, intercellular spaces are wider, and the barrier properties of the skin are less than "ordered" areas. Recently it has been suggested (Allen and Potten, 1975) that in "ordered" stratum corneum, the desmosomal linkages seen in great abundance between cells of the basal, prickle and granular layers (Breathnach, 1971) are normally broken down by hydrolytic enzymes derived from the keratinosomes (Weinstock and Wilgram, 1970) (these are intracellular organelles that are seen in the electronmicroscope to secrete their contents into the extracellular spaces of the stratum granulosum, and appear to coat the horny cell membranes: they were termed "membrane-coating granules" by Matoltsy and Parakkal, 1965). Adherence of the individual squames within individual columns and to adjoining columns is thought to be maintained by the deposition of material from the keratinosomes called "squamosome", that ensures tight cell contact and absence of channels between cells and columns. It is not unreasonable to imagine that certain chemicals coming in contact with the stratum corneum may interact with these specialized cell contacts, with resultant impaired barrier function and mechanical strength.

Allen and Potten (1975) have suggested that in mouse skin, for example, stimulated to divide faster than normal by experimental wounding, the horny cells are no longer stacked in ordered columns and a stratum corneum with impaired function results. Therefore, irritant chemicals that stimulate the epidermis to divide and turnover at accelerated rates may thereby elicit non-ordered squame stacking, impaired squame adhesion, and abnormal function. Thus, certain irritants may also modify the structure of the stratum corneum both directly and immediately, and indirectly, by altering the processes of cell renewal.

B. Chemistry of the Stratum Corneum

The stratum corneum is the end-product of differentiation and controlled degeneration of the viable cells of the epidermis. By the time that these cells have reached the relatively anhydrous stratum corneum metabolic activity (such as respiration) has ceased as all their intracellular organelles and components (nuclei, mitochondria, ribosomes, lysosomes) have been degraded or recycled, leaving flattened cellular envelopes containing an amorphous intracellular matrix. Thus, irritant chemicals contacting the stratum corneum will exert solely physico-chemical interactions with the constituent molecules, such as sorption and binding (non-covalent) or extraction.

The constituent molecules of the stratum corneum (reviewed recently by Mershon, 1975) include proteins, lipids, nitrogenous and acidic small-molecular weight compounds, polysaccharides and minerals, and they can be considered collectively, but in four discrete compartments.

1. *The skin surface film* or "acid mantle" is a mixture of water, lipids, proteins and salts derived from apocrine and eccrine sweat and sebum. It plays either a very limited or, indeed, no part at all in the regulation of flexibility and barrier function of the stratum corneum (Kligman, 1963). Removal of surface film by chemicals may influence the "feel" of the skin or its gross appearance to a degree. For example, removal of skin surface lipids by contact with a non-irritant solvent such as diethyl ether may produce a "whiteness" of the stratum corneum due to the presence of air between the outermost horny cells, thereby altering their light-reflecting properties, but such changes will always be short-lived due to the rapidity with which surface film is restored by continuing secretions of the sweat and sebaceous glands. Functional changes in the stratum corneum due to chemical irritants arise from interactions with the other components.

2. *The membranes of the horny cells* constitute about 5% by weight of the stratum corneum and comprise about 2/3 proteins, 1/3 lipids and small amounts of carbohydrates (Plewig and Marples, 1970). The membrane proteins contain about 13% proline, thereby preventing an helical arrangement, together with about 8% half-cystine units, allowing disulphide bridges and accounting for their insolubility and strength (Mershon, 1975). The lipids of the horny cell membranes, presumably derived from lipids of the differentiated cells that were not recycled or oxidized for energy, have been suggested to be different in composition from the lipids of the skin surface film (derived from sebum), and comprise about 65% triglycerides, 20% sterol esters and 15% free sterols (Downing and Strauss,

1974), although phospholipids have also been indicated (Spearman and Hardy, 1973).

3. *The intracellular matrix of the horny cells* (up to 85% of the stratum corneum) is an homogenous complex of filaments up to 90 nm in diameter that are themselves associations of low-sulphur containing, sulphur-rich and histidine-containing proteins. These filaments are coated with keratohyalin, nucleoproteins, non-fibrous proteins and lipids. About 10% of the stratum corneum that is part of the intracellular matrix is a mixture of water-soluble, dialysable small molecular weight molecules (Spier and Pascher, 1957). These are hygroscopic, and have also been termed the "Natural Moisturizer Factor" (Jacobi, 1959). They are probably end-products of epidermal nitrogen metabolism (i.e. urea from the ornithine cycle, lactic acid from glycolysis), and Middleton (1968) proposed their involvement in the binding of water in the stratum corneum, that ensures plasticity (Blank, 1952). The spatial arrangement of the components of the intra-cellular matrix has been discussed in detail by Mershon (1975).

4. *The intercellular material* (about 10% of the stratum corneum) is comprised of lipids, proteins, polysaccharides and some minerals (Brody, 1966), derived, at least in part, from the keratinosomes or membrane-coating granules (see above). This material ensures the tight attachment of individual squames, and the absence of discrete diffusion channels between the cells.

C. Impaired Stratum Corneum Function as a Result of Contact with Irritant Chemicals

1. *Barrier Function*

It is now widely accepted that the whole of the stratum corneum constitutes the barrier between the living cells of the organism and the external environment (Scheuplein and Blank, 1971). Barrier function has been measured in various ways, such as by the direct determination of the amount of a topically applied substance that penetrates to the blood, major organs or excretia (of live animals) (Howes, 1975; Prottey and Ferguson, 1975), by measuring the rate of transepidermal water loss *in vivo*, using man or animals (Matoltsy *et al.*, 1968), or by an indirect means such as conductivity (Dugard and Scheuplein, 1973).

(a) *The role of lipids in barrier function, and the action of solvents*   Skin lipids have long been considered to play an indisputable role in regulating barrier function, and so organic solvents, which can dissolve lipids, should be expected to have marked effects. Following the first report by Berenson and Burch (1951) that lipid removal enhanced penetration (i.e. barrier function was impaired) many others have subsequently appeared, such as the work of Onken and Moyer (1963), Vinson *et al.* (1965), Blank *et al.* (1967). Sweeney and Downing (1970) extracted human and mouse skin with a variety of lipid solvents of differing polarity (acetone, diethyl ether, chloroform and dimethyl sulphoxide). The first three solvents extracted cholesterol, wax alcohols, free fatty acids, triglycerides, wax and sterol diesters and wax monoesters, whereas dimethyl sulphoxide extracted only cholesterol, free fatty acids and triglycerides. In terms of effect upon varrier function, the activity of these solvents, in decreasing ability to enhance water diffusion, was chloroform > > dimethyl sulphoxide > ether > acetone ≥ no effect, but there were no correlations between the types or quantity of lipids removed and damage to the barrier. Exposure of the stratum corneum to non-polar solvents, such as petroleum ether or hexane, will readily cause the skin surface film of lipid to be removed, but there will be no effect upon the more polar lipids that are associated with proteins of the stratum corneum architecture. Indeed, non-polar solvents have been widely used in non-invasive techniques for sampling skin surface lipids (Downing and Strauss, 1974).

For solvents to affect barrier function they must chemically interact with, or extract, the structural lipids, that are distinctly different both in location and composition from skin surface film. Spearman and Hardy (1973) differentiated between the action of polar (pyridine, ethanol) and non-polar (petrol ether) solvents. The former act by disrupting phospho-lipid-protein hydrogen bonds, and pyridine, for example, removes phospholipids from unkeratinized cell membranes and cytoplasm, from keratohyalin granules (revealing a fine fibrillar structure), and from the interior of horny cells, leaving intact the more resistant plasma membranes. These authors suggested that non-polar solvents had minimal effect upon polar lipids bound to proteins unless linkages are disrupted by prior action of a polar solvent. This is well illustrated by reference to the action of mixtures of chloroform and methanol on the skin. Chloroform alone on the skin is sufficiently non-polar to remove only non-polar surface lipids, and cannot disrupt lipid-protein associations. Methanol, on the other hand, is sufficiently polar to break such links but is a poor solvent for lipids. When a mixture of chloroform–methanol (2:1 v/v) contacts the skin, the resultant actions of both include extensive extraction and dissolution of lipids, loss of barrier function and (as many hapless investigators will testify) considerable pain, not produced by either chloroform or methanol alone.

It has been generally accepted for many years (Malkinson, 1964; Scheuplein and Blank, 1971) that barrier function of the stratum corneum is maintained by the constituent cells *per se*, and not the intercellular spaces (as described above, the area of the intercellular space is far less than that of the flattened horny cells). However, recent evidence has been supplied by Elias (1975; Elias and Daniel, 1975) that lipid solvents reduce the barrier properties of the corneum by extraction of the lipid-rich material of the intercellular spaces of the stratum corneum. At the present time it is technically impossible to determine the discrete lipids of the horny cell interior, membranes, and the intercellular material, in order to evaluate their relative involvements in barrier function, but it is likely that lipids of all three sites are important. Electron microscopic studies on the action of kerosene and acetone (Lupulesco *et al.*, 1973) and pyridine (Spearman and Hardy, 1973) confirm the complex changes occurring in the stratum corneum. Recently, several instances of a precise role for linoleic acid in the maintenance of barrier function of certain laboratory animals have been reviewed (Prottey, 1976).

(b) *The actions of surface active materials upon barrier function—the role of proteins* There is much evidence that various surface active materials (including some soaps and synthetic detergents) may exert deleterious actions on the stratum corneum, and morphological studies in the light- and electron microscope have been reported (Kirk, 1966; Loomans and Hannon, 1970; Lansdown and Grasso, 1972). Their effects upon barrier function have been extensively studied. Bettley and Donohue (1960) showed that contact of the skin *in vitro* with a commercial soap or pure potassium palmitate caused marked increases in permeability to water, and a synthetic detergent, Teepol, had a much smaller effect. However, as these changes were reversible (disappearing when the surfactants were removed) it was thought that extraction and removal of lipids during contact could not be the prime cause of impaired barrier function. Further studies by Bettley (1961, 1965) and Smeenk and Polano (1965) demonstrated the enhanced permeability of human skin to various ions and chemicals as a result of exposure to solutions of surface active materials. Dugard and Scheuplein (1973) have described the use of conductance for measuring permeability of the skin. This is a very sensitive method, more so than those utilizing gravimetry, tritiated water, or determination of ion concentrations chemically, and these authors found relationships of chemical structure of various surfactants and their effects on barrier function. At low surfactant concentrations the changes in barrier function were reversible, and un-related to their detergency properties, ruling out extraction of lipids from the stratum corneum as a major, or sole cause of the effects. Only when such materials were used at higher concentrations were irreversible changes in skin permeability observed.

It is likely that both proteins and lipids contribute to the maintenance of barrier function, and surface-active substances have received particular attention with respect to the denaturation of proteins. Following the early work describing the interactions of anionic surfactants with soluble proteins, leading to complex formation and denaturation (reviewed by Putnam, 1948), relationships of protein denaturation by surfactants and their skin irritation potential were sought by numerous investigators. Van Scott and Lyon (1953) showed that when keratin powder was treated with various soaps and detergents, there was liberation of sulphydryl groups indicating unfolding of proteins. Similar studies were reported by Harrold (1959) who suggested that liberation of sulphydryl groups of keratin after contact with surfactants was due to breakage of weak hydrogen bonds and salt linkages (not the breakage of covalent disulphide bridges) between the polypeptide chains of keratin. Anionic surfactants were more potent than soap, and non-ionic surfactants had no effect upon sulphydryl release. Smeenk and Polano (1965) and Smeenk (1969) obtained similar results for different types of commercial surfactants. Recently, Wood and Bettley (1971) and Prottey and Ferguson (1975) have studied pure surfactants. In both studies, incomplete correlation between the ability to denature the skin and to irritate the skin were found. Nonetheless, there is ample evidence that certain surfactants (principally anionic synthetic detergents) are able to bind to and interact with stratum corneum proteins, causing swelling and uncoiling of them. Studies by Blohm (1957), with alkyl sulphates and soluble ovalbumin, and those of Harrold (1959), showed that sulphydryl group liberation was reversible, after removal of the surfactant, the proteins would re-align and reform original tertiary structures.

(c) *The effects of other solvents*   The action of dimethyl sulphoxide on the stratum corneum has received attention following the finding that this solvent enhanced percutaneous absorption (Stoughton and Fritsch, 1964; Kligman, 1965). Typical of numerous studies, Elfbaum and Laden (1968) showed that enhanced penetration of compounds depended upon the concentration of dimethyl sulphoxide, which required to be greater than about 60% in water in order to facilitate penetration. This was thought to be due to the unfolding and expansion of proteins, as demonstrated with albumin and keratin of skin and hair. Dioxan, which also swelled keratin, similarly enhanced skin penetration. The phenomenon was found to be reversible, and Elfbaum and Laden also suggested the participation of lipid removal in the action of this solvent. Baker (1968) reported that the application of three aprotic solvents, dimethyl sulphoxide, dimethyl formamide and dimethyl acetamide, profoundly influenced transepidermal water loss. Up to 10-fold increases in the rate were seen within two hours of application to the skin, which had returned to normal by twenty four hours. Although erythema was also elicited by these chemicals, Baker suggested that this did not influence barrier function.

Wright and Winer (1966) and Montes *et al.* (1967) described morphological changes in the stratum corneum exposed to dimethyl sulphoxide that suggested it acted by dissolving the intracellular contents of the horny cells and altered the fibrillar components, but had no effect upon the cell membranes. Embery and Dugard (1971) showed that extraction of human stratum corneum membranes with dimethyl sulphoxide removed substantial amounts of unidentified lipids and water-soluble components. This was offered as a possible explanation of how the solvent reduced barrier function. But it is difficult to reconcile how extraction (i.e. removal or translocation) of such important structural components as lipids could induce changes in barrier function, when such changes were reversible after the solvent had been removed (Baker, 1968). Embery and Dugard also considered that reversible conformational changes in proteins of stratum corneum might result from the direct substitution by dimethyl sulphoxide molecules of water required for the integrity of the lipoprotein membranes: at high concentrations of dimethyl sulphoxide, substitution of water (solvation) is known (Rammler and Zaffaroni, 1967).

(d) *Extraction of non-lipid material from the stratum corneum*   In 1952 Blank showed that the plasticity of stratum corneum was due to the presence of water, without which it would become dry and brittle. The work of Spier and Pascher (1957) identified a number of water-soluble and strongly hygroscopic substances in the stratum corneum (free amino acids, lactic, urocanic and pyrollidone carboxylic acids, urea, ammonia and sugars) that were shown to be responsible for the binding of water in the stratum corneum (Blank and Shappirio, 1955; Spier and Schwartz, 1962). Jacobi (1959) collectively described these components as the "natural moisturizer factor". Middleton (1968) proposed that the mechanism of water binding involved these hygroscopic substances that were held within the stratum corneum cells by semi-permeable lipoprotein membranes, and that treatment of the skin with lipid solvents dissolved the lipids of the semi-permeable membranes, thus allowing the hygroscopic substances to be leached out and lost. Moreover, Middleton (1969) suggested that certain detergents (e.g. sodium lauryl sulphate) could dissolve these lipids and allow the intracellular hygroscopic substances to escape, with resultant loss of water-binding ability. Indeed, detergents such as sodium lauroyl isethionate, which removed less lipids from the corneum, also had markedly less effect upon water binding capacity than sodium lauryl sulphate.

Smeenk and Polano (1965) and Smeenk (1969) showed that when human forearm skin was washed with various synthetic detergent solutions in a "washing simulator" (Vermeer *et al.*, 1963), free amino acids, soluble and insoluble proteins (i.e. horny cells) were all present in the wash liquors, in greater amounts than with just water washes. Brehm (1966) identified albumin and γ-globulin among the soluble proteins extractable from human skin with water.

Further studies with a Vermeer washing simulator have been described by Prottey and Ferguson (1975) with guinea pigs *in vivo*. Here, greater quantities of soluble protein and amino acids were removed with the more polar, anionic surfactants than with soap or water alone. Homologous series of alkyl sulphates and alkyl carboxylates (soaps) were studied, and it was found that the C_{12} (lauryl) and C_{14} (myristyl) moieties extracted far more of both fractions than higher or lower homologues. Thin-layer chromatographic separation of the amino acid fraction identified pyrollidone carboxylic acid, urocanic acid, alanine, citrulline, serine, glycine, arginine and ornithine as major components (C. Prottey, unpublished observations). Increased extraction by surfactants was only seen above their critical micelle concentrations, however.

It is probable that the water-soluble metabolites extracted by surface-active materials are not critical to the barrier properties of the skin, as they are almost certainly intracellular materials, and vestigial products of metabolism of the epidermal cells prior to cornification. Their presence in wash liquors, however, is probably an indication of disrupted horny cell membranes, as their extraction would only be possible if these membranes were damaged.

(e) *Determinants of barrier function in the skin*   Matoltsy *et al.* (1968) evaluated the respective roles of lipids, soluble proteins, insoluble cytoplasmic proteins (keratin) and insoluble plasma membrane proteins in the maintenance of barrier function. The effect of application of various organic solvents (including diethyl ether, dimethyl sulphoxide, acetone and ethanol), all increased the rate of transepidermal water diffusion, confirming the importance of lipids in barrier function. Extraction of soluble proteins with buffers in the range pH 4–10 did not produce significant alterations, suggesting that these components were not involved. Use of keratolytic agents showed that insoluble cytoplasmic proteins contributed to the barrier, but the proteins of the plasma membranes of horny cells seemed to be most important. Scheuplein and Ross (1970) precisely summarized the effects of different substances upon permeability. Lipid solvents remove large quantities of stratum corneum lipids, opening membrane interstices, that leads to loss of water-binding capacity but not impairing the structural elements or the mechanical strength. The result is an irreversibly increased permeability of the stratum corneum. Hydrogen-bonding solvents, such as water, dimethyl sulphoxide, not only may remove lipids, but solvate the membrane, interacting with proteins, causing swelling, with greater membrane permeability. Permeability is increased, usually reversibly when the solvent is removed, but some permanent damage may result. Surfactants, such as the anionic sodium lauryl sulphate, bind strongly to keratin filaments within the horny cell cytoplasm as well as the plasma membrane proteins. Reversible (at low concentration) denaturation or uncoiling occurs, with expansion of the tissue and loss of water binding capacity. Permeability is increased reversibly, but may become irreversible after prolonged treatment.

2. *Mechanical Properties*
In fulfilling its function as a barrier, the stratum corneum necessarily must be flexible, in order to withstand physical forces encountered during body movement and contact with surfaces. Equally, the smoothness and flexibility of the stratum corneum are important to cosmetic aspects. In particular, the stratum corneum must be plastic and elastic, and these physical properties are determined at the molecular level by the three-dimensional matrix of fibrillar proteins, lipids, polysaccharides and small molecular weight compounds. Chemicals that may come in contact with the stratum corneum and interact with its structural components, as well as affecting barrier function (as has already been discussed), may also considerably alter its mechanical properties. Reports such as those of Singer and Vinson (1966), Middleton (1968, 1969) and Park and Baddiel (1972) are representative of many that indicate how water binding by the stratum corneum, and, *ipso facto*, plasticity or rheology, may be altered by chemicals. Also Wildnauer and co-workers have extensively investigated the mechanical properties of the stratum corneum and the ways in which these are affected by various means (for a recent review, see Wildnauer *et al.*, 1975, to which the reader is also referred for general references to this aspect).

III. THE ACTIONS OF CHEMICAL IRRITANTS ON THE LIVING CELLS OF THE EPIDERMIS

The stratum corneum is non-living, metabolically inactive, and composed of a variety of structural molecules, and the effects of chemical irritants are physico-chemical interactions that are quickly manifested and readily observable or measurable. This is not so for the interactions of irritants with the underlying living cells of the epidermis, namely, the stratum basale (basal layer), the stratum spinosum (prickle cell layer) and the stratum granulosum (granular layer). Irritants that penetrate to the living epidermal cells can exert two broad categories of effects: on the one hand there may be direct toxic or cytolytic actions, producing cell death immediately, or soon after contact, or, on the other hand, there may be minor or moderate interactions that take much longer times to be manifested. These latter interactions range in magnitude from mere metabolic stimulations, that results in cellular hyperproliferation (hyperplasia), to metabolic disturbances, that release mediators of subsequent tissue reactions and tissue damage, resulting in grossly accelerated or maybe imperfect stratum corneum production. The extents to which the living cells of the epidermis so respond depend upon many factors, principally the chemical properties of the irritant and the mode of application to the skin, but body site and general health status of the organism are also important.

A. Morphological Changes

There are many references to structural changes produced in the epidermis by chemical irritants. The effects of soaps and detergents have been described by Skog (1958), Rebello and Suskind (1963), Mezei et al. (1966), McOsker and Beck (1967), Loomans and Hannon (1970), Lansdown and Grasso (1972), Prottey et al. (1973), Tovell et al. (1974). Of many descriptions of the effects of organic liquids and solvents, Steele and Wilhelm (1966, 1970) studied xylene, benzene, chloroform, carbon tetrachloride, acetic acid and phenol. Pyridine and chloroform have been studied by Spearman and Hardy (1973). Paraffins such as hexadecane have received detailed study (Kirk and Hoekstra, 1974; Rossmiller and Hoekstra, 1965; Christophers and Braun-Falco, 1970; Cowan and Mann, 1971; Hoekstra and Phillips, 1973), as have dimethyl sulphoxide (Wright and Winer, 1966; Montes et al., 1967), kerosene and acetone (Lupulesco et al., 1973). Nagao et al. (1972) described the ultrastructural changes following application of acid and alkali to human epidermis, and Lansdown (1973) by light microscopy has shown epidermal damage by aluminium salts.

Certain irritants elicit rapid epidermal responses. For example, within minutes of applying solvents such as xylene to the skin, Steel and Wilhelm (1970) observed loss of basophilic—and increased eosinophilic staining, particularly in the region of hair follicles, indicative of rapid initial penetration of the irritant via the appendigeal route (or "shunt"), as suggested by Scheuplein and Blank (1971). Nagao et al. (1972) described early changes due to alkali associated with presumed follicular entry of the irritant. Within the first hour, changes included more overt signs of cell damage, such as loss or clumping of nuclear chromatin, degeneration of mitochondria and dissociation of tonofilaments. At early stages the epidermal reaction is focal, later extending to the whole epidermis underlying the treated surface.

Later changes in irritated epidermis are probably mediated by the release of local hormones, hydrolytic enzymes, lower pH etc., rather than by the direct action of the irritant upon the cells. Such changes include shrinkage and pyknosis of nuclei, perinuclear vacuolation, intercellular oedema and spongiosis, rupture of dermosomal linkages, and extracellular deposition of cytoplasmic debris. Some of these features have been described by Lupulesco *et al.* (1973) for certain solvents, and Tovell *et al.* (1974) for sodium lauryl sulphate. Generally, when severe epidermal responses result, after a day or so outgrowth of new epidermal cells may be seen progressing outwards from epidermal appendages such as hair follicles, and as monolayers of cells extending under the degenerated epidermis. When dermal damage has also resulted, these epidermal outgrowths extend under the affected areas such that all damaged tissue is eventually sloughed off.

This sequence, from initial cell derangement to complete epidermal replacement is an extreme reaction and only occurs after grossly exaggerated application of irritants (e.g. grossly exaggerated application of sodium laurate to rats, as described by Prottey *et al.*, 1973; treatment of guinea pigs with 10% dinitrochlorobenzene in acetone, reported by Medenica and Rostenberg, 1971), and, as such, is not representative of the usual reactions of cosmetic ingredients upon human epidermis.

B. Cellular Injury and Cell Death in the Epidermis in Molecular Terms

Chemical irritants that penetrate to the living cells of the epidermis elicit specific biochemical responses. Epidermal metabolism in the epidermis is normally under very precise control, in that the rate of mitosis in the basal layer is matched by an equivalent rate of cell maturation (differentiation) and ultimately the rate of desquamation of the stratum corneum. This control ensures that within a finite range of hormonal, dietary or environmental alterations there will be either no excessive thinning or thickening of the skin. However, irritant stimuli may disrupt epidermal homeostasis, and to various degrees. There may be transient alterations that may or may not stimulate the basal cells to divide faster, that lead to eventual adaptation and recovery, or, in the extreme, there may be chronic alterations leading to cell death and necrosis. Necrosis is the subsequent degradation of dead cells into component molecules (fatty acids, peptides etc.) and this process is autolytic, i.e. the result of action of hydrolytic enzymes, normally confined within lysosomes, that are released upon injury (Lazarus *et al.*, 1975). Many of the morphological changes that have been observed in irritated epidermis may be characterized in biochemical terms.

A possible early effect of irritants that come in contact with living epidermal cells will be an interference of the supply or uptake of nutrients and oxygen from the dermis, such that aerobic respiration is impaired, with resultant reduction of cellular ATP concentration. Stimulation of anaerobic glycolysis may follow, with increased lactate production that results in lower intracellular pH. This may be associated with an observed clumping of nuclear chromatin, followed in turn by loss of nuclear RNA synthesis. Changes follow in the activity of plasma membrane ATPase-dependent ion pumps, with resultant alterations of cell surface microvillae, shrinkage of mitochondria and oedema of the endoplasmic reticulum. These changes are probably reversible, but if further cell damage is elicited, the changes become irreversible. These include permeability changes of mitochondrial and plasma membranes, loss of protein synthesis in the endoplasmic reticulum and phospholipase breakdown of membrane lipids. Necrosis then ensues, with swelling and leaking of mitochondria, loss of cell sap and the uptake of vital dyes by the cells. Lysosomal swelling and release of contents into the cell sap occurs, followed by rapid digestion of intracellular structures and macromolecules, and karyolysis of nuclear chromatin. Other than lysosomal hydrolases, all other cellular enzymic processes are lost. Cells are faintly discernible by their residual cell membranes and by strong eosinophilic staining.

This progression of changes for insulted cells in general has been described in detail by Trump and Mergner (1974). From the standpoint of chemical irritation of the skin, specific biochemical aspects have received particular attention by numerous investigators.

1. *Effect of Irritants upon Epidermal Metabolism*

The most striking morphological feature of the epidermis following mild to moderate irritation is hyperplasia, that is, increased epidermal thickness due to increased numbers of cell layers throughout the whole epithelium, as a result of stimulated cell division in the basal layer exceeding the rate of differentiation and/or desquamation. Most reports have concerned hyperproliferative skin diseases (such as psoriasis) or experimentally wounded animal skin (e.g. incision wounds, tape-stripped skin), although recently Fisher and Maibach (1975) have described the different effects of various chemical irritants upon mitosis in human skin. It is likely there is much in common mechanistically between accelerated cell division in experimental wounding and skin irritation by chemicals.

(a) *Chalones* Until relatively recently, much of what was known on the control of epidermal cell division originated from the work of Bullough (for a review, see Bullough, 1972). It was proposed that epidermal thickness in normal skin is under the control of a tissue-specific anti-mitotic messenger molecules called chalones, which are glycoprotein hormones synthesized within the cells concerned, that inhibit both mitosis and cell differentiation of the skin. Under normal conditions, despite varying fluctutations (due to dietary or diurnal factors) in the concentration of chalones and epinephrine (required for the full expression of chalone action), changes in mitotic rate are matched by similar changes in the rate that post-mitotic cells differentiate. The ratio of mitotic rate to the rate of cell ageing remains constant, and changes in mitotic rate have no effect upon epidermal thickness. In various regions of the body, or in certain animal species, higher mitotic rates result in increased rates of differentiation of the post-mitotic cells, and so epidermal thickness is controlled by the post-mitotic ageing process, and this in turn depends upon chalone concentration in these cells. In the case of mild, transient trauma (e.g. tape-stripped mouse skin), it was proposed that chalone concentration falls, mitosis is enhanced, leading to more post-mitotic cells with a shorter time of differentiation (due to the lower chalone concentration). The epidermis thickens in response, with an ultimate rise to normal of chalone in these cells, and mitosis and differentiation proceed as in normal skin. In chronic damage, however, the epidermis thickens to a point determined by the length of the post-mitotic ageing process. The chalone theory has come under closer scrutiny of late, however, and Elgjo *et al.* (1971) have suggested that cell division is regulated at different stages by different substances, basal cells producing a substance that regulates cells at the G_2 phase of mitosis, and differentiating cells producing a substance regulating the entry of basal cells from G_1 to S phase.

(b) *Cyclic nucleotides* During the past five years a deeper insight of the molecular control of epidermal homeostasis has been gained from the work of Voorhees and colleagues (1974) upon cyclic nucleotides. Epinephrine, suggested from Bullough's work to be involved in the inhibitory action of chalones on cell division, is known to raise the level of cyclic AMP in many tissues (Robison, Butcher and Sutherland, 1971) and the importance of cyclic AMP in the control of epidermal homeostasis has received close attention accordingly. Voorhees has generalized that hyperproliferative states of the skin (e.g. psoriasis, or skin neoplasms) are caused by aberrations in the control mechanisms of both mitosis and differentiation. Norepinephrine has been shown to cause the accumulation of cyclic AMP in the epidermis by the β-adrenergic stimulation of adenylate cyclase, which synthesizes it from AMP. It is postulated by Voorhees that high intracellular cycle AMP inhibits the entry of epidermal cells from the G_2 phase of the cell cycle into mitosis, as well as possibly affecting cells prior to DNA synthesis. Furthermore, Voorhees has suggested that the regulation of homeostasis in the skin is via the dual participation of cyclic AMP and cyclic GMP, as originally put forward by Goldberg *et al.* (1973). In normal epidermis the effects of cyclic AMP and cyclic GMP are balanced, such that the rate of mitosis is matched by the rates of differentiation and desquamation, with resultant normal skin thickness and structurally normal stratum corneum. However, in hyperproliferating skin the balance between cyclic AMP and cyclic GMP is altered, the former being abnormally low, the latter being raised. Under such conditions mitosis occurs at such a rate, and differentiation of the post-mitotic cells is so modified, that a thickened, hyperplastic epidermis with abnormal stratum corneum may result. Another aspect of hyperproliferative skin diseases, the deposition of glycogen in the epidermis (Braun-Falco, 1958), is also cited by Voorhees as being due to abnormally low levels of cyclic AMP in the epidermis, as is known to occur in other organs (Robison *et al.*, 1968). Furthermore, prostaglandin metabolism has been shown to be related to the regulation of tissue levels of cyclic AMP and cyclic GMP in many aspects of cutaneous physiology.

Voorhees has attempted to explain the various abnormalities in psoriasis in terms of aberrations of the various molecules described above, but reservations in some of the inconsistent data available have been voiced (Marks, 1972; Halprin *et al.*, 1975). Nonetheless, this approach has greatly augmented our understanding of the control of epidermal events in normal and abnormal states. In terms of chemical irritants that affect mitosis, much remains to be studied in terms of the way that the fine control is altered, but it is likely that there are many similarities between hyperproliferative skin diseases, physical wounding and chemical irritation.

(c) *Nucleic acids* There are numerous reports of the effects of injurious stimuli upon cell division in the epidermis, and many of these utilize the technique of measuring the uptake of radioactive thymidine into epidermal DNA. The effect of incision wounding upon cell-division in guinea-pig ear skin was examined by Hell and Cruickshank (1963). As early as 4 hours after injury there was an increase in the number of cells synthesizing DNA in the epidermis, and this was followed by a temporary synchrony of the cell cycle in the region of the injury. This study confirmed that a very early cellular event following injury was stimulation of G_1 cells to enter S phase.

In the case of primary irritation of skin, Prottey *et al.* (1973) and Prottey and Hartop (1973) demonstrated stimulation of DNA synthesis in rat skin following application of surfactants. In these studies maximum stimulation was seen after 1 day of application, which was before the morphological changes were fully developed. Mezei (1970) has shown that cutaneous application of polysorbate and polyoxyethylene surfactants stimulated the uptake of [^{32}P]-orthophosphate into phospholipids, DNA and RNA of the epidermis of rabbits, as well as increasing the net tissue content of these compounds. The increases were suggested to be a reflection of increased biosynthesis of membranes during the repair and acanthosis of the treated skin.

Tabachnick and LaBadie (1970) reported the increase in DNase activity in guinea pig skin after mild clipping injury and strong irradiation. In both cases the increases occurred prior to the stimulation of epidermal pro-liferation, and suggest that this enzyme, rather than being released from cellular organelles (e.g. lysosomes), was rapidly synthesized. As such, the appearance of enhanced DNase activity may be important to the stimulation of cellular events by injury, rather than participating in degradative change, and may well be an observable early phenomenon in chemically irritated skin.

Although there is much evidence that even after mild irritant stimuli, increased epidermal mitosis and hyperplasia result, the structural con-sequences in the resultant stratum corneum will depend upon the actual severity of the stimulus. When damage (such as marked cell loss) is incurred in the stratum corneum, it is likely that the ordered squame packing seen in normal epidermis (MacKenzie, 1969) is lost. This has been shown by Christophers (1971). When the ears of mice were damaged by moderate compression, DNA synthesis in the stratum basale was greatly stimulated (the labelling index with tritiated thymidine rose from about 4–20%) by the second day, and subsequently by day 10 the whole epidermis was thickened. But the ordered structure of stacks of stratum corneum cells was retained. However, following incision damage, although there was increased mitotic activity, there was complete loss of order in the rapidly forming new horny layer. Similar observations have been made by Allen and Potten (1975).

With chemically irritated skin, as far as is known, such studies have not yet been made. Clearly, the degree of stimulated cell division will depend upon the nature of the irritation. Mezei (1970) showed that for relatively non-irritant non-ionic surfactants there was enhanced DNA labelling, whereas Prottey et al. (1973) showed after grossly exaggerated application of sodium laurate to rats, an early stimulation of DNA synthesis was soon followed by complete loss of metabolic activity due to the epidermal necrosis. It is not known at what degree of epidermal stimulation the altered squame packing of the stratum corneum develops, but the chemical structure or properties and the method of application will be important.

(d) *Respiration* Other aspects of altered epidermal metabolism have been described. Decker (1971) reviewed energy metabolism in the epidermis, and pointed out that the mechanisms for regulating glycolysis, respiration, glycogen and fatty acid metabolism lay in the reactions catalyzed by phosphofructokinase, pyruvate dehydrogenase and isocitrate dehydrogenase, with secondary control by hexokinase and the glyceraldehyde-3 phosphate dehydrogenase—phosphoglycerate kinase complex. The most important molecular regulators were the adenine nucleotides. Thus, if an initial aberrant reaction were the elevation of ATP concentration, due, for example, to enhanced cellular respiration, one would anticipate blocking of phosphofructokinase, with glucose 6-phosphate being funnelled into glycogen, which is known to accumulate in the hyperplastic skin of psoriasis and in wounds.

Mezei *et al.* (1966) studied the effects upon the skin of rabbits of some non-ionic surfactants at various dilutions and for various periods of application. Routinely, the application of the surfactants resulted in increased respiration of the epidermis, in some cases up to four times as much O_2 was consumed compared with control skin, but no direct correlations were seen between these metabolic changes and the degree of epidermal hyperplasia and dermal inflammation produced. Polyoxyethylene ethers were seen to be consistently quite irritant under the conditions of application, compared with the relatively mild polysorbates and sorbitan surfactants, both of which caused greater stimulation of respiration. These authors suggested that the surfactants affected the permeability of the epidermal cells to nutrients, and thereby influenced respiration.

(e) *Lipid synthesis*   The responses of epidermal lipid metabolizing enzymes to irritants have been recently studied. Prottey and Hartop (1973) showed that soap irritation of rat skin produced a stimulated turnover of phospholipids after two days (i.e. subsequent to increased DNA synthesis), and the degree of this change closely corresponded to morphological alterations in the skin (Prottey *et al.*, 1973). When the epidermis was extensively damaged, due to grossly exaggerated treatments, phospholipid metabolism ceased. Other instances of stimulated epidermal phospholipid metabolism in cutaneous irritation include the reports of Mezei (1970) and Takasu (1975). Stimulated triglyceride synthesis in epidermis following soap irritation has also been described (Prottey *et al.*, 1973; Prottey and Hartop, 1973), such changes matching reciprocal alteration of phospholipid synthesis: some phospholipids are precursors of triglycerides. Increased triglyceride formation may be a general epidermal reaction to injurious stimuli, as Tovell *et al.* (1974) have shown that in the spongiotic, acanthotic epidermis of rats following repeated applications of sodium lauryl sulphate there is accumulation of fatty droplets in the cytoplasm of epidermal cells at each stage of maturation. These authors suggested that the sublethal cell damage by the irritant may cause local cellular hypoxia, when anaerobic glycolysis rather than fat oxidation would be favoured, with the tendency to deposition of intracellular fat. Trump and Mergner (1974) have reviewed the phenomenon of lipid accumulation in injured tissues generally, and suggest that factors leading to the deposition of lipid droplets in the liver include defective fatty acid metabolism, protein and phospholipid synthesis and the combination of phospholipids with proteins. Any or all of these metabolic disturbances may be possible in irritated epidermis. Indeed, the presence of intracellular droplets of lipid may prove to be diagnostic for sublethal effects of irritants upon epidermal metabolism, in the same manner that stimulated DNA synthesis seems to be.

(f) *Arginase*   The activity of the enzyme arginase (L-arginine amidino hydrolase) has received considerable attention in hyperplasia of the epidermis caused by solvent application. This enzyme is probably quite important in the epidermis as it converts arginine into urea and ornithine, both of which occur freely in the pool of water-soluble components of the stratum corneum. Following earlier reports of enhanced arginase activity in certain hyperplastic skin diseases, Rossmiller and Hoekstra (1965) showed a correlation between an up to 50-fold increase in epidermal arginase activity with the development of hyperkeratosis due to hexadecane in guinea pigs. Increased arginase activity did not precede, but rather accompanied elevated hyperkeratinization of the skin. That this method could be utilized as an index of epidermal change due to the action of primary irritants such as hydrocarbon solvents, has been suggested by Brown and Box (1970, 1971). These authors confirmed that maximum thickening and scaliness of the epidermis was accompanied by maximum stimulation of arginase activity in the epidermis.

(g) *Keratinization*   Detailed studies are lacking on the biochemistry of keratinization in irritated skin, a process that may be modified as a result of the hyperplasia observed microscopically. Bernstein and his group (Bernstein, 1971) have been concerned with the metabolism of the "histidine-rich protein" that is localized in the keratohyalin-containing granular cells of the epidermis. Bernstein has applied his studies to the disease psoriasis in order to examine how the failure to observe both keratohyalin and the histidine-rich protein is affected biochemically. Indeed, much of the impetus for elucidating the mechanism of keratin production has been provided by clinically oriented investigators, and this may be counter-productive to a degree, for the aetiology of this distressing disease is very complex. It may be that if actions of selected chemicals upon keratin production were studied more intensely, our understanding of the phenomenon might be more readily enhanced. This would probably aid not only our understanding of epidermal irritation, but the discrete biochemical aberrations of skin diseases also.

2. *Mediation of Altered Metabolism in Irritated Epidermis—the Participation of Lysosomes*

Although it is widely recognized (Jarrett, 1973) that epidermal lysosomes are vital to the normal metabolic economy of cell generation, differentiation and keratinization, these organelles, by virtue of the degradative enzymes contained therein, also play integral roles in the development of pathological changes in the skin (Trump and Mergner, 1974). Thus, the early release of lysosomal enzymes in irritated skin, with their subsequent secondary action upon the metabolic apparatus of the skin, is not unlikely (Lazarus et al., 1975).

Various degradative enzymes found in lysosomes generally have been listed by Hirschhorn (1974), with hydrolytic activity towards proteins, peptides, lipids, carbohydrates, nucleic acids and phosphate- or sulphate-containing molecules. Olson and Nordquist (1966) detected acid phosphatase in epidermal lysosomes, Dicken and Decker (1966) identified in addition, β-glucuronidase, aryl sulphatase and cathepsins (acid proteases). Mier and Van Den Hurk (1975) have characterized seven distinct epidermal glycosidases of lysosomal origin as well as indicating that phosphatases, sulphatases, ester hydrolases and peptidases are also present. Lazarus et al. (1975) have described the identification of cathepsins and neutral proteinases of epidermal lysosomes.

The specific susceptibility of epidermal lysosomes to an injurious stimulus was shown by Johnson and Daniels (1969) using strong ultraviolet irradiation of human skin (ten times the minimum erythemal dose). In normal skin, the enzyme acid phosphatase was found to be weak and diffuse throughout the upper region of the stratum granulosum and lower stratum corneum, but within the first hour following irradiation there was release of the enzyme from lysosomes throughout the whole of the epidermis but mainly in the upper regions. These authors concluded that epidermal lysosomes gradually acquired greater fragility as the differentiating cells moved up into the stratum corneum, and thus were more prone to leakage.

Furthermore, lysosomes isolated from irradiated skin were shown to be more fragile than normal skin, indicating that early damage to their limiting membranes occurred as a result of irradiation. A decrease of RNA in spinosum cells after irradiation also suggested the release of RNase from lysosomes. As no simultaneous increase of succinate dehydrogenase activity was observed (a non-lysosomal enzyme), this suggested that lysosomes were particularly liable to injurious stimulus compared with other cell organelles. Wolff and Schreiner (1970) also showed that lysosomes in the epidermis responded to ultraviolet irradiation of the skin by forming autophagic inclusions that contained residues of cellular debris. Equivalent studies of chemically irritated skin have not been reported, but Lazarus *et al.* (1975) have proposed a general mechanism of lysosomal enzyme release in damaged skin. The irritant stimulus damages epidermal cells such that their lysosomes leak hydrolases into the tissue. As well as exerting damaging effects in the epidermis, it has been proposed that the lysosomal enzymes diffuse into the dermis where they are chemotactic for neutrophils, with consequent tissue degeneration. Such activity could also be self-limiting, as the vascular permeability so induced would allow plasma proteinase inhibitors such as α2-macroglobulin and α1-antitrypsin to diffuse throughout the tissues and inhibit the lysosomal proteases. Rutherford and Pawlowski (1974) have provided indirect evidence that membrane coating granules (Matoltsy and Parakkal, 1965) which are probably functionally similar to lysosomes (Weinstock and Wilgram, 1970), may also be involved in the release of hydrolytic enzymes in skin irritation. Using a superficial biopsy technique, the presence of acid phosphatase activity was demonstrated in human stratum corneum. These authors suggested that this enzyme was located in the membrane coating granules (Wolff and Schreiner, 1970), and treatment of the skin by detergents caused the permeability of the granules to be increased to the histochemical stain for acid phosphatase. With stronger irritant stimuli, however, damage to the membrane coating granules would result, with loss of the hydrolases into the interstices of the stratum corneum. This approach is particularly valuable, for it may indicate initial changes in the skin by sub-irritant doses of chemicals, that subsequently trigger off more dramatic events.

3. *The Effects of Repeated Chemical Irritation upon the Epidermis*

The epidermal response to irritants will depend upon the frequency of exposure: an irritant that elicits only minor responses after few applications may exert strong action if repeated applications prevent the normal recovery of the metabolically stimulated cells between times. For example, it was found (Prottey *et al.*, 1973) that two successive applications of soap solutions to the skin of rats doubled the rate of DNA synthesis in the epidermis, whereas eight successive washes almost totally inhibited metabolic activity. None the less, when the skin is repeatedly exposed to irritants, the epidermis may eventually adapt, both structurally and metabolically, to the irritant stimuli by becoming "accommodated". This was described by Rothman and Lorincz (1963) for skin exposed to ultraviolet irritation or mechanical stimuli as a protective response whereby the skin became thicker, and these authors used the expression "superkeratinization". McOsker and Beck (1967) produced data for guinea pigs that had been exposed repeatedly to solutions of soap and synthetic detergents. When exposed up to eight successive times the skin developed increasingly severe irritation responses, in particular, erythema and epidermal hyerplasia were observed that led to complete epidermal necrosis. Thereafter, however, despite continued exposure to the irritants, new epidermis grew out from hair follicles. The resultant new epithelium was much thicker in all cell layers and the stratum corneum, and the mitotic index was three times higher than in untreated animals. Sebaceous glands were also hypertrophic. The thickened skin appeared macroscopically as scaly, hardened, shiny, but less elastic than untreated skin. Although the permeability of the skin was greater, it was more resistant to irritation. The accommodated animal skin was thought by McOsker and Beck to resemble more closely human skin, which presumably also becomes accommodated over the years due to repeated forces of friction and compression and exposure to water and other common chemical stimuli during daily life. Indeed, one may ponder whether animal application tests of skin products to evaluate irritancy or efficacy might be more representative of human skin if the animals were first "accommodated" to mild physical and chemical stimuli.

4. Dermo-Epidermal Interactions

A final aspect of epidermal metabolism in irritated skin involves its inter-actions with the dermis, as is briefly described in Fig. 1. It is accepted that the epidermis is closely related metabolically to the dermis in normal skin, not only from the point of supply of nutrients, oxygen, hormones etc., by diffusion from the dermal circulatory system, but also with regard to embryological dermo-epidermal interactions (Cohen, 1969). The dermis is believed to modulate the differentiation of the epidermis and, by feed-back control, the epidermis informs the dermis of epidermal change. Interactions of the epidermis and dermis also extend to the appendages, the blood supply and the nerves. These dermo-epidermal interactions are dependent upon the maintenance of equilibrium, as exemplified by studies of Billingham and Silvers (1967), and Dodson (1967), and whenever an irritant stimulus is experienced by one component of the skin, its effects will also be expressed in the other. This has been demonstrated by numerous investigators. Ryan et al. (1971) proposed that following the action of physical traumata or chemical irritants on the skin, when actual direct damage to the epidermis has been sustained, the epidermis releases an inhibitor of fibrinolysis that diffuses to the dermis, causing fibrin to be deposited (see below), which then mediates the subsequent dermal in-flammatory response. Similarly, Steele and Wilhelm (1970) suggested that the erythema and permeability increase rapidly following application of xylene to the skin was preceded by the release of specific mediators from the damaged epidermal cells. Dermo-epidermal interactions may operate in the reverse direction, as best exemplified by experimental models. Examples of stimulated epidermal mitosis overlying dermal granulomata have been reported by Schellander and Marks (1973), and Spearman and Garretts (1966) observed a similar epidermal response to saline injected into the dermis.

The chemical nature of these mediators of dermo-epidermal interaction is unknown, but histamine, "leucotoxins", collagenase, nerve impulses have been suggested (Malak and Kurban, 1971). It is likely that the precise chemical nature of the irritant will determine the types and amounts of any such release.

IV. THE ACTIONS OF CHEMICAL IRRITANTS ON THE DERMIS—THE INFLAMMATORY RESPONSE

A. Components of the Dermal Inflammatory Response

The inflammatory response of tissues to injurious stimuli has been extensively studied. Indeed, since the time of Celsius some two thousand years ago, four diagnostic signs of inflammation have been known, namely, swelling (oedema), redness (erythema), local heat and pain. Movat (1971) and Ebert and Grant (1971) have reviewed historical developments of this subject.

As already described for the stratum corneum and the living cells of the epidermis, the stimuli that elicit inflammation are numerous, and include physical traumata (heat, cold, ionizing and ultraviolet irradiation, abrasion, compression), microorganisms, antigens and immunological skin diseases, and chemicals that come in contact with the skin. This lattermost category includes the effects of cosmetics. There is no general inflammatory reaction, rather, there are as many different varieties of a total response as there are stimuli that can elicit them. There are numerous reactions that produce similar results but by varied molecular means, (for example, the generation of molecules that increase permeability of blood vessels, or the various complex pathways that produce molecules that are chemotactic for leucocytes), and some types of inflammation involve reactions not present in others (differences between various types of immunologic inflammations illustrate this). Much recent research on inflammation has been geared to inflammatory skin diseases, and utilizing by and large, laboratory animals and experimental systems *in vitro*, and the resultant scientific literature is vast and often conflicting. However, non-allergic cutaneous inflammatory responses as a result of chemicals are possibly among the least complex in aetiology, and in many instances produce less dramatic tissue changes, yet they have also been the least studied in detail. There are numerous detailed reviews of discrete aspects of inflammation, including those of Spector and Willoughby, 1968; Houck and Forscher, 1968; Bertelli and Houck, 1969; Winkelmann, 1971; Weissmann, 1974; Cochrane, 1975; Goldyne, 1975). By far the most comprehensive treatise, however, is "The Inflammatory Process", edited by Zweifach, Grant and McCluskey (1974) which accurately covers all aspects of inflammation. Below, some of the overall aspects that are relevant to chemical inflammation are discussed, but more detailed accounts will be found amongst these reviews cited.

Cutaneous inflammation is a basic defence reaction of the body; it commences with modification of specific structural components of the dermis, and terminates with tissue repair and restoration of normal functions. The overall reaction to chemicals applied to the skin may be described conveniently in terms of five components that are individual but, none the less, interdependent biological reactions. These are shown in Fig. 2.

1. *Vascular Events*

Irritant stimuli appear to exert their initial effects upon the small blood-vessels situated in the upper regions of the dermis. The first indication of cutaneous inflammation is local erythema, due to increased blood flow through these vessels. Steele and Wilhelm (1966) described the rapid appearance of erythema within minutes of applying xylene to guinea-pig skin, that rapidly faded within 30 min, but reappeared after about 4 h and was maximal at 10–20 h. This biphasic erythema has been shown for other chemicals (Wilhelm, 1973), and the phasic nature of the response seems to depend upon the type of irritant and the mode of application. Morphologically, within minutes there is a transient constriction of the sub-epidermal capillary plexus that is rapidly followed by dilatation of the post-capillary venules, resulting in increased blood flow. Majno *et al.* (1969) showed by electron microscopy that under normal circumstances the cells of the venular endothelium are closely interdigitated, separated by only 100–200 nm, preventing the leakage of humoral proteins. But early in inflammation these cells contract and separate somewhat, forming small "pores" such that the vessels become more permeable to components of the blood.

For chemical irritants or physical traumata such as experimental burns or ultraviolet irradiation (Steele and Wilhelm, 1966; Logan and Wilhelm, 1966), three types of permeability increase have been described, namely "immediate", "delayed", and "early" permeability changes. These may occur singly (monophasic) or in combination (diphasic). "Immediate" permeability responses are those occurring within minutes of injurious stimuli and last for up to 30 min. The small venules with diameter of

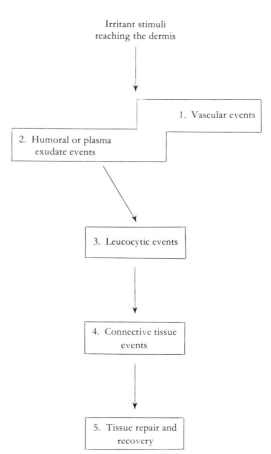

Fig. 2. Sequential aspects of dermal inflammation.

20–100 μm leak proteins as a result of mild irritant stimuli, such as mild burns. "Delayed" permeability responses (due to stronger burns, ultra-violet radiation or chemicals) are of two main types, either beginning 1/2–1 h after irritation and reaching a maximum in about 4 h, or beginning 2–10 h after irritation and being maximal in 12–24 h. Delayed responses are seen in both venules and capillaries. "Early" permeability responses are induced by strong stimuli (strong burns and chemicals), beginning 10–30 min after application and maximal by 20–60 min. It is not possible to classify accurately irritants according to their ability to elicit permeability changes without reference to their mode of application. Some strong irritants elicit both early and delayed permeability changes after a single application, but often frequent multiple applications cause direct damage to the vascular system, with formation of thrombi and the arrest of blood flow.

2. Humoral or Plasma-Exudate Events

With increased permeability of blood vessels, plasma proteins and fluid exude into the surrounding dermis, which becomes oedematous. The involved area may appear turgid or whealed. Indeed, measurement of the increased tissue volume produced in experimental inflammations has been utilized for assessing the extent of the response (Bonta et al., 1974).

Permeability changes of vessels have been demonstrated extensively by the use of specific markers for the blood proteins, and Evans Blue dye has been particularly popular. This complexes with plasma proteins and their presence outside the vessels is manifested by blueing of the tissues at the site of protein exudation. Wilhelm (1973) described this technique for chemical irritants. Blood proteins labelled with radioactive tracers have also been used (Morley et al., 1973).

Increased permeability of venules is an important feature of the total inflammatory response, as it allows exudation into the dermis of blood components (albumin, globulins, fibrinogen, etc.) that subsequently participate in the development of the leucocytic phase. In particular, some of these proteins are modified enzymes that are activated to produce polypeptide fragments with various functions in subsequent stages. The most important function of these fragments is the attraction of leucocytes, and the generation of the various polypeptides in this phase of inflammation is by a sequence of controlled proteolytic reactions. But the initiation of the sequence is not known for chemical irritation (unlike immediate hypersensitivity reactions, where antigen/antibody complexes probably do so), although direct damage to dermal structures by the irritants may be responsible for this triggering.

3. Leucocytic Events

Following the early vascular dilatation, leucocytes come into prominence and perform functions that are by far the most important to the overall inflammatory process. The roles of the vascular system and blood components are to set the scene for the expression of the complex and potent actions of the leucocytes. In acute inflammation neutrophils (polymorphonuclear leucocytes) are the predominant cells, but in chronic inflammation, macrophages assume prominence, and in various allergic inflammatory conditions, eosinophils, basophils, platelets and lymphocytes may actively participate. From the standpoint of acute non-allergic inflammation due to chemicals, only the neutrophils will be discussed here.

Soon after applying irritants to the skin, leucocytes accumulate in the cutaneous blood vessels. Steele and Wilhelm (1970) observed up to 20 times more neutrophils in venules within 20 min of applying xylene to guinea-pig skin compared with untreated controls: more eosinophils and monocytes were also seen. The neutrophils then align along and adhere to the inner walls of the vascular endothelium, probably involving changes in the electronegativity of the plasma membrane glycoproteins. These cells then move between the overlapped adherent cells of the endothelium and through the basement lamina of the vessels into the surrounding tissues, a process known as diapedesis. Neutrophils are highly locomotory cells and the process takes about 30 min. Steele and Wilhelm (1970) reported that maximum diapedesis of neutrophils occurred 2–6 h following application of xylene, but with stronger irritants such as phenol this continued for up to 26 h. Medenica and Rostenberg (1971) reported maximum leucocytic infiltration 16–24 h after application of dinitrochlorobenzene to guinea pigs, but the precise timing depended upon the concentration used.

The accumulation of neutrophils in inflammatory foci is not a fortuitous occurrence: they are specifically attracted from the blood by certain molecules specifically synthesized locally for the purpose. This phenomenon is known as chemotaxis. Although the subject of chemotaxis has been widely studied (reviewed by Ramsey and Grant, 1974), precise molecular mechanisms are not clear. Components of the activated plasma complement system (see below) are known to be chemotactic, but also, neutrophils themselves can generate chemotactic substances. Studies of experimental inflammations *in vitro* using a method first described by Boyden (1962) have provided most of what is known, but the reactions *in vivo* warrant more investigation, certainly for instances involving non-allergenic chemicals.

In general terms, in inflammation neutrophils migrate to the site in order to encounter and inactive the irritant stimulus. This is achieved by phagocytosis, a process of engulfment of the irritant, which is then broken down by lysosomal enzymes within the neutrophils, and subsequently transported away. Phagocytosis has been reviewed by Elsbach (1974) and Hirsch (1974), and the types of enzymes contained within the lysosomes are detailed in recent reviews of Goldstein (1974) and Hirschhorn (1975). During phagocytosis of foreign materials, neutrophils are often killed (especially those arriving first at the scene of the inflammation). The neutrophils degenerate and may be recognized by the loss of their characteristic PAS staining, and bizarre nuclei shapes: Steel and Wilhelm (1970), in severe solvent inflammation, and Modenica and Rostenberg (1971) described such features. Such neutrophils spill out the degradative enzymes of their lysosomes, and damage to the surrounding tissue results. In this process new substances that are chemotactic for neutrophils are generated, so that more of these cells emigrate from the blood to the site. A vicious circle can arise resulting in significant damage to the dermal connective tissue and blood vessels. At a certain point, however, the process is terminated, and tissue repair then commences.

The release of tissue-damaging enzymes and chemicals from leucocytes in inflammation is somewhat paradoxical, in that cells that are recruited to deal with the noxious substances eliciting the inflammation, themselves cause extensive tissue damage. When the irritant stimuli persist (such as in gout, with toxic crystals of urate in the tissues; in the Arthus reaction, with precipitated antigen–antibody complexes; or when bacteria are present in the tissues), chronic inflammations often develop, with much neutrophil death and severe tissue damage, continuing until the stimuli have been removed or inactivated. With acute chemical inflammation these extremes do not develop usually. It is not clear in such cases, however, whether the leucocytic events terminate with engulfment of the last traces of the irritant chemicals that have penetrated as far as the dermis to elicit the response.

That neutrophils are fundamental to the development of various types of immediate inflammation may be shown by using as models animals that are depleted of neutrophils before irritation (such as by treatment with nitrogen mustard). In such instances damage to the vascular and connective tissue elements is mild, or is not seen, unless normal neutrophils are re-introduced to the animals. This has been shown by Parish (1969) for the Arthus reaction in rabbits, and by Willoughby and Girond (1969) for non-allergic inflammation of rats.

It has been suggested by Weissmann (1974) that the inflammatory responses of vasodilatation, capillary leakage, chemotaxis and accumulation of leucocytes are essentially reversible, and merely set the scene for the irreversible phases, namely the cleavage of covalent bonds of the connective tissue. In the absence of leucocytes the true inflammatory response, of eventual removal of the irritant stimulus by phagocytosis and tissue destruction, cannot develop.

4. *Connective Tissue Events*

Early structural changes in the dermis as a result of chemical irritation have been reported by Steele and Wilhelm (1970). Within 2 h of application of solvents such as chloroform, benzene and carbon tetrachloride to guinea pigs, separation of collagen fibrils was seen in the upper regions of the dermis. Such changes probably arose from the oedema in the dermis, rather than the direct action of the irritants that had penetrated. Steele and

Wilhelm (1970) also observed small basophilic globules throughout the upper dermis, suggested to be either nuclear debris carried from the epidermis by the irritant, or the pyknotic nuclei of damaged fibroblasts. This would suggest direct action of the irritant upon the dermis, as such features were observed within 5 min. of application of chloroform to the skin. At this early time there would be no leucocytic action.

As mentioned above, neutrophils may also release degradative enzymes from their lysosomes into the tissues (collagenases, elastases, glycosidases etc., see below) which dissolve the acellular components of the connective tissue. Also, indirectly, when vascular elements are severely damaged, blood flow to the inflamed dermis may cease, causing anoxia and degeneration of the surrounding tissues.

5. *Tissue Repair and Recovery*

The repair phase following inflammation is complex. Leucocytes engulf debris and move away via lymphatics. Dead leucocytes form an exudate that is sloughed off when a new epidermis regrows. "Holes" that have been made in dermal connective tissue by lysosomal enzymes of neutrophils are filled by deposition of fibrin, the activation of which is by neutrophils interacting with plasma fibrinogen (Ryan *et al.*, 1971). The polymerized fibrin serves as a scaffold for subsequent tissue repair, as fibroblasts can migrate within, divide and produce new collagen. Tissue repair processes have been described by McMinn (1969), and are not further discussed here.

B. The Molecular Basis of Information—Mediators

Acute cutaneous inflammation is a cascade, a chemical chain reaction that, once initiated, develops step by step up to a certain point (determined by the nature of the irritant stimulus), and, thereafter, abates in stepwise fashion as tissue recovery and repair take over. Although direct penetration of an irritant chemical to the dermis may occur in an inflammatory response, its direct action upon components of the total reaction will be limited, and is usually only transitory (i.e. the irritant will initiate the first steps). Thereafter, subsequent steps are triggered off by endogenous substances or "mediators", that are generated locally, act locally, and are usually rapidly inactivated locally once their function has been expressed.

Mediators of inflammation are molecules, products of enzymic sequences, enzymes themselves, or substances released from cells, that initiate or control discrete aspects of the response. Prior to their involvement, mediators exist as inactive precursors (such as the kinin-, complement-, fibrinolytic- or coagulation systems of the blood, or as fatty acids in membranes) or are sequestered within cells. There are three groups of cell-bound mediators:

(i) bound ionically within intracytoplasmic granules, such as histamine or 5-hydroxytryptamine in mast cells, basophils and platelets;

(ii) within lysosomes of phagocytic cells that emigrate into the inflammation: neutrophils are predominant in acute inflammations, macrophages feature in chronic inflammations;

(iii) generated by lymphocytes that emigrate to the sites of certain types of allergic inflammation. These are the lymphokines (they are not further discussed here, but see David and David, 1972).

Following the initial irritant stimulus, mediators are activated, synthesized or released by specific biological mechanisms, and the various aspects of the inflammatory response come into play. There is no one general mediator of the total response (although cyclic nucleotides are now thought to participate in many of the discrete steps, see below), and each reaction or sequence is characterized by discrete mediators. However, there are multiplicities of action, and more than one type of mediator can elicit a specific reaction (e.g. vascular permeability, chemotaxis of leucocytes), and individual mediators may be involved in more than one reaction (e.g. histamine, complement, Hageman factor, prostaglandins).

Spector and Willoughby (1968) enumerated four criteria that should be satisfied before accepting that a substance be considered as a mediator of inflammation:

(i) the substance should be demonstrably present during the inflammatory reaction and absent when it subsides;

(ii) the substance should possess properties which qualify it as a mediator (e.g. it should be a permeability factor, or be leucotactic etc.);

(iii) inhibition of the action of the substance by specific antagonists should lead to a diminished action for which that substance is assumed to be responsible, and;

(iv) depletion of the tissues of the putative mediator prior to the irritant stimulus should suppress that part of the inflammatory reaction for which the substance is assumed to be responsible.

C. Mediator Molecules in Chemical Inflammation of the Skin

Various types of molecules have been found to participate in the generation, maintenance and termination of the non-allergic inflammatory response.

Table I
Mediators of chemical inflammation

Mediator	Structure and origin	Function
1. Histamine	Amine. Ionically bound in granules of mast cells, basophils, platelets, neutrophils	Contracts smooth muscle. An early mediator of vascular permeability. May control leucocyte functions. May promote tissue repair
2. 5-hydroxy-tryptamine	Amine. Ionically bound in granules of mast cells and platelets of some species	Contracts smooth muscle. An early mediator of vascular permeability, overlapping with, or following action of histamine in some species. Controls normal tonus of blood vessels
3. Kinins (kallidin, bradykinin)	Polypeptides. Produced from plasma glycoprotein precursors (kininogens) by specific enzymes (kallikreins) of plasma or leucocytes, or by trypsin	Produce slow contractions of smooth muscle, dilate arterioles, permeability factors following action of histamine and 5-hydroxytryptamine. Chemotactic for neutrophils
4. Prostaglandins	Acidic lipids. Derived from essential fatty acids of cell membrane phospholipids by enzymic cyclization. Probably in most (all?) cells	Contract smooth muscle. Delayed mediators of vasopermeability following kinin action. Chemotactic for neutrophils. Modulate various aspects of inflammation in conjunction with cyclic nucleotides. Initiate collagen synthesis in tissue repair
5. Hageman factor (factor XII of blood clotting)	Element of blood clotting system, normally inactive, but when activated exhibits limited proteolytic activity. Also can be cleaved to fragments enzymatically, with similar activities	Initiates (either intact or as fragments) activation of three plasma proenzymes: (i) prethromboplastin activator, that itself initiates intrinsic clotting mechanism, (ii) plasminogen proactivator, leading to plasmin (see 6), (iii) prekallikrein, leading to kinin formation (see 3)
6. Plasmin	Protease, from plasma protein substrate by proteolytic cleavage by activated Hageman factor	Directs progression of inflammation by; (i) Breaking down fibrin, (ii) activates Hageman Factor (iii) activates complement system (iv) indirectly stimulates kinin formation
7. Complement System	Multiglycoprotein complex of blood, when activated producing sequence of fragments and adducts with numerous functions, some enzymic	Components have varied functions: (i) release histamine from mast cells, (ii) chemotactic for leucocytes (iii) vasoactive (iv) promote phagocytosis and lysosome release
8. Lysosomal enzymes	Acidic and neutral hydrolytic enzymes, derived from lysosomes of neutrophils	(i) Damage connective tissue elements, (ii) inactivate certain irritant stimuli, (iii) chemotactic for leucocytes (iv) produce or break down kinins (v) generation or inactivation of complement components, (vi) various other duplicate roles of some mediators

Table I—*continued*

Mediator	Structure and origin	Function
9. Cationic proteins	Non-enzymic basic proteins, derived from lysosomes of neutrophils	Various functions: (i) Enhance vascular permeability, (ii) release histamine, (iii) chemotactic for neutrophils, (iv) pro- and anti-coagulant, (v) antibacterial, (vi) pyrogenic
10. Epidermal factors	Suggested to be readily diffusible molecules derived from epidermis (e.g. lysosomal proteins, histamine, prostaglandins)	(i) Initiate inflammatory response (vasoactivity), (ii) Inhibit fibrinolysis
11. Cyclic nucleotides	Cyclic AMP and cyclic GMP, produced by nucleotide cyclases in plasma membranes of cells	Regulation of cellular events, (e.g. phagocytosis, mediator release)—controlling or terminating activities as well as initiating them

Although most have not yet been shown to fulfil all of the criteria of mediators stated by Spector and Willoughby (1968), all are generally regarded as mediators of the process. Table 1 summarizes the most common mediators. But it must be stressed that this list is not exhaustive, and does not include specific mediators of various allergic responses (such as the slow-reacting substances of anaphylaxis; bacteriocidal proteins; the lymphokines etc.), and detailed accounts may be found in comprehensive reviews listed on p. 303.

1. Histamine (β-aminoethyl imidazole)
This participates in the earliest stage of inflammation, probably as the first mediator. Spector and Willoughby (1968) summarized earlier observations with X-rays, turpentine and thermal burns that showed histamine to be a permeability factor that acts consistently before 5-hydroxytryptamine or kinins in the rat. Willoughby (1973) described phases of permeability increase in various types of non-allergic inflammation that suggested sequential participation of more than one mediator. But there are species variability: in the rat histamine is not so potent as 5-hydroxytryptamine, unlike man or guinea pigs.

Majno *et al.* (1969) showed that histamine acts as the venules, contracting the endothelial cells and allowing leakage of plasma constituents. Capillaries are not affected by histamine, rather, they respond to the kinins produced later. Also, the action of histamine is expressed before diapedesis of neutrophils, and this amine is not chemotactic, but it may influence their subsequent functions (see below). Ash and Schild (1966) postulated two types of histamine receptors (H_1 and H_2), and Powell and Brody (1974) have shown that the peripheral vascular system of the dog possesses both types, and the released histamine binds to those sites and initiates permeability increase.

Histamine is mainly found in mast cells, bound ionically as a tertiary complex with zinc and heparin. Rat mast cells are particularly rich in histamine, as well as containing other mediators (5-hydroxytryptamine, a chymotrypsin-like protease). Tissue concentrations of histamine closely reflect the number of mast cells in the skin, which are found throughout the dermis, but predominantly associated with small blood vessels. Further details of the chemistry and morphology of mast cells are given in various reviews, including those by Riley (1959), Parish (1964), Keller (1969), Uvnäs (1969), Wilhelm (1973) and Henson (1974).

It is generally thought, but has not been fully substantiated, that in non-allergic inflammation such as due to chemicals, the histamine that acts upon venules arises from neighbouring mast cells, but the mechanism of its release is not known. Much more is known of the release of histamine from rat peritoneal mast cells (that may not be fully representative of those in the skin) by certain drugs and allergens. Bach (1974) proposed a theory of allergic histamine release invoking a sequence of esterases and phospholipases, membrane ATPase and nucleotide cyclases, linked with structural changes in the mast cell, and Cochrane (1925) has suggested a general mechanism that is common to many types of mediator release (amine release from mast cells and platelets, lysosomal enzymes from leucocytes). Here, the organelles (lysosomes) or granules containing the mediators move to and fuse with the plasma membranes of the cells and are released by a mechanism involving serine esterases, ATP generation, divalent cations, intact microtubules, low intracellular cyclic AMP and high cyclic GMP. It is proposed that specialized cell-surface receptor sites bind specific extracellular activators of mediator release. In the case of chemical-induced vasopermeability, the nature of the activator of histamine release is not known, although components of the complement system (see below, and Willoughby, 1973) may be involved. It may also be, moreover, that irritant chemicals directly lyse mast cells *in vivo*, as this has been shown for potentially irritant surfactants in contact with peritoneal mast cells *in vitro* (Prottey and Ferguson, 1975).

Histamine is formed by the enzyme histidine decarboxylase (see Fig. 3), and Schayer (1966) suggested that the amine was rapidly formed close to its site of action. On the other hand, Steele and Wilhelm (1970) speculated that in chemical irritation histamine from the epidermis might diffuse to the dermis and thus elicit inflammation. This latter suggestion is attractive as it supports the microscopic observations of these authors, that in chemical

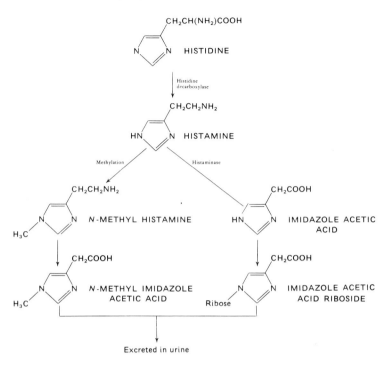

Fig. 3. Metabolism of histamine.

irritation morphological changes are seen in the epidermal cells immediately overlying the dilated vessels of the dermis. But corroboration is still required. Söndergaard and Glick (1971) measured endogenous histamine and its formation by histidine decarboxylase, and confirmed that mast cells were the chief site of its synthesis. However, neither endogenous epidermal histamine nor that formed by histidine decarboxylase could be confirmed as that which acted on the venules.

Histamine is rapidly inactivated close to its site of action after expression of its activity, by the action of diamino oxidase (histaminase) to imidazole acetic acid, or, following ring methylation, to N-methyl imidazole acetic acid. These compounds, which are not pharmacologically active, are then excreted in the urine, the former often as the riboside conjugate (Fig. 3). In man histaminase is the predominant reaction.

Histamine undoubtedly qualifies as a mediator of inflammation under the criteria of Spector and Willoughby (1968), but its action is rapid and transitory, and subsequently, other mediators of vasopermeability come into force. When the action of histamine in inflammation is prevented (by blocking specific binding sites on the blood vessels with drugs, or if laboratory animals are first depleted of their stores of histamine before inducing experimental inflammation) the overall inflammatory process always develops (albeit delayed in some instances, or with some diminished vasopermeability), and the infiltration of leucocytes is unaffected. Thus the role of histamine is as one of the substances that initiate release of plasma constituents into the interstices of the dermis, and these molecules mediate subsquent events. There may be other functions of histamine related to the inflammatory process: Kahlson and Rosengren (1968) described a role in wound healing; recently, histamine has been postulated to act in the control of leucocyte activity (Bourne *et al.*, 1974).

5. *5-Hydroxytryptamine (serotonin)*
This is a mediator of inflammation, particularly in the rat. Spector and Willoughby (1968) have described the release of 5-hydroxytryptamine in non-allergic inflammation of this species, subsequent to the release of histamine, but before that of kinins. Thus it may have a transitory role in the rat that overlaps with that of histamine, sustaining the initial permeability increase. In the rat, but not in man, 5-hydroxytryptamine is a potent venular permeability factor, ten times more active than histamine. In guinea pigs and rabbits it is much less active than histamine. At low dosage it is vasodilatory, but at higher levels it is constrictory. Use of specific antagonists of 5-hydroxytryptamine in rats has shown its action may be blocked without influencing the subsequent development of inflammation.

5-Hydroxytryptamine is formed from tryptophane by the action of a hydroxylase and a decarboxylase. Following its release and pharmacologic action it is broken down by monoamine oxidase to indole acetic acid (Fig. 4). The mast cells of the rat and the mouse have been found to contain 5-hydroxytryptamine (Keller, 1969; Unväs, 1969), but it is also found in the platelets of most mammals, where it may be involved in the intravascular mediation of circulation. Further discussions are given in reviews by MacFarlane (1974), Rodman (1974) and Cooper *et al.* (1976).

There is no great evidence suggesting that 5-hydroxytryptamine is an important mediator of inflammation, other than its properties as a permeability factor in the rat or mouse, although a role in the regulation of the normal tonus of blood vessels in many species cannot be overlooked.

3. *Kinins*
Kinins are thought to be the most likely mediators of the capillary permeability that occurs subsequent to the venular effects elicited by histamine (Spector and Willoughby, 1968). Their effects coincide with diapedesis of

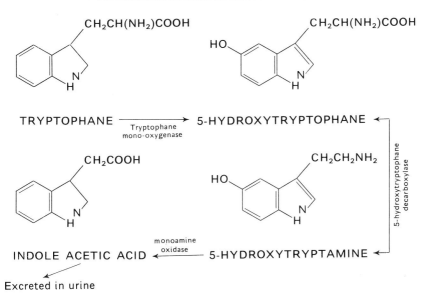

Fig. 4.   Metabolism of 5-hydroxytryptamine.

neutrophils, but it is thought that kinins are not directly responsible for their emigration. In addition to contracting smooth muscle, kinins produce pain when applied to blister bases.

Kinins are a family of polypeptides, the basic member of which is bradykinin. This is a nonapeptide, and other kinins are structural derivatives of it, for example, kallidin is N-lysyl bradykinin (Fig. 5). Kinins are formed from inactive α_2-globulin substrates (called kininogens), by various enzymes (collectively called kininogenases) and these include the highly substrate-specific and active kallikreins, as well as trypsin and other proteases from leucocytes. In addition to the two major kinins, kallidin and bradykinin, many other polypeptide and protein permeability factors have been reported (reviewed by Wilhelm, 1973). Some of these are derived from activated complement components (C3a, C5a), but they may exert their permeability effects by the prior release of histamine from mast cells. There is great species variability of the action of kinins.

The kininogenases or kallikreins are widely distributed throughout the body, existing as inactive precursors (prekallikreins) and may be subdivided into tissue- and plasma kallikreins, which have different physical characteristics. Tissue kallikreins may be activated by proteases such as trypsin. Kallikreins are also strongly chemotactic for neutrophils.

The formation of kinins is one of the numerous sequences of limited proteolysis that occur in the plasma or fluid phase of the dermal oedema.

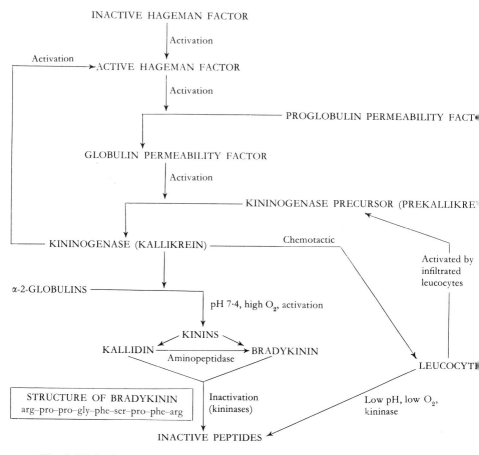

Fig. 5. Kinin formation.

The sequence for kinins (see reviews by Wilhelm, 1973; Spragg, 1974) is one of three initiated by activated Hageman factor, or factor XII of blood clotting (*Lancet*, 1972) and is summarized in Fig. 7. Activated Hageman factor itself can activate proglobulin permeability factor (prekallikrein activator), which also possesses vasoactivity in its own right. In turn, this activates kininogenase precursor (prekallikrein) to kininogenase (kallikrein). Kininogenases have numerous actions: they are vasoactive, chemotactic for neutrophils, and they can activate more Hageman factor. They also convert α_2-globulins to kinins (kallidin and bradykinin) which are vaso-active. Kallidin may also be converted to bradykinin by plasma amino peptidase which cleaves off the N-terminal lysine. Activated Hageman factor may also be hydrolysed by plasmin to Hageman factor pre-albumin fragments (see Fig. 7). These are even more effective than Hageman factor itself in forming kininogenase. Kinins are very short lived ($t_{1/2}$ of about 20 s), being broken down to inactive peptides by kininases from various sources.

Leucocytes participate in kinin generation and Melmon and Cline (1968) described the activating role of neutrophils and eosinophils in kinin formation and destruction. Following damage to the vascular endothelium, and activation of the plasma reactions, neutrophil emigration was observed. At high oxygen tension and neutral tissue pH, the leucocytes promoted further kinin formation by activating plasma kallikrein. As the oxygen tension and pH decreased in the inflamed area, kinin-generation by the cells diminished and kinin-destroying activity predominated. Zacharie and Oates (1967) also showed that kinin formation in rats was favoured at high pH, and kininase activity at low pH. Thus, changes in tissue pH as inflammation ensues may be a controlling factor.

4. *Prostaglandins*

There are a family of 20-carbon fatty acids, synthesized from essential fatty acids (Fig. 6). Goldyne (1975) has lucidly reviewed current knowledge of the structures of prostaglandins and their participation in inflammation and indicates their importance in modulating many of the discrete facets of the total response.

The presence or release of prostaglandins (principally the E and F structures) has been detected in skin as a result of various types of inflammatory stimuli, including ultraviolet irradiation (Greaves and Søndergaard, 1970), thermal burning (Arturson *et al.*, 1973), scalding (Anggard and Jonsson, 1971), cantharidin (Goldyne *et al.*, 1973), carageenin (Velo *et al.*, 1973), immunologic stimuli such as contact dermatitis (Greaves *et al.*, 1971) and bullous skin diseases (Goldyne, 1975). Recently, Søndergaard *et al.* (1974) have detected E and F prostaglandins in the perfused skin of man following primary irritation by the detergent benzalkonium chloride. The vascular activity of E prostaglandins, and to a lesser degree F prostaglandins, in man, namely, the production of erythema and whealing, has been described by Søndergaard and Greaves (1971) and several others (listed by Goldyne, 1975), and Weiner and Kaley (1969) showed increased vascular permeability in rats by the E prostaglandins. Studies on experimental inflammation by carageenin (Di Rosa *et al.*, 1971) have shown a triphasic vascular response, the first related to histamine release, the second associated with kinins and the third with prostaglandins. These data support the view that presence of prostaglandin activity is a common

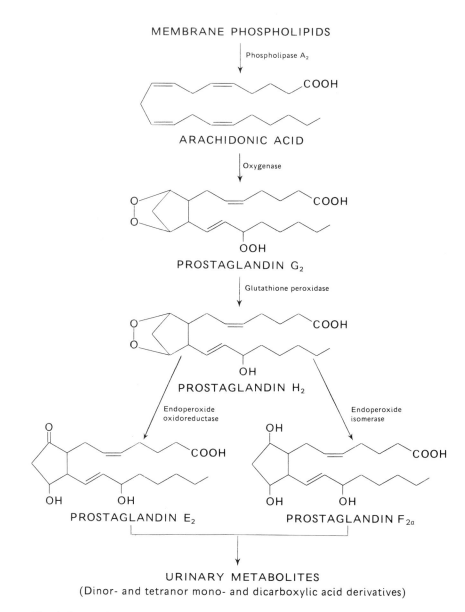

MEMBRANE PHOSPHOLIPIDS

Phospholipase A_2

ARACHIDONIC ACID

Oxygenase

PROSTAGLANDIN G_2

Glutathione peroxidase

PROSTAGLANDIN H_2

Endoperoxide
oxidoreductase

Endoperoxide
isomerase

PROSTAGLANDIN E_2

PROSTAGLANDIN $F_{2\alpha}$

URINARY METABOLITES
(Dinor- and tetranor mono- and dicarboxylic acid derivatives)

Fig. 6. Prostaglandin metabolism.

denominator in vascular permeability increase resulting from all types of stimuli.

In addition to possessing vasoactivity, prostaglandins also seem to modulate certain cellular activities in inflammation. Goldyne (1975) has summarized the participation of prostaglandins in certain functions of cells derived from the blood by infiltration during inflammation. The chemotactic attraction of neutrophils, the release of their lysosomal enzymes, the release of basophil histamine, the secretion of lymphokines and the production of antibody by sensitized lymphocytes, the participation of platelets in clotting, have all been studied by numerous groups from the standpoint of prostaglandins. A general feature of these data is that prostaglandins E_1 or E_2 are involved with the prevention of a leucocytic activity, whereas the F prostaglandins seem to initiate that activity, and this regulation is expressed in conjunction with cyclic nucleotides (see below). It seems that alteration in the relative production of the E and the F prostaglandins determines whether a specific reaction proceeds or not. Velo *et al.* (1973) showed that during the development of a carageenin-induced exudate in rats, at 6 h the ratio of E to F prostaglandins was $1:2$; as the response waned (by 24 h) the ratio had altered to $1:6$, and by 40 h it was $1:40$. These authors postulated that the prostaglandins liberated had arisen from the infiltrated neutrophils, and reflected changes in cellular function at different phases of the inflammation. Prostaglandins have also been shown to alter collagen biosynthesis (Blumenkrantz and Søndergaard, 1972), and so may feature in the repair stages.

The precise stimuli that initiate prostaglandin synthesis have not been characterized, although phospholipase A_2 is required for the initial release of dihomo-γ-linolenic or arachidonic acid from membrane phospholipids, and this reaction is known to be rate limiting in overall prostaglandin synthesis (Samuelsson, 1970). Prostaglandins have potent biological activity and are synthesized on demand close to their site of action, and are rapidly inactivated. Most processes which disturb membrane function activate the hydrolysis of arachidonic acid from phospholipids (Gilmore *et al.*, 1969), and so it is not unlikely that phospholipase A_2 is activated by a limited proteolysis reaction (serine esterase?), as have been proposed for various mediator release mechanisms (Henson, 1974).

5. *Hageman Factor and the Fibrinolytic System (Plasmin)*

These are both protease enzymes derived from elements of the blood-clotting system, that exert important effects in launching and amplifying early inflammation in the vascular and plasma phases. Hageman factor is normally present in the blood in an inactive form, but it may be activated by contact with various components of the vessels and connective tissues, such as collagen, elastin and cartilage. In chemically-induced inflammation, however, it is not known whether the actual presence of the irritant molecules directly effects activation (it is known that in gout the urate crystals may do so), or whether contact of the exuded plasma proteins with tissue damaged by the irritant is responsible. Activated Hageman factor is a protease that may act upon three plasma proteins that are themselves proenzymes, converting each to the active form. These are: preplasma thromboplastin anticedent (clotting factor XI) of the intrinsic coagulation system, secondly, the plasmin or fibrinolytic system is initiated by activation of plasminogen proactivator, and thirdly, prekallikrein is activated, leading to kinin formation, as described above. These reactions are summarized in Fig. 7. The three activation steps also possess positive feed-back loops, as products of each activation can also activate more Hageman factor. Furthermore, activated Hageman factor can be hydrolysed by plasmin to Hageman factor prealbumin fragments, and these may also act in similar fashion to intact Hageman factor, but with differences in specificity. For example, intact Hageman factor activates prethromboplastin activator and the coagulation system much better than the fragments, whereas the fragments are more effective than the intact molecule in activating kinin formation. Thus, this is a controlling mechanism that determines whether clotting or kinin formation ensue. Furthermore, various endogenous inhibitor molecules operate at numerous points to effect further control. Spragg (1974) has described Hageman factor in inflammation.

Plasmin is also a protease derived from a plasma substrate that has numerous controlling influences in the fluid milieu of inflammation. Plasmin formation is activated by activated Hageman factor, but it may also further activate more Hageman factor (positive feedback). Plasmin may direct the progress of inflammation somewhat by hydrolysing Hageman factor to fragments, that then initiate kinin formation. Furthermore, plasmin can activate the first component of the complement system and release mediators by a non-immunologically initiated process. Plasmin also breaks down fibrin. A feature of tissue damage that may occur as a consequence of an irritant stimulus is the deposition of fibrin in the tissue. Fibrin is important in tissue repair, as it forms a scaffold for migrating cells, and the fabric in which fibroblast proliferation, collagen production and capillary regeneration occur. Fibrin is ultimately broken down into soluble peptides and removed. Hageman factor is involved, thus, in the formation and the breakdown of fibrin.

In the process initiated by Hageman factor various protein mediators are generated and some of these are shown in Fig. 7. They are responsible

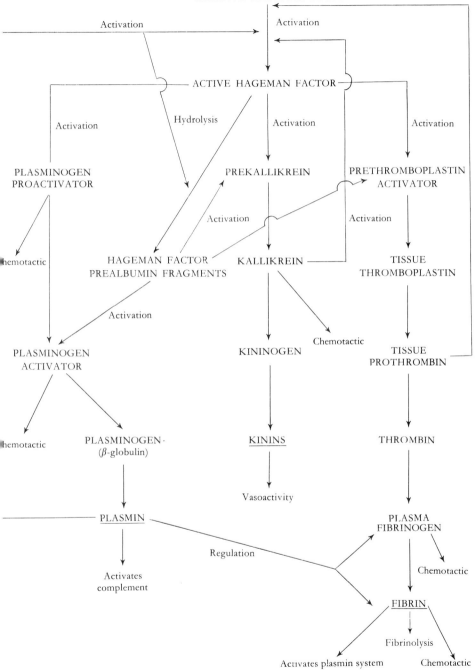

Fig. 7. Role of Hageman factor in inflammation.

for the chemotaxis of leucocytes, and so the subsequent leucocytic phase and resultant tissue damage of inflammation may be triggered off.

6. The Complement System

The complement system describes 11 serum glycoproteins (representing about 10% by weight of the globulin fraction of human serum), of molecular weights ranging from about 80 000 to 400 000, which, when activated and associated as discrete macromolecular components, produce a reversible sequence of proteolytic reactions. For example, complement is activated in the presence of antigen–antibody complexes, and the resultant series of reactions of the components culminates in irreversible damage to membranes and cytolysis. Also some of the components of the activated complement system mediate humoral and cellular reactions of inflammation, such as the release of histamine from cells, the contraction of smooth muscle, increased vascular permeability, chemotaxis of neutrophils, phagocytosis and lysosomal enzyme release. Much of what is known pertains to human complement, mainly in the context of immediate hypersensitivity and skin disease (for reviews Müller-Eberhard, 1969; Ruddy, 1974) but there are numerous similarities with animal species. There is evidence that complement is important in non-allergic, primary inflammation (Hurley, 1964; Müller-Eberhard and Lepow, 1965; Willoughby and Giroud, 1969; Willoughby et al., 1969; Willoughby and Spector, 1969).

The "classical" (immunological) pathway for activation of complement involves the interaction of the first component, C_1, with an antibody that has been aggregated or altered by combination with antigen and bound to a cell surface. Binding of complement activates C_1 esterase, and this then catalyses the binding of C_4 and then the C_2 components to the cell, which form an enzyme C_{42}. This activates C_3, cleaving off the C_{3a} fragment (anaphylatoxin I) which, in some species, releases histamine from mast cells and is chemotactic for neutrophils. The C_{423b} can induce immune adherence and phagocytosis of lymphocytes. The fifth component, C_5, is cleaved by C_{423b}, forming a fragment C_{5a} (anaphylatoxin II) which in some species is chemotactic for neutrophils and also promotes release of lysosomal enzymes. The remainder, C_{5b}, then activates C_6 and C_7 to form the C_{5b67} complex which is chemotactic for neutrophils. The penultimate step is the uptake and activation of C_8 by the cell surface to form a complex that makes the cell prone to protracted, low grade lysis. Finally, the binding and activation of C_9 enhances the membrane damage by the complex to the cell, which then lyses. This sequence may be modulated at various stages. There are natural inhibitors which combine with or destroy the activated forms of certain components.

Non-immunological cytolysis by complement has been described by Götze and Müller-Eberhard (1969). The mechanism is different from the immune-activated process in that C_1 esterase is activated in the absence of cell-bound antibodies and occurs in solution and not at the cell surface. It is thought that the initial stages involving the first four components all occur in the fluid phase, but the C_5 component upon activation, and subsequently, $C_{6,7,8,9}$, all bind to the target cell and induce lysis. Components C_1 to C_4 constitute the activation mechanism in solution, and the membrane damage to the cell is not initiated until C_5 has bound. The binding and activation of C_6 and C_7 components do not cause membrane damage *per se*, but their presence is prerequisite for the subsequent cytolytic action of C_8 and C_9.

The participation of the activated complement system in non-allergic inflammation was shown by Willoughby and Spector (1969) and Willoughby *et al.* (1969) for thermal injury and turpentine oedema. The total serum complement titre was reduced in both rats and guinea pigs by various means (by pretreatment with anti-lymphocyte serum, anti-complement serum or carrageenin up to 24 h beforehand) and a strong positive correlation between this and the diminished inflammatory response (oedema) was observed. On the basis of this Willoughby suggested that following the injurious stimulus there is some leakage into the tissue of plasma protein which becomes aggregated and bound to cells, such that the complement cascade is activated, or, inactive complement coming in contact with damaged tissue protein as a result of the irritant is activated. This leads to the sequential formation of histamine liberators, permeability factors and chemotactic factors for leucocytes.

The complement system represents another example of sequential, limited proteolytic actions within the inflammatory response, which may be related to others, forming, overall, a very complex network of reactions. For example, there are by-pass mechanisms in which lysosomal enzymes can cleave C_3 and C_5 fragments from complement, plasmin can activate complement, there are amplification reactions, in that C_{5a} can enhance the release of lysosomal enzymes that cleave more C_{5a}. Whether all or none of these interactions occur in chemical inflammation is not known, but it is likely that the irritation responses generated by individual chemicals will all vary greatly in this respect.

7. *Lysosomal Enzymes and Cationic Proteins*

These two groups of mediators are derived from the lysosomes of the neutrophil leucocytes that emigrate to the site of various types of inflammation, including the non-allergic response of the skin to irritant chemicals.

Lysosomes are intracellular organelles and were originally identified in rat liver about 20 years ago (for a review, see de Duve, 1964), and their importance in neutrophils in inflammation has been well established (Hirsch and Cohn, 1960), particularly with respect to the process of phagocytosis. Lysosomes contain potent hydrolytic enzymes, usually in latent form, and other molecules that participate in inflammation.

Phagocytosis (or endocytosis) is the process by which neutrophils ingest foreign materials (irritant molecules, bacteria) in the dermis or debris resulting from tissue damage. In phagocytosis the plasma membranes of neutrophils surround material to be ingested, forming invaginations and eventually intracytoplasmic vacuoles, or "phagosomes", in which the material is surrounded by a limiting membrane and not in contact with the cytoplasm of the neutrophils. These vacuoles then coalesce with the lysosomes and form "phagolysosomes" or "secondary lysosomes" within which the enzymes of the lysosomes exert their activity. Within these digestive sacs the pH is quite low and degradation and inactivation of the engulfed material proceeds. If the ingested materials are toxic, susceptible tissues are thereby protected, but at the expense of the phagocyte.

In the process of phagocytosis, some lysosomal enzymes may leak out into the surrounding tissues, phagolysosome vacuoles or their contents may be released into the extracellular space, or the neutrophils are killed, and their contents spill out due to cell lysis. The hydrolytic enzymes so released may then cause tissue damage, as is characteristic of the leucocytic phase of inflammation.

Various types of enzymes have been identified in neutrophil lysosomes: these have been shown to be present in inflammatory foci, or, have been found to produce reactions typical of those seen in inflammation upon experimental injection. There are several recent reviews that have listed these enzymes, for example, Baggiolini, 1972; Hirsch, 1974; Hirschhorn, 1974; and Goldstein, 1974, and the types of enzymes included are: phosphatases; polysaccharidases (amylase, dextranase, glucosidases, mannosidases, galactosidases, N-acetylglucosaminidase, glucuronidases); amino peptidases; neutral and acid proteases (cathepsins); elastases; collagenases; sulphatases; peroxidase; various lipases, ribo- and deoxyribonuclease etc. These enzymes are able to exert damaging effects upon various vascular and connective tissue elements of the dermis, such as the basement membranes and elastic tissues of vessels, collagen and mucopolysaccharides of the dermal matrix. Some of the products of this broad spectrum of hydrolytic activity may also function in the mediation and limitation of other reactions of inflammation (for example, some products of collagenolysis are chemotactic).

In addition to the potentially damaging action of lysosomal enzymes upon the dermal structures, there is also considerable action with components of the plasma exudate—indeed, there appear to be several alternative reactions for mediator production, in addition to those known to occur early on in the plasma exudate phase. Lysosomal enzymes also appear to control or direct certain reactions in preference to others. The fifth component of the activated complement system is chemotactic for neutrophils, and the neutrophil lysosome also possesses enzymes that can cleave yet more of this specific mediator, as well as possessing enzymes that can inhibit the complement cascade at several points. Fibrin can be broken down by leucocyte enzymes, plasminogen may be activated, leading to fibrinolysis. Kinins may be generated by specific leucokininogens (that are different from the plasma kininogens), or broken down by kininases, as described above. Leucocytes are attracted to prostaglandins, as well as possessing the enzymes for synthesizing or inactivating them.

Neutrophil leucocytes also contain a group mediator without enzyme activity. These are the lysosomal cationic proteins and they exhibit numerous functions, including, enhancement of vascular permeability, histamine release from mast cells, chemotaxis of leucocytes, pro- and anti-coagulation properties, pyrogenic and antibacterial functions.

A brief description of lysosomal components, as given here cannot do justice to the enormous amount of research devoted to the neutrophil leucocyte in inflammation, or its central role in the process. There are several detailed discussions of this field in the volumes edited by Zweifach *et al.* (1974), to which the reader is directed. Figure 8, however, attempts to summarize some of the functions of neutrophils in inflammation.

8. *"Epidermal" Factors*

In Fig. 1 and at other points in the text above, references are made to the possible release of factors in the epidermis that mediate dermal inflammation subsequently. In the absence of direct proof, this must remain an attractive hypothesis. Steele and Wilhelm (1970), in a detailed study of chemical inflammation, remarked that areas of the dermis in which inflammation developed were always those overlaid with structurally modified, or "irritated" epidermis. In terms of the short time-scale these authors employed, it seems somewhat unlikely that sufficient quantities of irritant molecules *per se* are able to penetrate directly to the dermis without undergoing immense dilution, whereas if "epidermal" mediators were released, and these were able to percolate to specific receptors on, for example, the venules, this would be consistent with the sequential activation of steps in the overall inflammatory response. This idea is reiterated in a recent review of Lazarus *et al.* (1975) with regard to epidermal lysosomes. Work of Ryan and colleagues also supports this (Turner *et al.*, 1969; Ryan *et al.*, 1971).

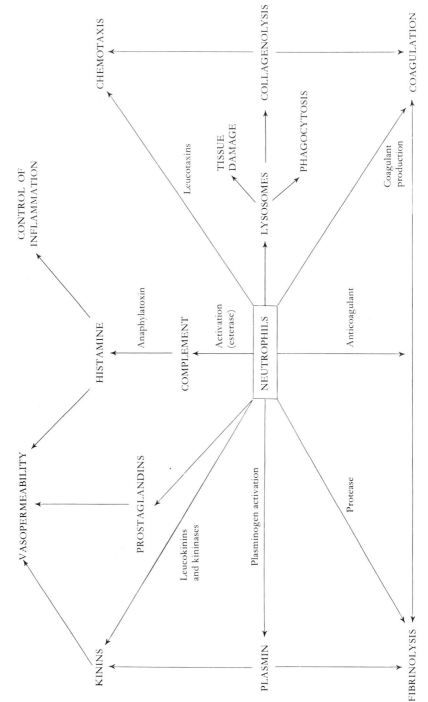

Fig. 8. Possible roles of neutrophil leucocytes in inflammation.

In skin irritation where damage to the epidermis has occurred, and where there is a delayed permeability response of the capillaries and leucocyte emigration, fibrin can be deposited in the dermis due to the inhibition of fibrinolysis. It is suggested that specific inhibitors are released from the epidermis, preventing the breakdown of the fibrin. In instances of mild damage to the dermis, where there is an immediate venular permeability response, but no leucocytic infiltration or damage to the epidermis, fibrinolysis is not inhibited. The inhibitors of fibrinolysis detected in the epidermis may be either antiplasminogen activators or inhibitors of the enzyme plasmin. Fibrin deposition is thought by these investigators to be characteristic of the delayed phase of irritation, and may be important in controlling whether an irritation persists or not. In a similar fashion, the participation of, for example, histamine or prostaglandins produced earlier in the epidermis might be involved in the generation of inflammation of the dermis.

9. Cyclic Nucleotides

Following the elucidation of cyclic AMP as an intracellular "second messenger", responsible for translating the specific cell surface activity of a hormone (the "first messenger") into the characteristic target tissue response (Robison et al., 1968, 1971) there is much evidence that this nucleotide is involved in numerous aspects of the mediation of inflammation (Henson, 1974; Goldyne, 1975). Furthermore, the concept of a dualistic regulation of tissue responses has appeared, invoking the opposing effects of cellular concentrations of cyclic AMP and cyclic GMP, as a result of studies by Goldberg and colleagues (Goldberg et al., 1972). This has been called the "Yin Yang" concept (from the oriental idea of a dualism between two opposing forces). In general it is proposed that synthesis or accummulation of cyclic AMP in a cell or tissue maintains the status quo, and prevents a new cellular activity from progressing, whereas a decrease in the amounts of this nucleotide permits that activity. Simultaneously, there are reciprocal alterations in cyclic GMP. Furthermore, there is much evidence that prostaglandins are intimately linked to these cyclic nucleotides, namely, that the E prostaglandins induce or maintain synthesis of cyclic AMP, and the F prostaglandins do likewise for cyclic GMP. Goldyne (1975) has described various examples of this dualism of inflammation, in which prostaglandin E synthesis induces increase of cellular cyclic AMP (suppressing the requisite function), and prostaglandin F induces increase of cyclic GMP (and activation of that function), including the expression of venoconstriction and dilatation, lysosomal enzyme release, chemotaxis of neutrophils and various lymphocyte functions in allergic inflammation. In this regard the work of Velo *et al.* (1973), described in Section 4 of Table I above is particularly interesting. These investigations showed that as an experimental inflammation developed, and leucocytes exerted their action, the relative proportions of E and F prostaglandins in the exudate altered: these changes may be reflections of altered cyclic AMP and cyclic GMP concentrations in the tissue at various stages of the reaction. A recent publication (Braun *et al.*, 1974) has covered in greater detail various examples of the action of cyclic nucleotides in the inflammatory response.

Much remains to be resolved in this research area, the involvement of cyclic nucleotides, prostaglandins and general cellular metabolism in various aspects of inflammation, especially as there are numerous quite different physiological responses of cells (e.g. vascular endothelial cells contract; infiltrating leucocytes physically move appreciable distances; phagocytozing leucocytes engulf and expel materials; mast cells degranulate, etc.). Henson (1974) has indicated certain unifying mechanisms in the release of mediators, however, that involve cyclic nucleotides as controlling influences.

Recently, also, the importance of histamine as a control factor together with cyclic AMP has been suggested. Bourne *et al.* (1974), studying the control of intracellular cyclic AMP synthesis in leucocytes, have proposed that histamine (and other substances) regulates the intensity of the inflammatory response. Histamine, released from mast cells by antigen–antibody reactions or trauma not only initiates vascular permeability, but also limits the extent of inflammation by binding at basophil cell surfaces, enhancing the production of cyclic AMP, and thereby preventing further release from those cells at the periphery of the inflammation. This proposal adds a new dimension, not only to the function of histamine in inflammation (see Section 1 of Table I, above) but also to the general mechanisms of limitation of inflammation and the onset of tissue recovery.

[The importance of cyclic nucleotides and prostaglandins in the control of epidermal homeostasis (Voorhees *et al.*, 1974) has been briefly discussed in Section III above, also.]

D. Sequences in Inflammation due to Chemicals

Instances of acute, non-allergic inflammation of the skin by chemicals show numerous general similarities to other types of irritant stimuli, such as microbial infections and immediate-type allergic responses, in so far that some of the mediators that participate in the numerous steps may be common, some of the cells involved may be similar, and the macroscopic indications of the inflammations may be barely indistinguishable. However, the relative importance and participation of individual reactions of the response are different. In particular, in bacterial infections or certain immune responses the stimulus (i.e. bacteria, antigen–antibody complexes) may remain in the affected areas for appreciable portions of the total duration of the inflammation. This is not the case for chemically induced inflammation. Antigen–antibody complexes, for example, may directly activate the various proteolytic steps, or be chemotactic for leucocytes etc., but there is no evidence that irritant chemicals persist in acute inflammation. Rather, it is thought that chemicals that can elicit inflammation do so by causing direct structural modification or frank tissue damage, and these in turn activate the inflammation. This has been discussed by Willoughby and Di Rosa (1971). It has been suggested that the earliest reactions of the dermis in chemical inflammation is the direct involvement of the chemical with the vascular system, such that some leakage of plasma proteins can occur. Various components (e.g. Hageman factor, complement) are activated by coming in contact with proteins damaged or modified by the irritant. Such a scheme of irritation is in line with the observations of Hurley et al., (1967) by electron microscopy of direct damage to the venules and capillaries, and leakage of plasma into the tissues, in solvent-induced pleurisy. The preliminary activation of plasma constituents is a prerequisite, for if the complement system is activated, pharmacologically active mediators of mast cell histamine release are generated, and histamine then elicits increased vasopermeability to plasma proteins that react further. With irritant stimuli such as crushing or burning there may also be direct damage to the mast cells, such that they lyse and spill out histamine, with resultant vascular permeability, but this probably does not occur in chemical inflammation, as insufficient of that applied to the skin surface could penetrate within the time span of the appearance of erythema.

With the generation of the histamine-mediated vasopermeability, the "classical" mechanism of inflammation is triggered. In addition, however, Willoughby and Di Rosa suggest that the initial activation of Hageman factor upon contact with damaged proteins activate the extrinsic blood coagulation system. Thereby, platelets may discharge their stored 5-hydroxytryptamine which sustains the earlier histamine-mediated vasopermeability, and fibrinogen, which has leaked from the damaged vessels can be converted to fibrin (see Fig. 7). Furthermore, the plasmin, kinin, and complement system are activated in the plasma exudate. Various components of these activated protease systems are chemotactic for neutrophils. After accumulating and marginating in the blood vessels from the earliest stages of the response, these then emigrate to the site of the plasma exudate. Prostaglandins may also be generated by the activation of proteases that generate phospholipase responsible for the release of precursors of prostaglandins, and later permeability increase of the vessels is maintained. As neutrophils participate in phagocytosis of tissue debris, and, in the process, release enzymes and proteins from their lysosomes, numerous amplification and by-pass reactions of mediator generation may occur, such that certain reactions are attenuated or repressed, and the overall inflammatory response is controlled and directed towards further tissue damage or recovery. Cyclic nucleotides, prostaglandins, histamine, and various other mediators interact in these controlling steps.

The inflammatory response of the skin to chemicals is a complex, highly interrelated phenomenon. The precise reaction sequence has not been established, as this must depend upon the chemical properties of the irritant, the method of application and the animal species in question—there are notable inter-species differences, such as in properties of components of the complement system, the potency of the amines that elicit vasopermeability, the constituents of mast cells, properties of the lysosomes etc. Furthermore, much of the information pertaining to inflammation has been obtained from instances quite different from chemically-induced responses, and so some extrapolations have been made. However, Fig. 9 is a brief summary of some of the mediated events thought to be important in the response to chemicals, and, if nothing else, illustrates the complexity of the phenomenon.

V. PRIMARY SKIN IRRITATION BY CHEMICALS

A. Factors that Determine Primary Skin Irritation

The foregoing sections have described how certain chemicals when applied to the skin may elicit reactions in three morphologically distinct compartments, namely the stratum corneum, the living cells of the epidermis, and the cells and blood vessels of the dermis. The responses of these components are collectively called skin irritation. There are three important factors that determine whether, and to what extent, a chemical may interact with these compartments and irritate the skin.

1. *Chemical Structure*
This determines whether the compound can interact with the chemical constituents and the biochemical apparatus of the skin: without such interactions there can be no irritation response.

2. *Penetration Through the Stratum Corneum*
This is fundamental, for even if the most toxic chemicals cannot reach the living cells and tissues, there can be no responses of the epidermis and

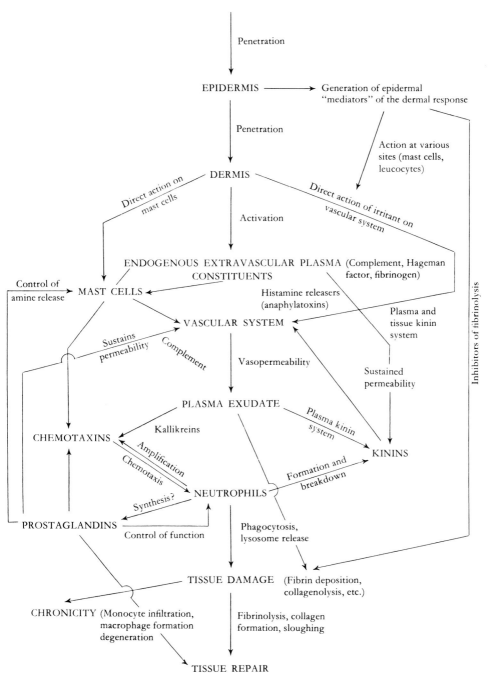

Fig. 9. Possible molecular reactions in primary cutaneous inflammation

dermis. The subject of skin penetration has received detailed attention by numerous investigators. Much of what is known of the kinetics, routes and physico-chemistry of penetration is due to the great contributions of Blank and Scheuplein (for a comprehensive review, see Scheuplein and Blank, 1971) and the work of Maibach and collaborators is also very significant (e.g. Feldmann and Maibach, 1970; Bartek et al., 1972).

There are numerous factors that determine whether a compound will penetrate the skin, and these have been reviewed by Grasso and Lansdown, 1972. Chemical structure is important, particularly with respect to ionization (and pH of the applied solution) and it is thought that all electrolytes and water penetrate relatively feebly, and to similar extents. Lipid solubility of the compound, or more exactly, the lipid/water partition coefficient, is a factor. This is the ratio of concentration of the applied compound in the stratum corneum to that in the solution. Due to the heterogenous composition of the stratum corneum it has been shown by several investigators that molecules with a partition coefficient in the region of unity penetrate most widely (e.g. Marzulli et al., 1965). The octanol/water partition coefficient is a reasonable estimate of the stratum corneum/water partition. Lipid-soluble materials tend to penetrate via the lipid components of the corneum, water-soluble materials via the aqueous phase, thus molecular diffusion mechanisms for extremely polar and non-polar molecules involve different molecular environments and interactions. Although molecular size may be a factor in penetration (molecules with small radii penetrate more readily than macromolecules), lipid solubility is of greater importance. The nature of the vehicle or solvent in which the compound is dissolved may be important, and Blank (1964) showed that polar alcohols penetrated faster from oily vehicles than from polar vehicles, whereas non-polar alcohols penetrated faster from aqueous rather than oily phases. This is due to the greater affinity for the stratum corneum than for the vehicle. Binding of the applied material to the stratum corneum will diminish penetrability, and this is probably one reason why, for example, strong anionic surfactants penetrate less than non-ionic surfactants (Prottey and Ferguson, 1975). The normal range of ambient temperature has a small effect on penetration, but there is a positive dependency. Hydration of the stratum corneum (e.g. due to occlusion) may increase penetration, and age of the skin may be a factor, as infant skin is more permeable than adult skin, whereas senile, atrophic skin is less so. Penetration varies according to body site, being higher, e.g. in scrotal skin than palmar skin, and this depends to a small extent upon the thickness of the stratum corneum. The role of the epidermal appendages (sweat glands, pilo-sebaceous units) have been particularly studied (Scheuplein and Blank, 1971). It is accepted that this route ("shunt" diffusion) is significant only in initial stages following cutaneous application, before steady state transcellular penetration ("bulk" diffusion) of the corneum has been established. In man the area of the skin appendages has been estimated to be about 0.1% of the total corneum, and so on a statistical basis, shunt diffusion is unlikely, except, perhaps for very feebly penetrating materials. The recent observations of Elias and Friend (1975), described above, add to the significance of the intercellular route for penetration through the stratum corneum for certain chemicals. Among various species (rats, rabbits, guinea pigs) the skin of man is the least permeable. The pre-existing condition of the skin is important, as in disease or following physical damage the stratum corneum may be abnormal or disrupted, such that the barrier function is impaired.

Many cosmetic ingredients, such as alcohols, soaps, detergents and emollients, may not penetrate the skin to any appreciable degree when applied initially, but their subsequent action upon the stratum corneum may sufficiently alter the barrier properties that their penetration (or that of an accompanying weakly penetrating ingredient) is increased, such that inflammation may yet result. Various references are cited above to the damaging effects of a wide variety of chemicals upon the stratum corneum, and this may be of greater importance in determining whether a compound causes irritation than knowledge of its precise rate of penetration through normal skin. The results of Matoltsy *et al.* (1968) and Scheuplein and Ross (1970) are representative of the effects of solvents, aqueous solutions of electrolytes, acids and detergents, and Scheuplein and Blank (1971) have summarized their actions in damaging the barrier to skin penetration.

3. *Mode of Application to the Skin*

This governs whether a potentially irritant chemical will, in fact, elicit cutaneous responses, by influencing the amount available for penetration, and whether permeability of the skin will be impaired. For the solvent hexadecane, for example, Kirk and Hoekstra (1964) showed that the degree of epidermal hyperplasia in guinea pigs receiving 1.5 mg/kg depended upon the frequency of treatment and the interval between treatments, and Cowan and Mann (1971) observed that a single application of 0.01 ml produced only minor epidermal changes, whereas multiple applications caused hyperkeratosis. Indeed, most materials applied to the skin in solution or as liquids can elicit irritation provided that appropriate treatments are employed, and even water itself cannot be excluded. Kligman and Wooding (1967) suggested that even water was irritant by causing sweat retention and by increasing permeability, and Willis (1973) showed that prolonged exposure of human skin to water caused swelling, hydration and maceration of the stratum corneum, which subsequently allowed water to penetrate to the living cells and cause inflammation, presumably by osmotic cytolysis.

B. The Prediction of Skin Irritation

The most popular and tested methods for determining whether skin products (or their ingredients) will elicit cutaneous irritation in man during normal usage employ the application of materials to the skin of laboratory animals and/or human test panels, at various concentrations and for various times of contact, followed by examination of the total skin reaction. From detailed examinations the treated skins may be "scored" under numerous criteria, such as oedema, erythema, cracking, exudation, at the visual, macroscopic level, and, by light microscopy, for features such as epidermal thickening, hyperkeratosis, parakeratosis, spongiosis, leucocytic infiltration etc. Ingram and Grasso (1975) have described such an approach, but the basic method has been utilized for many years (Draize *et al.*, 1944; Finkelstein *et al.*, 1968; Uttley and van Abbé, 1973; and others summarized by Lansdown, 1972). Shortcomings of such methods include that they are costly and time-consuming, they are susceptible to variability of response by animals or panellists, they are subjective assessments (albeit by trained assessors), and there are variabilities between different laboratories (Weil and Scala, 1971). This situation has prompted numerous investigators to study, by various laboratory investigative procedures, individual aspects of the overall phenomenon of skin-irritant interaction. The common goal has been to devise parametric methods yielding quantitative data of the irritation potential of chemicals applied to the skin.

1. *Correlations of Data of Laboratory Investigative Methods with Observed Skin Irritation*

There are numerous examples of laboratory procedures that have produced data directly correlating with the observed skin irritancy of surfactants. Gale and Scott (1953) studied the oral and intraperitoneal toxicity and the effect upon muscle of a series of sodium alkyl sulphates. In each case, sodium lauryl (dodecyl) sulphate exerted the most profound effect compared with higher and lower homologues. Van Scott and Lyon (1953) studied the denaturing effects of various commercial surfactants on keratin, following earlier observations of Anson (1941) that detergents uncoiled egg albumin and exposed sulphydryl were observed, and these authors suggested that this might be important "in the production of dermatitis from these substances . . ." Blohm (1957) studied the denaturation of egg albumin by a series of sodium alkyl sulphates, assuming that this protein was representative of the soluble proteins of the epidermis, and found that the lauryl moiety possessed the greatest denaturing ability. Harrold (1959) studied the denaturation of callus powder also by titrating sulphydryl groups. He found that thiol groups were liberated only above the critical micelle concentration, and sodium lauryl sulphate was more effective than alkyl benzene sulphonate. Both were far more effective than soap, and a non-ionic surfactant had no effect. Protein denaturation was found to be reversible. Choman (1963) utilized the swelling of discs of calf skin collagen in the hope of obtaining better understanding of interactions between chemicals and skin. When studied at or above the critical micelle concentrations, it was found that sodium alkyl soaps could be ranked: $C_{12} > C_{14} > C_{10} > C_8 > C_{16} =$ water, but sodium alkyl sulphates induced greater swelling than the soaps, and were ranked: $C_{12} > C_{10} > C_8 > C_{14} > C_{16} = C_{18} =$ water. Sodium alkyl isethionate, cationic and non-ionic surfactants had no effect. The relative trends observed reflected the relative irritancies of these surfactants. Dugard and Scheuplein (1973) studied reversible changes in ion conductance, which is a sensitive measure of skin permeability. The reversibility of these changes argued against extraction of lipids as the cause of permeability increase, but suggested other events were important, such as protein denaturation. The relative changes, reflecting the known skin irritancy of the surfactants studied, led these investigators to conclude that reduction of barrier function was an important factor in skin irritation. Prottey and Ferguson (1975) investigated various reactions of a series of soaps. With the extraction of soluble proteins and amino acids from the skin, the lauryl and myristyl moieties were most effective. When tested on mast cells *in vitro*, as a test for cytolytic activity, laurate was far more potent than either the C_{10} or C_{14} homologues. Howes (1975) measured the penetration of various alkyl soaps through human skin *in vitro* and rat skin *in vivo*: sodium laurate possessed the greatest penetrability of the series used.

Some of these data are summarized in Tables II and III, together with published rankings of the relative skin irritancies of these surfactants as determined by direct observation and assessment. Consistently, the C_{12} moiety of both the series of soaps and alkyl sulphates was the most potent in the individual laboratory procedures, exactly as seen in the direct determinations of irritancy. Schott (1973) analysed data of this type in an attempt to explain the particular effectiveness of the C_{12} moiety. This was thought to be due to the relationships of two factors of the surfactants in solution, namely, the oil-water partition coefficient and the upper limit of the concentration of unassociated (non-micellar) molecules. The oil-water partition coefficient gradually increases with increasing chain length, whereas the critical micelle concentration falls. Thus, from chain length of C_8 to C_{12}, with increasing partition coefficient there is increased ability of

Table II
Correlations of the structure of an homologous series of sodium alkyl carboxylates and their properties in various laboratory test methods, with observed irritant action on human and rat skin

Chain length of sodium alkyl carboxylate	HUMAN SKIN IRRITANCY (Emery and Edwards, 1940)	RAT SKIN IRRITANCY (Prottey et al., 1973)	COLLAGEN DISC SWELLING (Choman, 1963)	EXTRACTION OF STRATUM CORNEUM (Prottey and Ferguson, 1975)		ION CONDUCTANCE OF STRATUM CORNEUM (Dugard and Scheuplein, 1973)
	Positive reactions to 22·5 mM solutions (%)	Assessed score for irritancy (macroscopic and microscopic). 0·25 M solutions for 15 min, once daily for 3 days	Change in thickness, critical micelle concentration (%)	Increase relative to water	Proteins: Amino acids (%)	Rate of change of conductance $(\text{Mohm}/\text{cm}^2/\text{min} \times 10^{-3})$
C_8	2	2·5	62	126	0	0
C_{10}	19	13·5	94	197	43	1
C_{12}	70*	Reaction of skin* too strong for accurate assessment	136*	187	235*	45*
C_{14}	41	2·0	121	793*	148	40
C_{16}	4	1·0	19	148	161	2
C_{18}	0	2·0	0	ND	ND	ND

Table II—*continued*

Chain length of sodium alkyl carboxylate	HUMAN SKIN PENETRATION (Howes, 1975) Permeability constants (μcm.min^{-1}), 6mM solution for 6 h *in vitro*	RAT SKIN PENETRATION (Howes, 1975) Amount penetrating 7.5 cm^2 of skin, applied for 15 min 0.1 ml of 6 mM solution	INHIBITION OF DNA SYNTHESIS *in vitro* (Ferguson and Prottey, 1976) Conc. (mM) required to inhibit uptake of 3HTdR into fibroblasts *in vitro*	MAST CELL LYSIS *in vitro* (Ferguson and Prottey, 1976) Conc. (mM) to release histamine from mast cells *in vitro*	FIBROBLAST LYSIS *in vitro* (Ferguson and Prottey, 1976) Conc. (mM) to release ^{51}Cr-labelled cytoplasm from fibroblasts *in vitro*
C_8	ND	ND	0·6	>5·0	>10·0
C_{10}	5·4	1·8	0·4	1·0	>10·0
C_{12}	18·2*	5·1*	0·1*	0·4*	7·1*
C_{14}	1·6	2·0	0·2	0·5	7·7
C_{16}	0·1	0·5	0·3	1·0	>10·0
C_{18}	0·1	0·5	ND	ND	ND

ND = Not determined.　　　　* Denotes chain length with most potency in that test.

Table III
Correlations of the structure of an homologous series of sodium alkyl sulphates and their properties in various laboratory test methods, with their observed irritant action on human skin

Chain length of sodium alkyl sulphate	HUMAN SKIN IRRITANCY (Emery and Edwards, 1940)	DENATURATION OF PROTEIN (Blohm, 1957)	EXTRACTION OF STRATUM CORNEUM (Prottey and Ferguson, 1975)		ION CONDUCTANCE OF STRATUM CORNEUM (Dugard and Scheuplein, 1973)	CELL LYSIS in vitro (Prottey and Ferguson, 1975)	TOXICITY TO MICE (Gale and Scott, 1953)
	Positive reactions at 22·5 mM solutions (%)	Proportion of total sulphydryl groups liberated from ovalbumin (%)	Increase relative to water proteins : amino acids (%)		Rate of change of conductance (megohm/cm²/min $\times 10^{-3}$)	Conc. (mM) to release histamine from mast cells	Intraperitoneal injection mg/kg
C_8	5	0	ND	ND	0	ND	396
C_{10}	5	32	166	84	1	0·5	284
C_{12}	43*	93*	238*	195*	50*	0·03	250*
C_{14}	24	73	164	110	20	0·025*	342
C_{16}	5	21	ND	ND	4	0·05	356
C_{18}	0	ND	ND	ND	ND	ND	477

ND = Not determined.   * Denotes chain length with most potency in that test.

the surfactants to enter the "oily phase" of the skin (keratin, lipoprotein membranes), whereas from chain length C_{12} to C_{16}, with decreasing concentration of monomer molecules, the amount of surfactant available is also decreasing, producing lower responses. This approach may prove to be valuable in the future as it takes into account the solution properties of surfactants, but a shortcoming is that it applies only to dilute solutions, whereas in practice the concentrations of surfactants applied to the skin are greatly in excess of the critical micelle concentration. Furthermore, Schott has not extended his calculations to surfactants of widely differing structure and irritancy, when other significant physico-chemical factors may be important. Data such as those shown in Tables II and III suggest a value for laboratory procedures in quantifying irritancy for surfactants of similar chemical structure.

2. *Non-correlations*

In a collaborative study (Smeenk and Polano, 1969; Brown, 1971), a series of surfactants were examined by various laboratory and clinical methods in order to assess irritation potential and to see if they would provide a basis for the prediction of irritancy to human skin in normal usage. The surfactants studied were branched and unbranched chain sodium alkyl sulphates, soap, and various ethoxylated non-ionic surfactants. The laboratory procedures were: estimation of free amino acids in the wash liquors, titration of liberated horny layer sulphydryl groups, measurement of skin permeability. Clinical methods were the application to the skin of man, rabbits, rats, guinea pigs and hairless mice. For each procedure the surfactants were ranked according to potency of action, or total assessed irritancy. Overall, there was poor agreement between the individual methods. For example, the soap sample had a minimal effect upon liberation of sulphydryl groups but markedly influenced permeability, and a sodium alkyl sulphate surfactant was irritant when applied to rabbits at 1% or in an arm-immersion test, but relatively non-irritant when applied at similar concentrations to guinea pigs. It was concluded that although these approaches may be useful, caution should be exercised in attempting prediction of irritancy by such tests, as the methods of application and duration of treatment were so widely different in individual experiments. It was felt by the investigators that much greater research on the biochemical changes brought about by skin-surfactant interaction was necessary before such an approach to irritancy evaluation could be meaningful.

Bettley (1972) reviewed some of the problems associated with determining the irritancy of detergents by laboratory procedures tailored to examine discrete aspects of the total irritation response. The assumption was made that irritation potential depends both upon the ability to penetrate the skin and the toxicity of the penetrated compound to the viable skin cells. Various surfactants were studied by patch testing to forecast their skin irritancy in normal usage, and a numerical score was assigned for their degree of action. Also, these surfactants were examined for effects upon skin permeability and skin toxicity (by exposure to buccal mucosa cells *in vitro*), and numerical indices were assigned accordingly. The product of permeability and toxicity was thus taken to be representative of irritancy. By patch testing the observed irritancies were ranked, in decreasing order: cetyltrimethylammonium bromide > sodium lauryl sulphate > sodium laurate ≫ sodium sulpho succinate lauric monoethanolamide > sodium alkyl benzene sulphonate > sodium caprylate > sorbitan oleate polyoxyethylene; when ranked according to the product of permeability and toxicity, the order was: sodium lauryl sulphate ⩾ sodium alkyl benzene sulphonate ⩾ cetyltrimethyl ammonium bromide ≫ sodium laurate > sodium sulphosuccinate lauric monoethanolamide ⩾ sorbitan oleate polyoxyethylene = sodium caprylate.

Bettley stated that these results, although not without value, required cautious interpretation, as there were notable discrepancies. For example, sodium alkyl benzene sulphonate was observed to have a lower skin irritancy by patch test, yet by the laboratory procedures appeared to be a potent irritant.

Earlier studies on the use of liberated sulphydryl titration as a means of assessing skin permeability changes were also discussed by Bettley. Positive correlations were found for cetyl trimethyl ammonium bromide and sodium dodecyl benzene sulphate (both uncoiled insoluble proteins and greatly increased skin permeability). Sodium lauryl sulphate, however, gave a less conclusive correlation (markedly affecting sulphydryl but not equally influencing permeability), and sodium sulpho-succinate and lauric monoethanolamide were found to increase permeability without significantly affecting sulphydryl liberation, yet sodium lauroyl sarcosinate had the opposite effects. Bettley thus concluded that increased permeability does not necessarily correlate with denaturation of epidermal protein, when sulphydryl group liberation is the index.

That there are non-correlations of laboratory data with the clinical appearance of the treated skin indicates that inadequate comparisons have been made, rather than there being inaccurate data. It is not sufficient to attempt to solve the simple equation:

"Skin irritancy = a function of penetration
                × a function of cell toxicity",

for the following reasons. The amount of an irritant that may penetrate to the dermis during a finite time will not necessarily determine the ultimate irritation, as only traces may be required to initiate the first steps of a mediated cascade of reactions; also, absolute penetration data are meaningless for chemicals that alter the barrier properties of the stratum corneum in the process of penetrating through it. Furthermore, the "cytotoxicity potential" of a putative irritant, derived from an experiment utilizing cells *in vitro* will not necessarily correlate with the ability of that irritant to activate Hageman Factor or the complement system, for example.

If what is meant by "skin irritancy" is broken down to relevant constituent parts, such as: effects on barrier function; ability to alter water-binding capacity and flexibility; ability to elicit epidermal hyperplasia or hyperkeratinization; ability to elicit vascular events etc. it should not be too difficult a task, in the light of current knowledge of the skin irritation process, to select relevant laboratory procedures. Singly, such procedures would accurately quantify the discrete components of the response, and when suitably combined (presumably by computer) the total response would be accurately predictable. And such an approach would aid the process of determining whether cosmetics or their chemical ingredients can irritate the skin of man.

VI. CONCLUSIONS

This review describes many of the morphological and biochemical changes possible when a variety of irritants is applied to the skin. There are discrete molecular reactions in the stratum corneum, the epidermis and the dermis, and there are numerous possible interactions of these. A feature that is lacking from all of the studies performed to date, however, concerns the manner by which an irritant that has penetrated the stratum corneum initiates the biochemical and pharmacological events in the underlying living cells. We have a fair understanding of possible chemical reactions in the horny layer (although it must be added that the nature of the cutaneous barrier still awaits precise chemical definition), but the initial biochemical triggers to epidermal and dermal events are unknown. The participation of initially released lysosomal hydrolases is attractive, as these enzymes may then act as mediators of both epidermal and dermal reactions. Also, the release of "factors" from the epidermis that diffuse to the dermis and elicit inflammation may occur, but awaits full ratification. If chalones, cyclic AMP and GMP, prostaglandins etc. are fundamental to the mediation of homeostasis in both the epidermis and the dermis, one must still ask how they are first stimulated or repressed in the initial phase of irritation. The initiation of the primary inflammatory response is still unknown, although the prior activation of plasma components is likely. The biochemical control of many of the events in skin irritation are not yet fully understood. The prediction of skin irritancy by using specific laboratory procedures has not been adequately utilized.

In view of the recent advances made in research on the biochemistry of the skin in general, and the control of inflammation in particular, it seems likely that some of these problems will be solved in the foreseeable future.

REFERENCES

Allen, T. D. and Potten, C. S. (1975). *J. Ultrastruct. Res.* **51**, 94–105.
Anggard, E. and Jonsson, C.-E. (1971). *Acta Physiol. Scand.* **81**, 440–447.
Anson, M. L. (1941). *J. Gen. Physiol.* **24**, 399–421.
Arturson, G., Hamberg, M. and Jonsson, C.-E. (1973). *Acta Physiol. Scand.* **87**, 270–276.
Ash, A. S. F. and Schild, H. O. (1966). *Brit. J. Pharmacol.* **27**, 427–439.
Bach, M. K. (1974). *J. Theoret. Biol.* **45**, 131–151.
Baggiolini, M. (1972). *Enzymes* **13**, 132.
Baker, H. (1968). *J. Invest. Dermatol.* **50**, 283–288.
Bartek, M. J., LaBudde, J. A. and Maibach, M. I. (1972). *J. Invest. Dermatol.* **58**, 114–123.
Berenson, G. S. and Burch, G. E. (1951). *Amer. J. Trop. Med.* **31**, 842–853.
Bernstein, I. A. (1971). *In* "Psoriasis, Proceedings of the International Symposium" (Eds E. M. Farber and A. J. Lox), 287–295. Stanford University Press, Stanford.
Bertelli, A. and Houck, J. C. (1969). "Inflammation Biochemistry and Drug Interaction". Excerpta Medica Foundation, Amsterdam.
Bettley, F. R. (1961). *Brit. J. Dermatol.* **73**, 448–454.
Bettley, F. R. (1965). *Brit. J. Dermatol.* **77**, 98–101.
Bettley, F. R. (1972). *Trans. St. John's Hosp. Dermatol. Soc.* **58**, 65–74.
Bettley, F. R. and Donoghue, E. (1960). *Nature (Lond.)* **185**, 17–20.
Billingham, R. E. and Silvers, W. T. (1967). *J. Exp. Med.* **125**, 429–446.
Björnberg, A. (1968). "Skin reactions to primary irritants in patients with hand eczema". Thesis. Oscar Isacsons Tryckeri AB, Gothenburg.
Blank, I. H. (1952). *J. Invest. Dermatol.* **18**, 433–439.
Blank, I. H. (1964). *J. Invest. Dermatol.* **43**, 415–420.
Blank, I. H. and Shappirio, E. B. (1955). *J. Invest. Dermatol.* **25**, 391–401.
Blohm, S.-G. (1957). *Acta Dermatoven.* **37**, 269–275.
Blumenkrantz, N. and Sondergaard, J. (1972). *Nature New Biol.* **239**, 246.
Bonta, I. L., Chrispijn, H., Noordhoek, J. and Vincent, J. E. (1974). *Prostaglandins* **10**, 495–503.
Bourne, H. R., Lichtenstein, L. M., Melmon, K. L., Henney, C. S., Weinstein, Y. and Shearer, G. M. (1974). *Science* **184**, 19–28.
Boyden, S. (1962). *J. Exp. Med.* **115**, 543–466.

Braun, W., Lichtenstein, L. M. and Parker, C. W. (1974). "Cyclic AMP, Cell Growth, and the Immune Response". Springer-Verlag, Berlin, Heidelberg and New York.

Braun-Falco, D. (1958). *Ann. New York Acad. Sci.* **73**, 936–976.

Breathnach, A. (1971). "An Atlas of the Ultrastructure of Human Skin. Development, Differentiation and Post-Natal Features." J. and A. Churchill, London.

Brehm, G. (1966). *Arch. Klin. Exp. Dermatol.* **226**, 130–135.

Brody, I. (1966). *Nature Lond.* **209**, 472–476.

Brown, V. K. H. (1971). *J. Soc. Cosmet. Chem.* **22**, 411–420.

Brown, V. K. H. and Box, V. L. (1970). *Brit. J. Dermatol.* **82**, 606–612.

Brown, V. K. H. and Box, V. L. (1971). *Brit. J. Dermatol.* **85**, 432–436.

Bullough, W. S. (1972). *Brit. J. Dermatol.* **87**, 187–199 and 347–354.

Choman, B. R. (1963). *J. Invest. Dermatol.* **40**, 177–182.

Christophers, E. (1971). *J. Invest. Dermatol.* **57**, 241–246.

Christophers, E. and Braun-Falco, O. (1970). *Brit. J. Dermatol.* **82**, 268–275.

Christophers, E. and Kligman, A. M. (1964). *J. Invest. Dermatol.* **42**, 407–409.

Cochrane, C. G. (1975). *J. Invest. Dermatol.* **64**, 301–306.

Cohen, J. (1969). *Brit. J. Dermatol.* **81** Suppl. 3, 46–54.

Cooper, H. A., Mason, R. G. and Brinkhous, K. M. (1970). Annual Review of Physiology (Eds E. Knobil, R. S. Sonnenschein and I. S. Edelman), Vol. 38, 501–535. Annual Reviews, Inc., Palo Alto.

Cowan, M. A. and Mann, P. R. (1971). *Brit. J. Dermatol.* **84**, 353–360.

Cronin, E. (1967). *J. Soc. Cosmet. Chem.* **18**, 681–691.

David, J. R. and David, R. R. (1972). *Prog. Allergy* **16**, 300.

Decker, R. H. (1971). *J. Invest. Dermatol.* **57**, 351–363.

de Duve, C. (1964). *In* "Injury, Inflammation and Immunity" (Eds L. Thomas, J. W. Uhr and L. Grant), 283–311. Williams and Wilkins, Baltimore, Maryland.

Dicken, C. H. and Decker, R. H. (1966). *J. Invest. Dermatol.* **47**, 426–431.

Di Rosa, M., Giroud, J. P. and Willoughby, D. A. (1971). *J. Pathol.* **104**, 15–29.

Dodson, J. W. (1967). *J. Embryol. Exp. Morphol.* **17**, 83–105.

Draize, J. H., Woodard, G. and Calvary, H. O. (1944). *J. Pharmacol. Exp. Therapeutics* **82**, 377–389.

Downing, D. T. and Strauss, J. S. (1974). *J. Invest. Dermatol.* **62**, 228–244.

Dugard, P. H. and Scheuplein, R. J. (1973). *J. Invest. Dermatol.* **60**, 263–269.

Ebert, R. H. and Grant, L. (1974). *In* "The Inflammatory Process" (Eds B. W. Zweifach, L. Grant, R. T. McCluskey), 2nd Edn, Vol. I, 3–49. Academic Press, New York and London.

Elfbaum, S. G. and Laden, K. (1968). *J. Soc. Cosmetic Chem.* **19**, 119–127; 163–172; 841–847.

Elgjo, K., Laerum, O. D. and Edgehill, W. (1971). *Virchows. Arch. Abt. B. Zell Path.* **8**, 277–282.

Elias, P. M. (1975). *Clin. Res.* **23**, 90A.

Elias, P. M. and Friend, D. S. (1975). *J. Cell Biol.* **65**, 180–191.

Elsbach, P. (1974). *In* "The Inflammatory Process" (Eds B. W. Zweifach, L. Grant and R. T. McCluskey), 2nd Edn, Vol. I, 363–408. Academic Press, New York and London.

Embery, G. and Dugard, P. H. (1971). *J. Invest Dermatol.* **57**, 308–311.

Emery, B. E. and Edwards, L. D. (1940). *J. Amer. Pharm. Assoc.* **29**, 251–255.

Feldmann, R. J. and Maibach, H. I. (1970). *J. Invest. Dermatol.* **54**, 399–404.

Ferguson, T. F. M. and Prottey, C. (1976). *Food Cosmet. Toxicol.* **14**, 431–434.

Finkelstein, P., Laden, K. and Miechowski, W. (1963). *J. Invest. Dermatol.* **40**, 11–14.

Fisher, L. B. and Maibach, H. I. (1975). *Contact Dermatitis* **1**, 273–276.

Fregert, S. (1974). "Manual of Contact Dermatitis." Munksgaard, Copenhagen.

Gale, L. E. and Scott, P. M. (1953). *J. Amer. Pharmac. Assoc.* **42**, 283–287.

Gilmore, N., Vane, J. R. and Wyllie, J. H. (1969). *In* "Prostaglandins, Peptides and Amines" (Eds P. Mategazza and E. W. Horton), 21. Academic Press, London.

Goldberg, N. D., Haddox, M. K., Estensen, R., White, J. G., Lopez, C. and Hadden, J. W. (1973). *In* "Cyclic AMP, Cell Growth, and the Immune Response" (Eds W. Braun, L. M. Lichtenstein and C. W. Parker), 247–262. Springer-Verlag, Berlin–Heidelberg–New York.

Goldstein, I. M. (1974). *In* "Mediators of Inflammation" (Ed. G. Weissman), 51–84. Plenum Press, New York.

Goldyne, M. E. (1975). *J. Invest. Dermatol.* **64**, 377–385.

Goldyne, M. E., Winkelmann, R. K. and Ryan, R. J. (1973). *Prostaglandins* **4**, 737–749.

Götze, D. and Müller-Eberhard, H. J. (1969). *Fed. Proc.* **28**, 818.

Greaves, M. W. and Søndergaard, J. (1970). *J. Invest. Dermatol.* **54**, 365–367.

Grasso, P. and Lansdown, A. B. G. (1972). *J. Soc. Cosmetic. Chem.* **23**, 481–521.

Halprin, K. M., Adachi, K., Yoshihawa, K., Levine, V., Mui, M. M. and Hsia, S. L. (1975). *J. Invest. Dermatol.* **65**, 170–178.

Hardy, J. (1973). *J. Soc. Cosmet. Chem.* **24**, 423–468.

Harrold, S. P. (1959). *J. Invest Dermatol.* **32**, 581–588.

Harry, R. G. (1973). *In* "Harry's Cosmeticology" (6th Edn, revised by J. B. Wilkinson), 1–20. Leonard Hill Books, Aylesbury.

Hell, E. A. and Cruickshank, C. N. D. (1963). *Exp. Cell. Res.* **31**, 128–139.

Henson, P. M. (1974). *In* "Mediators of Inflammation" (Ed. G. Weissmann), 9–50. Plenum Press, New York.

Hirsch, J. G. (1974). *In* "The Inflammatory Process" (Eds B. W. Zweifach, L. Grant and R. T. McCluskey), 2nd Edn, Vol. I, 411–447. Academic Press, New York and London.

Hirsch, J. G. and Cohn, Z. A. (1960). *J. Exp. Med.* **112**, 1005–1014.

Hirschhorn, R. (1974). *In* "The Inflammatory Process" (Eds B. W. Zweifach, L. Grant and R. T. McCluskey), 2nd Edn, Vol. I, 259–285. Academic Press, New York and London.

Hoekstra, W. G. and Phillips, P. H. (1963). *J. Invest. Dermatol.* **40**, 79–88.

Houck, J. C. and Forscher, B. K. (1968). "Chemical Biology of Inflammation". Pergamon Press, Oxford.

Howes, D. (1975). *J. Soc. Cosmet. Chem.* **26**, 47–63.

Hurley, J. V. (1964). *Ann. New York Acad. Sci.* **116**, 918–935.

Hurley, J. V., Ham, K. N. and Ryan, G. B. (1967). *J. Pathol. Bact.* **93**, 621–635.

Hurley, J. V. and Spector, W. G. (1965). *J. Pathol. Bact.* **89**, 245–254.

Ingram, A. J. and Grasso, P. (1975). *Brit. J. Dermatol.* **92**, 131–142.

Jacobi, D. K. (1959). *Proc. Sci. Sect. Toilet Goods Assoc.* **31**, 22–24.

Jarrett, A. (1973). "The Physiology and Pathophysiology of the Skin". Academic Press, London and New York.

Johnson, B. E. and Daniels, F. (1969). *J. Invest. Dermatol.* **53**, 85–94.

Kahlson, G. and Rosengren, E. (1968). *Physiol. Rev.* **48**, 155–196.

Keller, R. (1969). *In* "Inflammation Biochemistry and Drug Interaction" (Eds A. Bertelli and J. C. Houck), 234–239. Excerpta Medica Foundation, Amsterdam.

Kirk, J. E. (1966). *Acta Dermatoven.* **46**, Suppl. 57.

Kirk, D. L. and Hoekstra, W. G. (1964). *J. Invest. Dermatol.* **43**, 93–98.

Kligman, A. M. (1963). *In* "Advances in Biology of Skin. The Sebaceous Glands" (Eds W. Montagna, R. A. Ellis and A. F. Silvers), Vol. 4, 110–124. Pergamon, Oxford.

Kligman, A. M. (1965). *J. Amer. Med. Assoc.* **193**, 140–148.

Kligman, A. M. and Wooding, W. M. (1967). *J. Invest. Dermatol.* **49**, 78–94.

Lancet (1962), **ii**, 437–438.

Lansdown, A. B. G. (1972). *J. Soc. Cosmet. Chem.* **23**, 739–772.

Lansdown, A. B. G. (1973). *Brit. J. Dermatol.* **89**, 67–76.

Lansdown, A. B. G. and Grasso, P. (1972). *Brit. J. Dermatol.* **86**, 361–373.

Lawrence, J. C. (1968). *Brit. J. Ind. Med.* **26**, 223–227.

Lazarus, G. S., Hatcher, V. B. and Levine, N. (1975). *J. Invest. Dermatol.* **65**, 259–271.

Logan, G. and Wilhelm, D. L. (1966). *Brit. J. Exp. Med.* **47**, 300–314.

Loomans, M. E. and Hannan, D. P. (1970). *J. Invest. Dermatol.* **55**, 101–114.

Lupulesco, A. P., Birmingham, D. J. and Pinkus, H. (1973). *J. Invest Dermatol.* **60**, 33–45.

MacFarlane, R. G. (1973). *In* "The Inflammatory Process" (Eds B. W. Zweifach, L. Grant and R. T. McCluskey), 2nd Edn, Vol. II, 335–362. Academic Press, New York and London.

Mackenzie, I. C. (1969). *Nature (Lond.)* **222**, 881–882.

Mackenzie, I. C. (1970). *Nature (Lond.)* **226**, 653–655.

Mackenzie, I. C. (1975). *J. Invest. Dermatol.* **65**, 45–51.

Majno, G., Shea, S. M. and Leventhal, M. (1969). *J. Cell Biol.* **42**, 647–672.

Malak, J. A. and Kurban, A. K. (1971). *Brit. J. Dermatol.* **84**, 516–522.

Malkinson, F. D. (1964). *In* "The Epidermis" (Eds W. Montagna and W. C. Lobitz), 435–452. Academic Press, New York and London.

Marks, R. (1972). *Brit. J. Dermatol.* **86**, 543–548.

Marzulli, F. N., Callahan, J. F. and Brown, D. W. C. (1965). *J. Invest. Dermatol.* **44**, 339–344.

Matoltsy, A. G., Downes, A. M. and Sweeney, T. M. (1968). *J. Invest. Dermatol.* **50**, 19–26.

Matoltsy, A. G. and Parakkal, P. F. (1965). *J. Cell Biol.* **24**, 297–307.

McMinn, R. M. H. (1969). "Tissue Repair". 1–36. Academic Press, New York and London.

McOsker, D. E. and Beck, L. W. (1967). *J. Invest. Dermatol.* **48**, 372–383.

Medenica, M. and Rostenberg, A. (1971). *J. Invest. Dermatol.* **56**, 259–271.

Melmon, K. L. and Cline, M. J. (1968). *In* "Chemical Biology of Inflammation" (Eds J. C. Houck and B. K. Forscher), 271–281. Pergamon Press, Oxford.

Menton, D. N. and Eisen, S. Z. (1971). *J. Ultrastruct. Res.* **35**, 247–264.

Mercer, E. H., Jahn, R. A. and Maibach, M. I. (1968). *J. Invest. Dermatol.* **51**, 204–214.

Mershon, M. M. (1975). *In* "Applied Chemistry at Protein Interfaces", 41–73, by R. E. Baier, *Advances in Chemistry*, Series 145 (Ed. R. F. Gonel). Amer. Chem. Soc., *Washington, D.C.*

Mezei, M. (1970). *J. Invest. Dermatol.* **54**, 510–517.

Mezei, M., Sager, R. W., Stewart, W. D. and De Ruyter, A. L. (1966). *J. Pharm. Sci.* **55**, 584–590.

Middleton, J. D. (1968). *Brit. J. Dermatol.* **80**, 437–450.

Middleton, J. D. (1969). *J. Soc. Cosmet. Chem.* **20**, 399–412.

Mier, P. D. and van den Hurk (1975). *Brit. J. Dermatol.* **93**, 1–10.

Montagna, W. and Parakkal, P. F. (1974). "The Structure and Function of Skin". 3rd Edn. Academic Press, New York and London.

Montes, L. F., Day, J. L., Ward, C. J. and Kennedy, L. (1967). *J. Invest. Dermatol.* **48**, 184–196.

Morley, J., Wolstencroft, R. A. and Dumonde, D. C. (1973). *In* "Handbook of Experimental Immunology" (Ed. D. M. Weir), 2nd Edn, Chapter 28. Blackwell's Scientific Publications, Oxford.

Movat, H. Z. (1971). "Inflammation, Immunity and Hypersensitivity". Hoebner Medical Division, Harper and Row, Publishers Inc., New York.

Müller-Eberhard, H. J. (1969). Annual Reviews of Biochemistry (Ed. E. Snell), Vol. 38, 389–414. Annual Reviews, Inc., Palo Alto.

Müller-Eberhard, H. J. and Lepow, I. H. (1965). *J. Exp. Med.* **121**, 819–833.

Nagao, S., Stround, J. D., Hamada, T., Pinkus, H. and Birmingham, D. J. (1972). *Acta Dermatoren.* **52**, 11–23.

Olsen, R. L. and Nordquist, R. E. (1966). *J. Invest. Dermatol.* **46**, 431–436.

Onken, H. D. and Moyer, C. A. (1963). *Arch. Dermatol.* **87**, 584–590.

Orfanos, C. E., Mahrle, G. and Ruska, H. (1971). *Brit. J. Dermatol.* **85**, 437–449.

Parish, W. E. (1964). *In* "Biological Aspects of Occlusive Vascular diseases" (Eds D. G. Chalmers and G. A. Gresham), 84–119. Cambridge University Press, Cambridge.

Parish, W. E. (1969). *Brit. J. Dermatol.* **81**, Suppl. 3, 28–35.

Park, A. C. and Baddiel, C. B. (1972). *J. Soc. Cosmet. Chem.* **23**, 3–21.

Plewig, G. and Marples, R. R. (1970). *J. Invest. Dermatol.* **54**, 13–18.

Powell, J. R. and Brody, M. J. (1974). *Fed. Roc.* **33**, 585.

Prottey, C. (1976). *Brit. J. Dermatol.* **94**, 579–587.

Prottey, C. and Ferguson, T. F. M. (1975). *J. Soc. Cosmet. Chem.* **26**, 29–46.

Prottey, C. and Hartop, P. J. (1973). *J. Invest. Dermatol.* **61**, 168–179.

Prottey, C., Hartop, P. J. and Ferguson, T. F. M. (1973). *J. Soc. Cosmet. Chem.* **24**, 473–492.

Putnam, F. W. (1948). *Adv. Protein Chem.* **4**, 79–122.

Rammler, D. H. and Zaffaroni, A. (1967). *Anal. New York Acad. Sci.* **141**, 13–23.

Ramsey, W. S. and Grant, L. (1974). *In* "The Inflammatory Process" (Eds B. W. Zweifach, L. Grant and R. T. McCluskey), 2nd Edn, Vol. III, 287–362. Academic Press, New York and London.

Rebello, D. J. A. and Suskind, R. R. (1963). *J. Invest. Dermatol.* **41**, 67–80.

Riley, J. F. (1959). "The Mast Cells". Livingstone, London.

Robison, G. A., Butcher, R. W. and Sutherland, E. W. (1968). *In* "Annual Reviews of Biochemistry" (Ed. P. D. Boyer), Vol. 37, 149–174. Annual Reviews, Inc., Palo Alto, California.

Robison, G. A., Butcher, R. W. and Sutherland, E. W. (1971). *In* "Cyclic AMP" 145–232. Academic Press, New York and London.

Rodman, N. F. (1973). *In* "The Inflammatory Process" (Eds B. W. Zweifach, L. Grant, R. T. McCluskey), 2nd Edn, Vol. II, 363–392. Academic Press, New York and London.

Rossmiller, J. D. and Hoekstra, W. G. (1965). *J. Invest. Dermatol.* **45**, 24–27.

Rothman, S. and Lorincz, A. L. (1963). *Ann. Rev. Med.* **14**, 215.

Ruddy, S. (1974). *In* "Mediators of Inflammation" (Ed. G. Weissman), 113–140. Plenum Press, New York.

Rutherford, T. and Pawlowski, A. (1974). *Brit. J. Dermatol.* **91**, 503–506.

Ryan, T. J., Nishioka, K. and Dawber, R. P. R. (1971). *Brit. J. Dermatol.* **84**, 501–515.

Samuelsson, B. (1970). Proc. Fourth Internat. Congress Pharmacol. Vol. IV, Schwabe, Basel-Stuttgart.

Schayer, R. W. (1966). *In* "Handbook of Experimental Pharmacology" (Eds O. Eichler and A. Farah), Vol. 18, 672–725. Springer-Verlag, Berlin, Heidelberg and New York.

Schellander, F. and Marks, R. (1973). *Brit. J. Dermatol.* **88**, 363–367.

Scheuplein, R. J. (1967). *J. Invest. Dermatol.* **48**, 79–88.

Scheuplein, R. J. and Blank, I. H. (1971). *Physiol. Rev.* **51**, 702–747.

Scheuplein, R. J. and Dugard, P. H. (1973). *J. Invest. Dermatol.* **60**, 252.

Scheuplein, R. J. and Ross, L. (1970). *J. Soc. Cosmet. Chem.* **21**, 853–873.

Schott, H. (1973). *J. Pharm. Sci.* **62**, 341–343.

Shelanski, H. A. and Shelanski, M. V. (1953). *Proc. Sci. Sect. Toilet Goods Assoc.* **19**, 46–49.

Singer, J. and Vinson, L. (1966). *Toilet Goods Assoc.* **46**, 29.

Skog, E. (1958). *Acta Dermatoren* **38**, 1–14.

Smeenk, G. (1969). *Arch. Klin. Exp. Dermatol.* **235**, 180–191.

Smeenk, G. and Polano, M. K. (1965). *Trans. St. John's Hosp. Dermatol. Soc.* **51**, 220–232.

Søndergaard, J. and Glick, D. (1971). *J. Invest. Dermatol.* **56**, 231–234.

Søndergaard, J. and Greaves, M. W. (1971). *Brit. J. Dermatol.* **84**, 424–428.

Søndergaard, J., Greaves, M. W. and Jorgensen, H. P. (1974). *Arch. Dermatol.* **110**, 256–258.

Spearman, R. I. C. and Garretts, M. (1966). *J. Invest. Dermatol.* **40**, 245–250.

Spearman, R. I. C. and Hardy, J. A. (1973). *Brit. J. Dermatol.* **89**, 265–276.

Spector, W. G. and Willoughby, D. A. (1968). "The Pharmacology of Inflammation." The English Universities Press, Ltd., London.

Spier, H. W. and Pascher, G. (1957). *Acta Dermatoven.* **11**, 14–22.

Spier, H. W. and Schwartz, E. (1962). Prox. XII. Inter. Cong. Dermatol. 389. Excerpta Medica Foundation, Amsterdam.

Spragg, J. (1974). *In* "Mediators of Inflammation" (Ed. G. Weissman), 85–111. Plenum Press, New York.

Steele, R. H. and Wilhelm, D. L. (1966). *Brit. J. Exp. Pathol.* **47**, 612–623.

Steele, R. H. and Wilhelm, D. L. (1970). *Brit. J. Exp. Pathol.* **51**, 265–279.

Stoughton, R. B. and Fritsch, W. (1964). *Arch. Dermatol.* **90**, 512–517.

Sweeney, T. M. and Downing, D. T. (1970). *J. Invest. Dermatol.* **55**, 135–140.

Tabachnick, J. and LaBadie, J. H. (1970). *J. Invest. Dermatol.* **55**, 89–93.

Takasu, H. (1975). *Jap. J. Pharmacol.* **25**, 41–45.

Tovell, P. W. A., Weaver, A. C., Hope, J. and Sprott, W. E. (1974). *Brit. J. Dermatol.* **90**, 501–506.

Trump, B. F. and Mergner, W. J. (1974). *In* "The Inflammatory Process" (Eds B. W. Zweifach, L. Grant and R. T. McCluskey), 2nd Edn, Vol. I, 115–257. Academic Press, New York and London.

Turk, J. L. (1967). *In* "Frontiers of Biology" (Eds A. Neuberger and E. L. Tatum), Vol. 4. North-Holland Publishing Co. Amsterdam.

Turner, R. H., Kurban, A. K. and Ryan, T. J. (1969). *J. Invest. Dermatol.* **53**, 458–462.

Uttley, M. and van Abbe, N. J. (1973). *J. Soc. Cosmet. Chem.* **24**, 217–227.

Uvnäs, B. (1969). *In* "Inflammation Biochemistry and Drug Interaction" (Eds A. Bertelli and J. C. Houck), 221–227. Excerpta Medica Foundation, Amsterdam.

Van Scott, E. J. and Lyon, J. B. (1953). *J. Invest. Dermatol.* **21**, 199–203.

Velo, G. P., Dunn, C. J., Giroud, J. P., Timsit, J. and Willoughby, D. A. (1973). *J. Pathol.* **111**, 149–158.

Vermeer, D. J. H., de Jong, J. C., Donk, L. and Leemhuis, J. (1963). *Ned. Tijdschr. Geneesek.* **107**, 1768–1769.

Vinson, L. J., Singer, E. J., Koehler, W. R., Lehman, M. D. and Masurat, T. (1965). *Tox. Appl. Pharmacol.* **7**, 7–19.

Voorhees, J. J., Duell, E. A., Stawiski, M. and Harnell, E. R. (1974). *In* "Advances in Cyclic Nucleotide Research" (Eds P. Greengard and G. A. Robison), Vol. 4, 117–162. Raven Press, New York.

Weil, C. S. and Scala, R. A. (1971). *Tox. Appl. Pharmacol.* **19**, 276–360.

Weiner, R. and Kaley, G. (1969). *Amer. J. Physiol.* **217**, 563–566.

Weiss, L. (1972). "Cells and Tissues of the Immune System". Prentice-Hall, New Jersey.

Weissmann, G. (1974). "Mediators of Inflammation". Plenum Press, New York.

Wildnauer, R. H., Miller, D. L. and Humphries, W. T. (1975). *In* "Applied Chemistry at Protein Interfaces" 74–124, by R. E. Baier, *Advances in Chemistry*, Series 145 (Ed. R. F. Govel). Amer. Chem. Soc., Washington, D.C.

Wilhelm, D. L. (1973). *In* "The Inflammatory Process" (Eds B. W. Zweifach, L. Grant and R. T. McCluskey), 2nd Edn, Vol. II, 251–301. Academic Press, New York and London.

Willis, I. (1973). *J. Invest. Dermatol.* **60**, 166–171.
Willoughby, D. A. (1973). *In* "The Inflammatory Process" (Eds B. W. Zweifach, L. Grant and R. T. McCluskey), 2nd Edn, Vol. II, 303–331. Academic Press, New York and London.
Willoughby, D. A., Coote, E. and Turk, J. L. (1969). *J. Pathol.* **97**, 295–305.
Willoughby, D. A. and Di Rosa, M. (1971). *In* "Immunopathology of Inflammation" (Eds B. K. Foscher and J. C. Houck), 28–38. Excerpta Medica, Amsterdam.
Willoughby, D. A. and Giroud, J. P. (1969). *J. Pathol.* **98**, 53–60.
Willoughby, D. A. and Spector, W. G. (1969). *In* "Inflammation, Biochemistry and Drug Interaction" (Eds A. Bertelli and J. C. Houck), 29–33. Excerpta Medica Foundation, Amsterdam.
Winkelmann, R. K. (1971). *J. Invest. Dermatol.* **57**, 197–208.
Wolff, K. and Schreiner, E. (1970). *Arch. Dermatol.* **101**, 276–286.
Wood, D. C. F. and Bettley, F. R. (1971). *Brit. J. Dermatol.* **84**, 320–325.
Wright, E. T. and Winer, L. H. (1966). *J. Invest. Dermatol.* **46**, 409–414.
Zacharie, H. and Oates, J. A. (1967). *J. Invest. Dermatol.* **47**, 493–495.
Zelickson, A. S. (1967). "Ultrastructure of Normal and Abnormal Skin". Henry Kimpton, London.
Zweifach, B. W., Grant, L. and McCluskey, R. T. (1974). "The Inflammatory Process". 2nd Edn. Academic Press, New York and London.

SUBJECT INDEX